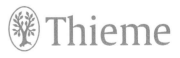

Spine Surgery in an Aging Population

Nathaniel P. Brooks, MD, FAANS
Associate Professor
Department of Neurological Surgery
University of Wisconsin School of Medicine and Public Health
Madison, Wisconsin

Andrea L. Strayer, MS, NP, CNRN
Neurosurgery Nurse Practitioner, Distinguished
Department of Neurological Surgery
University of Wisconsin School of Medicine and Public Health
Madison, Wisconsin

80 illustrations

Thieme
New York • Stuttgart • Delhi • Rio de Janeiro

Executive Editor: Timothy Y. Hiscock
Managing Editor: Nikole Y. Connors
Director, Editorial Services: Mary Jo Casey
Production Editor: Sean Woznicki
International Production Director: Andreas Schabert
Editorial Director: Sue Hodgson
International Marketing Director: Fiona Henderson
International Sales Director: Louisa Turrell
Director of Institutional Sales: Adam Bernacki
Senior Vice President and Chief Operating Officer: Sarah Vanderbilt
President: Brian D. Scanlan

Library of Congress Cataloging-in-Publication Data

Names: Brooks, Nathaniel P., author. | Strayer, Andrea L., author.
Title: Spine surgery in an aging population / Nathaniel P. Brooks,
MD, FAANS, Associate Professor, University of Wisconsin School
of Medicine and Public Health, Department of Neurological
Surgery, Madison, Wisconsin, USA, Andrea L. Strayer, MS, NP,
CNRN, Neurosurgery Nurse Practitioner (Distinguished), Univer-
sity of Wisconsin School of Medicine and Public Health, Depart-
ment of Neurological Surgery, Madison, Wisconsin, USA.
Description: New York : Thieme, [2019] | Includes bibliographical
references and index. |
Identifiers: LCCN 2019006686 (print) | LCCN 2019011479 (ebook) |
ISBN 9781626239159 (e-book) | ISBN 9781626239142 (print)
Subjects: LCSH: Spine–Surgery. | Spine–Aging. | Spine–Diseases–
Treatment.
Classification: LCC RD768 (ebook) | LCC RD768 .B72 2019 (print) |
DDC 617.4/71–dc23
LC record available at https://lccn.loc.gov/2019006686

© 2019 Thieme Medical Publishers, Inc.
Thieme Publishers New York
333 Seventh Avenue, New York, NY 10001 USA
+1 800 782 3488, customerservice@thieme.com

Thieme Publishers Stuttgart
Rüdigerstrasse 14, 70469 Stuttgart, Germany
+49 [0]711 8931 421, customerservice@thieme.de

Thieme Publishers Delhi
A-12, Second Floor, Sector-2, Noida-201301
Uttar Pradesh, India
+91 120 45 566 00, customerservice@thieme.in

Thieme Publishers Rio de Janeiro, Thieme Publicações Ltda.
Edifício Rodolpho de Paoli, 25º andar
Av. Nilo Peçanha, 50 – Sala 2508,
Rio de Janeiro 20020-906 Brasil
+55 21 3172-2297 / +55 21 3172-1896
www.thiemerevinter.com.br

Cover design: Thieme Publishing Group
Typesetting by Thomson Digital

Printed in the United States of America   5 4 3 2 1
by King Printing Co., Inc.
ISBN 978-1-62623-914-2

Also available as an e-book:
eISBN 978-1-62623-915-9

Important note: Medicine is an ever-changing science undergoing continual development. Research and clinical experience are
continually expanding our knowledge, in particular our knowledge of proper treatment and drug therapy. Insofar as this book
mentions any dosage or application, readers may rest assured that
the authors, editors, and publishers have made every effort to
ensure that such references are in accordance with **the state of
knowledge at the time of production of the book.**

Nevertheless, this does not involve, imply, or express any
guarantee or responsibility on the part of the publishers in respect
to any dosage instructions and forms of applications stated in the
book. **Every user is requested to examine carefully** the manufacturers' leaflets accompanying each drug and to check, if necessary
in consultation with a physician or specialist, whether the dosage
schedules mentioned therein or the contraindications stated by the
manufacturers differ from the statements made in the present
book. Such examination is particularly important with drugs that
are either rarely used or have been newly released on the market.
Every dosage schedule or every form of application used is entirely
at the user's own risk and responsibility. The authors and publishers
request every user to report to the publishers any discrepancies or
inaccuracies noticed. If errors in this work are found after publication, errata will be posted at www.thieme.com on the product
description page.

Some of the product names, patents, and registered designs
referred to in this book are in fact registered trademarks or proprietary names even though specific reference to this fact is not
always made in the text. Therefore, the appearance of a name
without designation as proprietary is not to be construed as a
representation by the publisher that it is in the public domain.

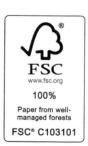

FSC
www.fsc.org
100%
Paper from well-
managed forests
FSC® C103101

Contents

Contents

Foreword

Brooks and Strayer, in teaming with Thieme, have amassed an amazing collection of scholarly works on the subject of spine surgery in the aging population. The book is masterfully crafted and illustrated. The information transmitted is relevant, comprehensive, and cleverly presented.

The content flows seamlessly from one chapter to the next. The topics comprehensively cover the field, without any gaps in the transmission of information.

This book functions as a great 'read', as well as an extraordinarily valuable reference for surgeons and for those who work with surgeons caring for the elderly.

The systematic approach to this book and the manner in which it is presented, facilitates the absorption of information. The acquisition of data, the amplification of skills, and the enhancement of the reader's foundation of knowledge are clearly facilitated by the editors' structured approach.

Please read and enjoy. Use this book as a 'great read' and also as a reference of the highest order. This book will remain relevant for years.

Edward C. Benzel
Emeritus Chairman
Neurosurgery Neurological Institute
Cleveland Clinic
Cleveland, Ohio

Preface

The world's population of older persons is expected to increase from 14% in 2017 to over 20% by 2050 (Figure 1).[1] The growth is attributed to a global increase in life expectancy, decreasing fertility rates, and aging of persons born in the post-World War II baby boom.[1] The high percentage of older persons now and in the future has significant implications for health care systems and spine care providers.

With longevity, has come a change in aging adults' activity level and functional expectations. For example, in the United States the retirement age of 65 is viewed as a new beginning for long awaited post-retirement activity.

The effects of aging on function and social factors has to be accounted for when providing spine care. Even in healthy older people, the evidence of aging is apparent. Loss of function can increase the risk of other conditions, such as falls, diminish quality of life, and decrease independence. Additionally, aging is associated with an increased risk of comorbidities such as osteoporosis, sarcopenia, frailty and poor social support that can impact treatment decisions.

Aging patients are not old children. In most cases the expectations of the older patient cannot be restored youth. The patient and family should be counseled that the goal is to restore function. This function may improve independence and quality of life. In very rare cases will interventions make your patient feel young again or entirely pain free.

Our role as physicians and medical providers is that of the teacher and guide. Only on rare occasion should we act as "mechanics." Time must be spent listening to patients, carefully diagnosing their problems, learning about their goals and finally teaching them in plain language about the risks, alternatives and expectations of treatment. The patient cannot be expected to have our experience with various treatment approaches nor an understanding of the natural history of disease processes. Therefore, our role as guides is critical so that patients travel down the safest treatment path.

In this textbook we have compiled information on the fundamentals of the aging patient, common pathologies of the aging spine, and surgical, as well as non-surgical, treatment options. This will provide you with a foundation of knowledge to help you to provide optimal treatment to your aging patients.

Use this book as a reference. Additional readings are highlighted in each chapter to provide further insight into the research on these topics.

We hope that you find this book to be helpful as you work to take care of your patients.

Sincerely,
Nathaniel Brooks
Andrea Strayer

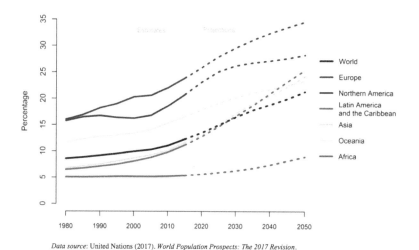

Data source: United Nations (2017). *World Population Prospects: The 2017 Revision.*

Reference

1. Department of Economic and Social Affairs, Population Division, 2017 Available: http://www.un.org/en/development/desa/population/publications/pdf/ageing/WPA2017_Report.pdf.

Acknowledgments

I would like to thank my loving wife for helping me "make" the time to work on this book. Without you I am nothing.

To my kids, "Do what gets you out of bed in the morning."

I would like to thank my parents for supporting me through my education and giving me enough common sense to know what I don't know.

Thank you to all of my mentors who have taught me to take care of the patient first and my ego last.

I would like to thank all of the English and writing teachers that I have had in my lifetime. Although the editors of this book would not believe it, I did learn something about punctuation, sentence and paragraph structure. Spellcheck takes care of the rest.

Nathaniel Brooks

Thank you to my loved ones and mentors for encouraging me to learn and grow, giving me unbelievable support and guidance.

Thank you to the authors of this text. You are all amazing. Without your depth of knowledge and altruism, this collection of thoughtful direction and insights would not be possible.

Last, but not least, thank you to Nikole Connors, Managing Editor and Timothy Hiscock, Executive Editor, Thieme Publishers. They have been extraordinary throughout the process.

My hope is all who read this book will translate their learning into improving the lives of the older adults they care for.

Andrea Strayer

Contributors

Ahmed A. AlBayar, MD
Research Scholar
University of Pennsylvania School of Medicine
Philadelphia, Pennsylvania

Paul A. Anderson, MD
Professor
Department of Orthopedic Surgery and Rehabilitation
University of Wisconsin
Madison, Wisconsin

Mohammad M. Alshardan, MD
Neurosurgery Resident
Faculty of Medicine
University of Ottawa
Ottawa, Ontario, Canada

Angela A. Auriat, PhD
Research Associate
Neurosciences
Ottawa Hospital Research Institute
Ottawa, Ontario, Canada

Steven Barczi, MD, FAASM
Program Director, Geriatric Medicine and VA Advanced
    Geriatrics Fellowships
Director, Geri-PACT and GRECC Connect, Wm S. Middleton
    VA Hospital
Director for Education & Eval & Clinical, Madison VA
    Geriatric Research, Education & Clinical Ctr
Professor of Medicine (Geriatrics and Sleep Medicine)
University of Wisconsin School of Medicine and Public
    Health
Madison, Wisconsin

Edward C. Benzel, MD
Emeritus Chairman of Neurosurgery
Neurological Institute
Cleveland Clinic
Cleveland, Ohio

Sigurd Berven, MD
Professor in Residence
Chief, Spine Service
Department of Orthopaedic Surgery
UC San Francisco
San Francisco, California

Neil Binkley, MD
Professor of Medicine
Divisions of Geriatrics and Endocrinology
Department of Medicine
University of Wisconsin School of Medicine and Public
    Health
Madison, Wisconsin

Nathaniel P. Brooks, MD, FAANS
Associate Professor
Department of Neurological Surgery
University of Wisconsin School of Medicine and Public
    Health
Madison, Wisconsin

Bjoern Buehring, MD
Division of Geriatrics and Gerontology
Department of Medicine
University of Wisconsin School of Medicine and
    Public Health
Madison, Wisconsin
Rheumazentrum Ruhrgebiet
Ruhr-Universität Bochum
Herne, Germany

Carli Bullis, MD
Resident
Department of Neurosurgery
Oregon Health and Science University
Portland Oregon

Daniel Burkett, MD
Resident
Department of Neurological Surgery
University of Wisconsin School of Medicine and
    Public Health
Madison, Wisconsin

Sigita Burneikiene, MD
Clinical Research Director
Neurosurgery
Justin Parker Neurological Institute
Boulder, Colorado

Suzan Chen, MD
Research Associate
Neurosciences
Ottawa Hospital Research Institute
Ottawa, Ontario, Canada

Darryl John DiRisio, MD
Professor
Department of Neurosurgery
Albany Medical Center
Albany, New York

Alexander B. Dru, MD
Resident Physician
Department of Neurosurgery
University of Florida
Gainesville, Florida

Daniel Eddelman, MD
Resident
Department of Neurosurgery
Rush University Medical Center
Chicago, Illinois

Bradley B. Gale, MD
Department of Physical Medicine and Rehabilitation
University of Colorado
Aurora, Colorado

Clayton L. Haldeman, MD, MHS
Resident
Department of Neurosurgery
University of Wisconsin Hospitals and Clinics
Madison, Wisconsin

Julie A. Hastings, MD
Clinical Instructor
Creighton University School of Medicine - Phoenix Campus
Phoenix, Arizona
Assistant Professor
University of Arizona College of Medicine
Tuscon, Arizona

Daniel J. Hoh, MD
Associate Professor
Lillian S. Wells Department of Neurosurgery
University of Florida
Gainesville, Florida

Lee S. Hwang, MD
Resident Physician
Department of Neurosurgery
The Center for Spine Health
The Cleveland Clinic
Cleveland, Ohio

John Paul G. Kolcun, BS
Medical Student
Miller School of Medicine
University of Miami
Miami, Florida

Ajit A. Krishnaney, MD, FAANS
Vice Chair
Department of Neurosurgery
Cleveland Clinic
Cleveland, Ohio

Jay Kumar, MD
Resident
Department of Neurosurgery and Brain Repair
University of South Florida
Tampa, Florida

Bryan S. Lee, MD
Chief Resident
Department of Neurosurgery
Cleveland Clinic
Cleveland, Ohio

Jason I. Liounakos, MD
Resident
Department of Neurological Surgery
University of Miami Miller School of Medicine
Miami, Florida

Eric A. K. Mayer, MD
Staff Physician
Seton Spine & Scoliosis
Austin, Texas

Vincent J. Miele, MD
Clinical Associate Professor
Department of Neurological Surgery
University of Pittsburgh
Pittsburgh, Pennsylvania

Thomas E. Mroz, MD
Director, Center for Spine Health
Director, Clinical Research
Neurological Institute
Departments of Orthopaedic and Neurological Surgery
Cleveland Clinic
Cleveland, Ohio

Adeolu Olasunkanmi, MS, MD
Assistant Professor
Virginia Tech Carilion Neurosurgery
Virginia Tech Carilion School of Medicine
Roanoke, Virginia

John E. O'Toole, MD, MS
Professor
Department of Neurosurgery
Rush University Medical Center
Chicago, Illinois

Samuel Overley, MD
Assistant Professor
Department of Orthopaedic Surgery
University of Arkansas for Medical Sciences
Little Rock, Arkansas

Paul Page, MD
Resident
Department of Neurosurgery
University of Wisconsin
Madison, Wisconsin

Matthew Pease, MD
Resident
Department of Neurosurgery
University of Pittsburgh Medical Center
Pittsburgh, Pennsylvania

Dominic W. Pelle, MD
Center for Spine Health
Cleveland Clinic
Cleveland, Ohio

Karen A. Petronis, ACNPc MS
Nurse Practitioner – Assistant Professor
Department of Neurosurgery
Albany Medical Center
Albany, New York

Ken Porche, MD
Resident Physician
Department of Neurosurgery
University of Florida
Gainesville, Florida

Sharad Rajpal, MD, FAACS
Boulder Neurosurgical & Spine Associates
Boulder, Colorado

Daniel K. Resnick, MD, MS
Professor and Vice Chairman
Department of Neurological Surgery
University of Wisconsin School of Medicine and
   Public Health
Madison, Wisconsin

Jianning Shao, BA
Medical Student
Cleveland Clinic Lerner College of Medicine at
   Case Western University
Cleveland, Ohio

John H. Shin, MD
Director, Spinal Deformity & Spine Oncology Surgery
Department of Neurosurgery
Massachusetts General Hospital
Boston, Massachusetts

Lauren N. Simpson, MD, MPH
Resident Physician
Department of Neurological Surgery
Oregon Health & Science University
Portland, Oregon

Casey A. Slattery, BS
Medical Student
Department of Orthopedics and Sports Medicine
University of Washington
Seattle, Washington

Samantha Sokol, PA-C
Surgical First Assist
CHI Franciscan Health
Tacoma, Washington

Michael P. Steinmetz, MD
William P. and Amanda C. Madar Endowed Professor
   and Chair
Department of Neurological Surgery
Cleveland Clinic Lerner College of Medicine
Neurologic Institute
Cleveland, Ohio

Andrea L. Strayer, MS, NP, CNRN
Neurosurgery Nurse Practitioner, Distinguished
Department of Neurological Surgery
University of Wisconsin School of Medicine and
   Public Health
Madison, Wisconsin

William Sullivan, MD
Associate Professor
Department of Physical Medicine and Rehabilitation
University of Colorado School of Medicine

Swetha J. Sundar, MD
Resident
Department of Neurological Surgery
Cleveland Clinic
Cleveland, Ohio

Khoi D. Than, MD
Assistant Professor
Department of Neurological Surgery
Oregon Health & Science University
Portland, Oregon

Eve C. Tsai, MD, PhD
Suruchi Bhargava Chair in Spinal Cord and
    Brain Regeneration
Assistant Professor
Department of Surgery
The Ottawa Hospital
Ottawa, Ontario, Canada

Kushagra Verma, MD, MS
Adult and Pediatric Scoliosis and Spine Deformity Surgeon
Volunteer, Global Spine Outreach
Member, Scoliosis Research Society
Department of Orthopaedic Surgery
Long Beach Memorial and Miller Children's Hospital
Long Beach, California

Michael Y. Wang, MD
Chief of Neurosurgery
University of Miami Hospital
Professor
Departments of Neurological Surgery and Rehabilitation
    Medicine
Miami, Florida

Ryan Zate, DO
Physician Southwest Sports and Spine, Clinical Preceptor
PM&R
Burrell College of Osteopathic Medicine
Tucson, Arizona

1 Assessing the Aging Patient

Bjoern Buehring and Steven Barczi

Abstract

Due to current demographic developments, more older adults will seek care for spine related diseases. This chapter emphasizes key geriatric concepts and approaches that will better equip spine health providers to deliver optimal care to this population. These approaches keep the patient's goals of care at the center, reduce complications of therapy yet can be delivered efficiently. First, epidemiological data and pathophysiological models are reviewed and an overview of geriatric syndromes is presented. Next, the structured geriatric assessment is highlighted as a way to systematically evaluate an older adult, and examples are given on how to perform such an assessment. Lastly, evidence-based examples of perioperative management of geriatric syndromes and society guidelines on the topic are discussed to emphasize the merits of endorsing and applying such an approach.

Keywords: Older adults, goals of care, physiology of aging, geriatric syndromes, multi-morbidity, frailty, delirium, structured geriatric assessment, perioperative outcomes, interdisciplinary team

Key Points

- The expanding demographic of older adults will lead to greater numbers of persons seeking care for spine disease and related conditions.
- Seniors may have different care preferences and goals of care that revolve more around function than longevity.
- Age-related changes in physiology lead to greater vulnerabilities and chances for decompensation in health and functioning.
- Geriatric syndromes may have multiple precipitating or causative factors and require management with multifaceted interventions.
- A structured systematic geriatric assessment targeted toward medically complex or frail older persons is an effective tool for addressing unrecognized risks and health issues that can influence perioperative outcomes.
- Geriatric care is best delivered by interdisciplinary teams.

1.1 Background

According to the United Nation's 2017 World Population Aging report, the number of adults aged 60 and older more than doubled from 1980 to 2017. The current number of 962 million adults in this age group is expected to grow to 2.1 billion in 2050. By 2050 there will be more older adults than those aged 10 to 24. These demographic changes are most pronounced in Europe and North America but are now also being observed in the rest of the world.[1] An aging population has many socioeconomic, political and health care implications. For example, as people get older, the number of patients with degenerative musculoskeletal disorders increases, including degenerative spine disease.[2,3,4,5] Additionally, the prevalence of persons 65 and older with injurious falls, osteoporosis, and resulting fractures rises.[6,7] It is important to note that with increased longevity, a person's expectations on quality of life can change. In Europe and North America, adults may focus more on "aging well" rather than "aging as long as possible." An integral part of the quality of life of older adults is to be pain free, mobile, and able to live independently.[8] Consequently, it is anticipated that older persons seeking care for spine diseases to maintain or improve their quality of life will significantly increase. As such, the knowledge of how to assess, counsel, and treat geriatric patients will become vital to health care providers treating spine disorders.

Geriatric patients are more than "old" adults. There is a great variation in biological and physical function among older adults. Therefore, chronological age cannot be used to estimate how well older individuals function from a biological, physical, or psychosocial perspective. A 75-year-old individual might still run marathons, work 60 hours a week or play in an orchestra. On the other hand, he or she might live in a nursing home and require help with relatively simple tasks such as using the phone, cooking meals or even cleaning themselves. Additionally, variations in organ system function within the same individual often exist. For example, an older adult might develop heart failure, diabetes mellitus, and depression but not suffer from osteoarthritis or dementia, while another might have renal insufficiency, skin cancer, and dementia.

Accepting this marked increase in the number and heterogeneity of older individuals seeking care for their spinal disease, it is vital for health care providers to take into account the overall health (biological, physical, cognitive, and psychological), support network, and goals of care of each particular aging individual when developing a treatment plan. This chapter aims to: a) summarize current aging epidemiology and knowledge of physiologic changes of aging, b) describe critical geriatric syndromes that might be particularly important for caring for patients with spine disease, and c) introduce the concept of the structured geriatric assessment.

1.2 Changes of Aging

A foundational understanding of the biology and physiology of aging is necessary to assess, counsel and adequately treat aging patients with spine disease. This chapter highlights a few important concepts regarding the physiology of aging. Foremost, it is critical to recognize that not all individuals age in the same manner. This leads to a diversity of biologic, physical, and cognitive function across older persons. These aging factors may lead to the loss of physiological buffer or homeostatic reserve that can in turn lead to earlier presentations of disease or more rapid deterioration in health status or function when stressors emerge. In an outstanding review of the hallmarks of aging, Lopez-Otin and colleagues[9] proposed a framework that groups nine aging factors into three categories. These three categories are: causes of damage (e.g., genomic instability), response to damage (e.g., mitochondrial dysfunction), and the integration of these two processes (e.g., altered intracellular communication). Clinically,

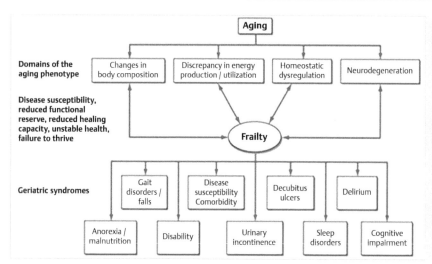

Fig. 1.1 A unifying model of aging, frailty, and the geriatric syndromes. Adapted from Kasper DL, et al. Harrison's Principles of Internal Medicine, 19th edition. McGraw-Hill Education.

this is observed as a phenotype (presentation) that is the result of a complex and variable combination of causes and responses to damage that manifests differently in various cell systems, tissues, and organs. This aging phenotype can be grouped into four different categories: body composition, energetics, homeostatic regulation and neurodegeneration. These domains of the aging phenotype are helpful because they can be assessed and quantified clinically (▶ Fig. 1.1, Table 1-1).[10]

In sum, the pattern of biological changes described through the hallmarks of aging and the resultant aging phenotype in a particular individual lead to a susceptibility for certain common age-related conditions, termed geriatric syndromes. This entire picture ultimately explains why there is so much variability in biological, physical, and cognitive function in older adults and why chronological age cannot be used to quantify the overall health of a geriatric patient. Instead, the comprehensive geriatric assessment was developed to systematically assess the domains of the aging phenotype, presence of geriatric syndromes, and level of frailty.

1.3 Geriatric Syndromes and Problems

When familiarizing oneself with geriatric health issues, it is important to understand the concept of geriatric syndromes. Although the term is somewhat vague, there are key aspects on which experts agree. In contrast to diseases that are common in geriatric patients (for example, cancer, diabetes mellitus, or heart disease), geriatric syndromes are not pathophysiologically linked to one organ or organ system. Rather, they have multifactorial etiologies.[11] Often in frail individuals, an insult to one organ system (for example, an orthopedic surgery of the hip), leads to multiple intermediate changes in other domains (e.g., increased adrenergic tone, fluid shifts, pain, and new medications) that leads to a deficit in an altogether different organ system (e.g., the development of delirium). As such, the clinically presenting symptom (in our example of delirium it could be confusion, agitation or apathy) is not as easily traced back to one inciting event that caused the symptom to develop. It is difficult to solve this puzzle by applying a "one cause and one outcome" mindset because of the multifactorial character of geriatric syndromes. The health provider has to look for interac-

tions of multiple factors. Our surgical patient might have had a prior trauma, received psychotropic medication such as opioids, and/or have comorbidities such as dementia that all contribute to or even cause delirium independently.

1.4 Fundamental Geriatric Syndromes

Fundamental geriatric syndromes are grouped into "The Body" (frailty, sarcopenia, cachexia, falls), "The Mind" (cognitive impairment, delirium, depression) and "Others" (polypharmacy, support network) in order to aid conceptualization of this multifactorial framework.

1.4.1 The Body

Frailty– Its Components and Outcomes

Frailty is one of the most global and ubiquitous, yet difficult to characterize, geriatric syndromes. Frailty is defined as multiple incremental factors that lead to loss of functional reserve to respond to internal and external stressors that results in difficulty regaining homeostasis after a physiological or medical challenge. Frailty is associated with an increased risk for adverse health outcomes such as disability, falls, delirium, morbidity, and mortality.[12,13,14,15] A common external stressor is a surgical intervention.[13] It is important to identify frail older adults prior to surgery to reduce the risk of postoperative complications such as delirium, delayed wound healing, and loss of ability to perform activities of daily living or live independently.[14,16,17,18] Optimizing the health of such an individual prior to surgery can reduce the risk of postoperative complications, and being aware of nonmodifiable risk factors will help to risk-stratify the surgery and put measures in place to recognize and treat complications as early as possible.[14]

Frailty is often considered the most important geriatric syndrome, as it underlies and contributes to many other geriatric syndromes such as delirium, falls, and incontinence. There are two common approaches to classify and diagnose frailty: a phenotype model which hypothesizes that frailty is based on distinct features (the phenotype) and a cumulative deficit model which

Table 1.1 Examples of assessment of the four domains of the aging phenotype
Adapted from Kasper DL, et al. Harrison's Principles of Internal Medicine, 19th edition. McGraw-Hill Education

Approach to Assessment	Body Composition	Energetics	Homeostatic Regulation	Neurodegeneration
Self report		Self-reported questionnaires investigating physical activity, sense of fatigue/exhaustion, exercise tolerance		
Physical examination	Muscle strength testing (isometric and isokinetic) Anthropometrics (weight, height, BMI, waist circumference, arm and leg circumference, skin folds)	Performance-based tests of physical function		Objective assessment of gait, balance, reaction time, coordination Standard neurologic exam, including assessment of global cognition[a]
Laboratory values	Biomarkers (24-h creatinuria or 3-methyl-histidine)		Nutritional biomarkers (e.g., vitamins, antioxidants) Baseline levels of biomarkers and hormone levels Inflammatory markers (e.g., ESR, CRP, IL-6, TNF-αN	
Imaging	CT and MRI, DEXA		Magnetic resonance spectroscopy	MRI, fMRI, PET, and other dynamic imaging techniques
Other	Hydrostatic weighing	Resting metabolic rate Treadmill testing of oxygen consumption during walking Objective measures of physical activity (accelerometers, double-labeled water)	Stress response Response to provocative tests, such as oral glucose tolerance test, dexamethasone test, and others	Evoked potentials Electroneurography and electromyography

[a]Mini Mental State; Montreal Cognitive Assessment.
Abbreviations: BMI, body mass index; CRP, C-reactive protein; DEXA, dual-energy x-ray absorptiometry; ESR, erythrocyte sedimentation rate; fMRI, functional MRI; IL-6, interleukin 6; PET, positron emission tomography; TNFα,tumor necrosis factor α.

proposes that frailty is based on the accumulation of a number of abnormal health conditions. There is no consensus as to which approach should be used, particularly clinically.[15] Regardless of the ongoing scientific debate, many clinicians have incorporated the assessment of frailty using the phenotype definition, often because it is easier to do in a busy practice. Text box 1 (p.3) shows this frailty definition proposed by Linda Fried.[19]

Reviewing these five criteria one can easily see that body composition (weight loss) and muscle function (weakness and walking speed) are key components of frailty according to this definition. As such, cachexia and sarcopenia often coexist and contribute to frailty but can also exist on their own. (▶ Fig. 1.2).

Fried Index (or Cardiovascular Health Study Index)

- Positive for frailty with ≥ 3 positive
  - **Weight loss** (≥ 5% of body weight in the last year)
  - **Exhaustion** (positive response to questions regarding effort required for activity)
  - **Weakness** (decreased grip strength)
  - **Slow walking speed** (> 6 to 7 s to walk 15 feet)
  - **Decreased physical activity** (Kcals/week: males expending < 383 Kcals and females < 270 Kcal)

Sarcopenia and Cachexia

Sarcopenia is the age-related loss of muscle mass. Most definitions include a measure of muscle mass (appendicular lean mass) and a measure of physical function (gait speed), muscle

function (grip strength) or both.[20] Cachexia is defined as the inflammation-associated weight loss seen in many chronic illnesses such as malignancy, chronic kidney disease, congestive heart failure, COPD or rheumatoid arthritis. Some authors also suggest an idiopathic, senile form of cachexia. Usually the loss of muscle mass is larger than the loss of fat mass. Due to the overlap in definitions, it should be no surprise that sarcopenia and cachexia are also associated with the adverse health outcomes of frailty.[21,22] It should be noted, however, that physical function and muscle function tests by themselves predict health outcomes such as falls, fractures, and mortality. As a matter of fact, studies have suggested that muscle function is a better predictor of health outcomes than appendicular lean mass.[23,24,25,26]

Falls

Falls and fractures in older adults often lead to injuries of the spine and skeletal system, so they are of particular relevance to spine providers. Approximately one-third of adults above 65 years of age fall once a year or more. This number significantly increases in older age groups, with the percentage increasing to over 50% in adults older than 90 years. Sixty to 70% of older adults who fall will fall again in the next 12 months. Ten to 20% of falls lead to an injury, with approximately 5% of these being a fracture. But even falls without significant injuries can lead to decrease in quality of life and loss of independence, with 70% of fallers developing a fear of falling that can result in a decrease in mobility and increased social isolation.[24,27] As seen in ▶ Table 1.2, the risk factors with the highest relative risk are linked to the musculoskeletal system. Additional risk factors

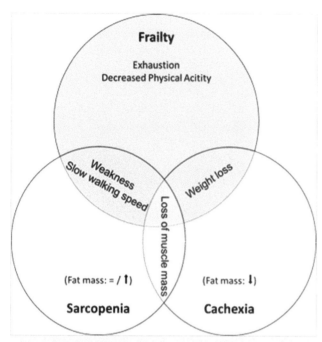

Fig. 1.2 The overlap between frailty, sarcopenia and cachexia definitions. Exhaustion and decreased physical activity are features only included in Fried's frailty definition. Weakness and slow walking speed are factors included both in frailty and sarcopenia definitions. Weight loss is included in cachexia and frailty, whereas loss of muscle mass is included in all three syndromes (explicitly in sarcopenia and cachexia and implicitly through weight loss in frailty). Although fat mass is not included in the definitions (and therefore listed in parentheses), it is a distinguishing feature between sarcopenia and cachexia. In cachexia, there is a loss of fat mass along with a decrease in muscle mass and body weight, whereas fat mass can be stable or even be increased in sarcopenia, often leading to no significant change in body weight.

involve vision, cognition, and the cardiovascular system. The table also reinforces that falls fit the paradigm of a geriatric syndrome, given their multifactorial nature.[24] This is important because the management of falls requires a multidisciplinary approach that can be best coordinated by a health provider with geriatric experience (▶ Table 1.2).

1.4.2 The Mind

Depression

Depression is common in the general population and increases further in older adults. Prevalence for current depression in many studies ranges between 5 and 15%, with prevalence of lifetime depression being significantly higher. A subclinical depression, whereby only some but not all of the criterion for major depression are met, is two to three times more frequent in older adults. It is important to note that the rate of suicidality is higher in older age groups compared to younger age groups and higher in men compared to females.[28,29,30] Geriatric patients may also present with a different constellation of symptoms, with more somatic and less psychological features than other populations. Specifically, there may be more complaints of pain, neurocognitive difficulties, or sleep disturbance and less endorsement of guilt, worthlessness and hopelessness.[29] A commonly used tool to assess depression in older

Table 1.2 Important individual risk factors for falls: summary of 16 studies. Weakness is the most significant risk factor.

Risk factor	Relative risk	Range
Weakness	4.9	1.9–10.3
Balance Deficit	3.2	1.6–5.4
Gait Deficit	3.0	1.7–4.8
Visual Deficit	2.8	1.1–7.4
Mobility limitation	2.5	1.0–5.3
Cognitive impairment	2.4	2.0–4.7
Impaired functional status	2.0	1.0–3.1
Postural hypotension	1.9	1.0–3.4

Adapted from: Rubenstein LZ. Falls in older people: epidemiology, risk factors and strategies for prevention. Age Ageing 2006;35 Suppl 2: ii37-ii41.

adults is the Geriatric Depression Scale (GDS), which consists of 15 questions. A score of five or above suggests mild or moderate depression, whereas a score of 10 or higher suggests a major depression. It is important to recognize depression in older adults, not only because of the significant rate of suicide but also because it is associated with poorer surgical results, postoperative complications, and decreased ability to participate in rehabilitation.[31,32]

Delirium

Delirium is one of the most common postsurgical complications, especially in individuals with coexisting dementia, depression, or polypharmacy. It has a substantial financial and individual cost, with longer hospitalizations, more hospital acquired complications, greater institutionalization rates postdischarge, and higher 30-day mortality rates.[31] It is characterized by problems with attention and typically one or more additional neurocognitive difficulties (such as memory, orientation, sensory perception, or language) which waxes and wanes.[33,34,35] Most providers taking care of older adults have encountered agitated, disoriented patients with delirium, but there are equal numbers of individuals with hypoactive delirium that may go unrecognized yet have equally negative outcomes. Where a hyperactive delirious patient will be recognized quickly, patients with hypoactive delirium might suffer significantly longer before it is diagnosed.[34] A tool to diagnose delirium is the Confusion Assessment Method (CAM).[34,35] This screening instrument is also available for patients who are unable to communicate verbally, for example because they are ventilated in the Intensive Care Unit (CAM-ICU).[35] As with falls (or any other geriatric syndrome), finding the underlying causes of delirium and developing a treatment plan requires a multidisciplinary approach often lead by a provider with geriatric experience.[36]

Dementia

Dementia is another cognitive disorder that influences an older adult's ability to function in their environment and interact with others. As the U.S. population is aging and safer surgical and anesthetic approaches are developed, older and more debilitated patients are now undergoing spine surgery, including those with dementia. Management of perioperative status and comorbid conditions is more challenging in the presence of dementia, due to the often-limited capability of the patient to communicate or adhere to treatment recommendations. There are established associations between a preoperative diagnosis of dementia and increased rate of discharge to a facility as well as length of stay, though not with case fatality.[37] Dementia is defined as a cognitive impairment that persists, involves at least two cognitive domains (decline in memory being a prominent one), and is a decline from previous cognitive abilities. The cognitive impairment must be severe enough to result in difficulties or inabilities to manage one's daily activities independently. If the cognitive impairment is present but does not limit daily function the individual is classified as mild cognitive impairment (MCI).[38,39,40,41] Before the diagnosis of dementia can be made, other causes which can lead to similar symptoms need to be excluded, important examples of which are depression and delirium. Several types of dementia exist which have different pathophysiological causes and present with different clinical features (i.e., different cognitive domains being affected) and different time lines. Alzheimer's dementia is the most common type of dementia, with vascular, frontotemporal, and Lewy body dementia being other common types.[38,39,40,41] Several screening tools for dementia exist. They vary in length of time to complete and sensitivity/specificity; also, not all are freely available. Two commonly used, free and validated tools are the St. Louis University Mental Status (SLUMS) and the Mini-Cog.[42,43] Ultimately, the provider assessing for dementia should use the tool she/he is most comfortable with and is broadly used in the health system the provider is working. Identifying individuals with dementia has the same importance as other geriatric syndromes such as frailty or depression, because dementia also increases the risk for postoperative delirium and falls and can result in more frequent rehospitalization and longer hospital stays.[44,45] As outlined above, it is fairly straightforward to screen an individual for dementia, but it is a lot more time intensive and requires experience to make the diagnosis of dementia. As such, a positive dementia screen should lead to a referral to a provider who has this experience.

1.4.3 Others

Polypharmacy

The presence of multiple concurrent health issues, termed multimorbidity, leads to polypharmacy. Older patients with many geriatric syndromes and other diseases often take more than five prescription medications, which is often the number suggested to be classified as polypharmacy. To some, this might be a surprisingly low number, considering that many patients take more than 10 or even 20 medications. Polypharmacy is associated with health problems such as gastrointestinal bleeding, hypotension, and liver and renal disease, but also several geriatric syndromes such as falls and delirium.[46,47] This can quickly turn into a vicious cycle in which the treatment of certain diseases and syndromes results in creation of new ones or worsening of already existing ones through side effects of medication. This increased morbidity causes decreased quality of life, more frequent and longer hospitalizations, hospital readmissions, and an increase in mortality. Certain medication groups such as anticholinergic drugs and psychotropic medications cause a particularly high risk for adverse events.[46,48]

Managing polypharmacy requires both the discontinuation of certain potentially inappropriate medications (PIMS), termed deprescribing, and ensuring that age-relevant medications are used. Several tools and approaches exist to address polypharmacy, including the American Geriatric Society's Beers criteria or the START/STOPP tool.[49,50,51,52] Again, the decision to remove PIMS is best accomplished by engaging a multidisciplinary geriatric team (particularly a pharmacist).

Support Network

Even after addressing and optimizing the many aforementioned health factors, the older adult may still have residual physical and psychological deficits. In such cases, the patient's social support network, access to home resources and care management serves as key determinants for the success or failure of that individual to safely return home and live independently. As such, it is essential for the spine provider to know how much help the cared-for patient has available.[53,54,55] The postdischarge care plan (e.g., medication administration, wound care, physical therapy) and care coordination (attending clinic appointments, etc.) will only be successful if the geriatric patient has the necessary support to follow these recommendations. However, many older adults are socially isolated and do not have a primary social support network anymore.[56] In such cases, the support cannot be provided through the patient's own social network. Evaluating and optimizing the social support network is often accomplished through comprehensive discharge planning and transitions of care programs, or as part of a comprehensive geriatric assessment during inpatient or outpatient visits.[57,58,59,60,61,62,63,64,65,66,67,68]

1.5 Structured Geriatric Assessment

A geriatric patient will present with his or her own aging phenotype and resulting geriatric diseases, syndromes, and concurrent psychosocial and psychological complexity. It is easy to miss important issues if a systematic approach is not employed in the patient's evaluation. The comprehensive geriatric assessment (CGA) was developed as a structured method with adequate time dedicated by an interdisciplinary team to properly define and examine the presence and severity of these health issues. Special emphasis is placed on addressing common age-associated illnesses, function, and patient care preferences. A number of controlled trials demonstrate the value of preoperative comprehensive geriatric assessment in reducing complications and improving postoperative outcomes in older patients undergoing elective surgery.[60] However, it is unrealistic to expect that a comprehensive geriatric assessment can be performed in a busy spine clinic. Rather, it will be important to build a network within one's own health system that engages geriatric specialists and other health care disciplines such as social work, nursing, pharmacy, and rehabilitation therapists to accomplish this task. This information ideally should be easily available in a structured format in the electronic health record.

It might not, however, be possible to create such a system quickly or to easily access a geriatrics care team, so the spine provider and team should understand the core elements of such an assessment. Ultimately, the spine provider should get a general idea of the patient's functional status, mobility, and level of independence. A basic screen for cognitive impairment and depression and the quality of the patient's social support network can predict the capacity for the patient to adhere to the postoperative care plan.[60,61] Having this information will make it much easier to be able to estimate whether a certain intervention has the potential to improve the particular patient's mobility, independence, and quality of life, whether the patient can understand the risks and benefits of such an intervention and consent to it themselves, how high the risk of potential complications are, and how well and quickly the patient will recover from the intervention.

There are many publications and guidelines on how to perform a geriatric assessment and which factors should be included.[59,61,62,63,64,65,66,67,68] In practice, it is helpful to focus on a few very common and clinically important geriatric problems. To start, determine the patient's degree of independence. There are several validated tools to assess Activities of Daily Living (ADLs) and Instrumental Activities of Daily Living (IADLs). Some examples of ADLs and IADLs are listed in ▸ Table 1.3. This information gives a broad overview of how a patient is functioning and how much assistance he or she needs. Several factors, including geriatric syndromes and diseases will impact ADLs and IADLs.

As mentioned above, there are many algorithms describing how to perform a comprehensive geriatric assessment and systematically assess the presence and severity of geriatric syndromes. Several common approaches warrant brief description. The first one, the MAGIC (Manageable Geriatric Assessment) approach, has been developed for primary care providers. It includes nine factors that were chosen out of a larger set.[66,67] A German guideline committee added five additional points that also are relevant to health providers taking care of older adults with spine problems.[69] All 14 are listed in ▸ Table 1.3 The table also lists reasons why addressing this problem might improve care during a spine health encounter.

Even addressing these 14 points will take some time, likely 10 to 30 minutes depending on the patient. As such, a provider might choose only to address a few in the encounter or have the patient go through these with the clinical team prior to the encounter. Ideally, this information is already available in the

Table 1.3 Geriatric syndromes and points to be considered by providers caring for older adults with spine problems

Geriatric Syndrome	Potential Impact for Encounter
Daily activities	ADLs and IADLs can give a "big picture" overview how well the patient is functioning in daily life.
Vision	Poor vision might impact the patient's ability to read instructions, consent forms etc. and also is a risk factor for confusion and delirium.
Hearing	Poor hearing also might impact the patient's ability to understand instructions, consent conversation etc. and also is a risk factor for confusion and delirium.
Falls	Frequent falls are one sign of frailty, risk factor for serious injuries like fractures and intracranial bleeds.
Urinary Incontinence	Urinary incontinence leads to social isolation and also is a risk factor for pressure ulcers.
Immunization	Likely more relevant for the primary care provider than the spine specialist. However up-to-date immunizations on tetanus, pneumococcal pneumonia and influenza could protect the patient for infections acquired during a trauma or a hospital stay.
Depression	Depression is an important factor for quality of life, goals in life and social isolation. Furthermore, it impacts cognition, pain, and adherence to therapy and rehabilitation.
Social Environment	The living situation and social support network play a key role for most geriatric syndromes. Older individuals with frailty and many other geriatric syndromes might still be able to live independently thanks to a good social environment. Conversely, healthier older adults still might not be able to live independently if they lack a good support network.
Cognition	Cognitive impairment, whether it is mild or a dementia, can impact a patient's ability to understand instructions, consent conversation, etc. and also is a risk factor for confusion and delirium. It is important to recognize that poor vision, poor hearing, insomnia, and depression all can make an individual appear as if they have cognitive impairment. Addressing these issues will often lead to a marked improvement in the patient's ability to understand and follow instructions and recommendations.
Pain	Pain already is routinely assessed in most encounters. It is a very common complaint in older adults and often the reason why patients come to a spine specialist. Pain and pain medication both can cause confusion and delirium.
Dizziness	Dizziness in older adults is often multifactorial rather than caused by a single organ system (such as benign paroxysmal positional vertigo). However, it can lead to fear of falling and falls themselves.
Mobility and Sarcopenia	Sarcopenia, the age-related loss of muscle mass and muscle function, is increasingly recognized as a major cause of frailty, loss of mobility and independence, and poor health outcomes such as increased morbidity, hospitalizations, surgical complications, and mortality.
Unintentional Weight Loss	Cachexia, poor appetite, and malnutrition are common in older adults and again a major contributor to frailty. Cachexia includes the loss of fat and muscle tissue, whereas sarcopenia can also be associated with obesity. Poor nutrition, especially inadequate protein intake, can negatively affect surgical outcomes and the rehabilitation process.
Medication	Polypharmacy (often described as five or more prescribed medications) is also associated with poor health outcomes, such as increased risk for hospitalizations. Furthermore, certain classes of medication (for example anti-cholinergic medication or benzodiazepines) significantly increase the risk for falls and delirium.

medical record, and the presence of geriatric syndromes is flagged and easily accessed by every provider. To structure and speed up the assessment, John Morley and colleagues developed the Saint Louis University Rapid Geriatric Assessment that focuses on frailty, sarcopenia, anorexia, cognition, constipation, incontinence, and advanced directives. Their approach provides simple screening tools and helpful mnemonics to identify older individuals at risk and potential causes of anorexia and cognitive impairment.[62] Regardless of how the information becomes available to the provider, it should then be used to tailor intervention to the particular patient in a patient-centered care fashion. This means identifying syndromes that may require preoperative intervention, such as nutrition or preoperative physical therapy. Or it could mean identifying problems that need to be organized postoperatively, such as a skilled nursing facility, home health, or planned assistance of family members for recovery. This could include asking the patient to bring glasses and hearing aids to clinic visits and/or potential hospital stays, and asking family members to be present at important appointments to help with understanding and decision-making. Furthermore, it may emphasize strategies to ensure good nutritional intake and appropriate rehabilitation interventions or to flag the patient as a high fall risk during a hospital stay or ensure regular checks for pressure ulcers if the patient is incontinent. A geriatric or internal medicine consult service could be engaged at the onset of the admission to minimize the risk of delirium, change potentially harmful medication, and help manage problems such as depression and pain. These targeted interventions can lead to better outcomes, less complications, shorter hospital stays, and better patient satisfaction, with many reviews and guidelines providing guidance regarding how to best implement them.[36,60,61,68,70]

1.6 Making the Difference: Outcomes of Addressing Geriatric Syndromes Perioperatively

As previously outlined, many geriatric syndromes have a negative impact on postoperative outcomes (e.g., frailty, depression, dementia, polypharmacy).[16,44,59,68] In this section, a few strategies to reduce the risk of these negative outcomes are introduced. Postoperative delirium and the need for reoperation will be used as examples. Several studies have demonstrated that geriatric syndromes such as frailty, depression and cognitive impairment are associated with postoperative delirium and need for reoperation. Brown and colleagues reported that the frequency of postoperative delirium was 40% after spine surgery.[35] Esamadicy found that the rate of postoperative delirium after elective spine surgery was twice as high in individuals with depression compared to those without that diagnosis.[31] Flexman and colleagues reported that the rate of frailty was 8% in all examined individuals older than 65 years of age undergoing surgery for degenerative spine diseases. The frequency was higher in older age groups when adults older than 65 were separated. In their study, the concurrent diagnosis of frailty increased the risk of reoperation for a surgical infection by 30% and prolonged the length of stay by 30%. It increased the 30-day mortality by almost 50% (odds ratio 1:48).[18] In sum, there are several studies that demonstrate that the presence of

geriatric syndromes leads to a higher frequency of negative postsurgical outcomes in older individuals undergoing spine surgery.

Less data is available on the effectiveness of interventions for geriatric syndromes to reduce the risk of postsurgical complications. A 2018 report by the Coalition for Quality in Geriatric Surgery on the hospital standards to promote optimal surgical care of the older adult recommends screening for many of the factors discussed in this chapter based on their analysis of the available data.[71] This panel recommended CGA or accessing assistance from a multidisciplinary service with geriatrics expertise as the most effective intervention if a screen is positive for any of these diagnoses. Additionally, they advocate for a multidisciplinary conference with the patient and/or the family present for high-risk patients. In 2018, Eamer and colleagues published a Cochrane review on the comprehensive geriatric assessment for older patients admitted to a surgical service.[59] In this systematic review, the authors examined the effect of a comprehensive geriatric assessment on several postsurgical outcomes, including delirium, readmission, length of stay, and mortality. Eight studies were included in the analysis, seven of which were on hip fracture patients. The authors concluded that the comprehensive geriatric assessment made little or no difference on readmission rates and delirium but did lead to decreased mortality (relative risk 0.85) and slightly decreased length of stay. In contrast, a study that was not included in this analysis (likely because of trial design and outcomes) showed significant improvements in postsurgical outcomes.[70] Specifically, the authors report a delirium frequency of 18.5% in 54 patients before their intervention and a rate of 5.6% in 54 different patients after the implementation of their intervention. There was no difference in the readmission rate. A systematic review examining a different type of intervention that focuses on improving the functional status prior to surgery, Prehabilitation, found no positive effect on outcomes such as function, quality of life, or pain.[72,73] In sum, one has to conclude that while the tools to identify risk factors for postsurgical complications have been established, evidence-based interventions to prevent the incidence of these geriatric syndromes are lacking and need to developed and/or validated. Ultimately, guidance from the American College of Surgeons and the American Geriatric Society in their best practice guideline,[61] and Oresanya and colleagues[68] from their evidence-based review can direct the choice of interventions for patients who present or develop geriatric syndromes.

1.7 Conclusion

Caring for the older patient can be very rewarding but often requires a different approach compared to younger adults due to important differences in age-related physiology and care preferences. Health care providers can easily find themselves overwhelmed by the pathophysiologic (multimorbidity, geriatric syndromes, polypharmacy) and psychosocial (depression, delirium, dementia, lack of social support) complexity present in many older patients. A structured geriatric assessment can assist in identifying significant issues and risks in a systematic and manageable approach. Although each patient will present with their own unique profile of problems, frailty, nutritional deficits, depression, dementia, and polypharmacy are of particular importance to the spine provider. Recognizing and addressing these common diagnoses can help in making better decisions as to which interventions to pursue for the sake of better surgical outcomes. No provider will be able to accomplish this task alone. By creating or accessing a multidisciplinary team that has geriatric expertise to manage these factors, the spine specialist can meaningfully reduce postsurgical complications. However, more research is needed to develop and validate evidence-based methods that can guarantee a quick and successful recovery from a necessary spinal intervention in older adults.

References

[1] World Population Ageing 2017 - Highlights. 2017. at http://www.un.org/en/development/desa/population/publications/pdf/ageing/WPA2017_Highlights.pdf

[2] O'Lynnger TM, Zuckerman SL, Morone PJ, Dewan MC, Vasquez-Castellanos RA, Cheng JS. Trends for Spine Surgery for the Elderly: Implications for Access to Healthcare in North America. Neurosurgery. 2015; 77 Suppl 4:S136–S141

[3] Hurwitz EL, Randhawa K, Yu H, Côté P, Haldeman S. The Global Spine Care Initiative: a summary of the global burden of low back and neck pain studies. Eur Spine J. 2018; 27 Suppl 6:796–801

[4] Fehlings MG, Tetreault L, Nater A, et al. The Aging of the Global Population: The Changing Epidemiology of Disease and Spinal Disorders. Neurosurgery. 2015; 77 Suppl 4:S1–S5

[5] Waldrop R, Cheng J, Devin C, McGirt M, Fehlings M, Berven S. The Burden of Spinal Disorders in the Elderly. Neurosurgery. 2015; 77 Suppl 4:S46–S50

[6] Costa AG, Wyman A, Siris ES, et al. When, where and how osteoporosis-associated fractures occur: an analysis from the Global Longitudinal Study of Osteoporosis in Women (GLOW). PLoS One. 2013; 8(12):e83306

[7] Odén A, McCloskey EV, Kanis JA, Harvey NC, Johansson H. Burden of high fracture probability worldwide: secular increases 2010–2040. Osteoporos Int. 2015; 26(9):2243–2248

[8] Nosraty L, Jylhä M, Raittila T, Lumme-Sandt K. Perceptions by the oldest old of successful aging, Vitality 90 + Study. J Aging Stud. 2015; 32:50–58

[9] López-Otín C, Blasco MA, Partridge L, Serrano M, Kroemer G. The hallmarks of aging. Cell. 2013; 153(6):1194–1217

[10] Kasper D, Fauci A, Hauser S, Longo D, Jameson JL, Loscalzo J. Harrison's Principles of Internal Medicine, 19e. New York: McGraw-Hill Education LLC

[11] Inouye SK, Studenski S, Tinetti ME, Kuchel GA. Geriatric syndromes: clinical, research, and policy implications of a core geriatric concept. J Am Geriatr Soc. 2007; 55(5):780–791

[12] Cooper C, Dere W, Evans W, et al. Frailty and sarcopenia: definitions and outcome parameters. Osteoporos Int. 2012; 23(7):1839–1848

[13] Partridge JS, Harari D, Dhesi JK. Frailty in the older surgical patient: a review. Age Ageing. 2012; 41(2):142–147

[14] Robinson TN, Walston JD, Brummel NE, et al. Frailty for Surgeons: Review of a National Institute on Aging Conference on Frailty for Specialists. J Am Coll Surg. 2015; 221(6):1083–1092

[15] Clegg A, Young J, Iliffe S, Rikkert MO, Rockwood K. Frailty in elderly people. Lancet. 2013; 381(9868):752–762

[16] Lin HS, Watts JN, Peel NM, Hubbard RE. Frailty and post-operative outcomes in older surgical patients: a systematic review. BMC Geriatr. 2016; 16(1):157

[17] Leven DM, Lee NJ, Kothari P, et al. Frailty Index Is a Significant Predictor of Complications and Mortality After Surgery for Adult Spinal Deformity. Spine. 2016; 41(23):E1394–E1401

[18] Flexman AM, Charest-Morin R, Stobart L, Street J, Ryerson CJ. Frailty and postoperative outcomes in patients undergoing surgery for degenerative spine disease. Spine J. 2016; 16(11):1315–1323

[19] Fried LP, Tangen CM, Walston J, et al. Cardiovascular Health Study Collaborative Research Group. Frailty in older adults: evidence for a phenotype. J Gerontol A Biol Sci Med Sci. 2001; 56(3):M146–M156

[20] Edwards MH, Buehring B. Novel Approaches to the Diagnosis of Sarcopenia. J Clin Densitom. 2015; 18(4):472–477

[21] Jeejeebhoy KN. Malnutrition, fatigue, frailty, vulnerability, sarcopenia and cachexia: overlap of clinical features. Curr Opin Clin Nutr Metab Care. 2012; 15(3):213–219

[22] Ali S, Garcia JM. Sarcopenia, cachexia and aging: diagnosis, mechanisms and therapeutic options - a mini-review. Gerontology. 2014; 60(4):294–305

[23] Studenski S, Perera S, Patel K, et al. Gait speed and survival in older adults. JAMA. 2011; 305(1):50–58

[24] Rubenstein LZ. Falls in older people: epidemiology, risk factors and strategies for prevention. Age Ageing. 2006; 35 Suppl 2:ii37–ii41

[25] Cawthon PM, Fox KM, Gandra SR, et al. Health, Aging and Body Composition Study. Do muscle mass, muscle density, strength, and physical function similarly influence risk of hospitalization in older adults? J Am Geriatr Soc. 2009; 57(8):1411–1419

[26] Cawthon PM, Fullman RL, Marshall L, et al. Osteoporotic Fractures in Men (MrOS) Research Group. Physical performance and risk of hip fractures in older men. J Bone Miner Res. 2008; 23(7):1037–1044

[27] Panel on Prevention of Falls in Older Persons, American Geriatrics Society and British Geriatrics Society. Summary of the Updated American Geriatrics Society/British Geriatrics Society clinical practice guideline for prevention of falls in older persons. J Am Geriatr Soc. 2011; 59(1): 148–157

[28] Busch MA, Maske UE, Ryl L, Schlack R, Hapke U. [Prevalence of depressive symptoms and diagnosed depression among adults in Germany: results of the German Health Interview and Examination Survey for Adults (DEGS1)]. Bundesgesundheitsblatt Gesundheitsforschung Gesundheitsschutz. 2013; 56 (5–6):733–739

[29] Taylor WD. Clinical practice. Depression in the elderly. N Engl J Med. 2014; 371(13):1228–1236

[30] Kok RM, Reynolds CF, III. Management of Depression in Older Adults: A Review. JAMA. 2017; 317(20):2114–2122

[31] Elsamadicy AA, Adogwa O, Lydon E, et al. Depression as an independent predictor of postoperative delirium in spine deformity patients undergoing elective spine surgery. J Neurosurg Spine. 2017; 27(2):209–214

[32] Wadhwa RK, Ohya J, Vogel TD, et al. Risk factors for 30-day reoperation and 3-month readmission: analysis from the Quality and Outcomes Database lumbar spine registry. J Neurosurg Spine. 2017; 27(2):131–136

[33] Inouye SK, Westendorp RG, Saczynski JS. Delirium in elderly people. Lancet. 2014; 383(9920):911–922

[34] Marcantonio ER. Delirium in Hospitalized Older Adults. N Engl J Med. 2017; 377(15):1456–1466

[35] Brown CH, IV, LaFlam A, Max L, et al. Delirium After Spine Surgery in Older Adults: Incidence, Risk Factors, and Outcomes. J Am Geriatr Soc. 2016; 64 (10):2101–2108

[36] Nazemi AK, Gowd AK, Carmouche JJ, Kates SL, Albert TJ, Behrend CJ. Prevention and Management of Postoperative Delirium in Elderly Patients Following Elective Spinal Surgery. Clin Spine Surg. 2017; 30(3):112–119

[37] Bekelis K, Missios S, Shu J, MacKenzie TA, Mayerson B. Surgical outcomes for patients diagnosed with dementia: A coarsened exact matching study. J Clin Neurosci. 2018; 53:160–164

[38] Sachdev PS, Blacker D, Blazer DG, et al. Classifying neurocognitive disorders: the DSM-5 approach. Nat Rev Neurol. 2014; 10(11):634–642

[39] Gale, S.A., Acar, D., Daffner, K.R. (2018). Dementia. The American Journal of Medicine, 131(10), 1161–1169

[40] Elahi FM, Miller BL. A clinicopathological approach to the diagnosis of dementia. Nat Rev Neurol. 2017; 13(8):457–476

[41] Livingston G, Sommerlad A, Orgeta V, et al. Dementia prevention, intervention, and care. Lancet. 2017; 390(10113):2673–2734

[42] Lin JS, O'Connor E, Rossom RC, et al. U.S. Preventive Services Task Force Evidence Syntheses, formerly Systematic Evidence Reviews. Screening for Cognitive Impairment in Older Adults: An Evidence Update for the US Preventive Services Task Force. Rockville (MD): Agency for Healthcare Research and Quality (US); 2013

[43] Long LS, Shapiro WA, Leung JM. A brief review of practical preoperative cognitive screening tools. Can J Anaesth. 2012; 59(8):798–804

[44] Culley DJ, Flaherty D, Fahey MC, et al. Poor Performance on a Preoperative Cognitive Screening Test Predicts Postoperative Complications in Older Orthopedic Surgical Patients. Anesthesiology. 2017; 127(5):765–774

[45] Levinoff E, Try A, Chabot J, Lee L, Zukor D, Beauchet O. Precipitants of Delirium in Older Inpatients Admitted in Surgery for Post-Fall Hip Fracture: An Observational Study. J Frailty Aging. 2018; 7(1):34–39

[46] Lu WH, Wen YW, Chen LK, Hsiao FY. Effect of polypharmacy, potentially inappropriate medications and anticholinergic burden on clinical outcomes: a retrospective cohort study. CMAJ. 2015; 187(4):E130–E137

[47] Hayes BD, Klein-Schwartz W, Barrueto F, Jr. Polypharmacy and the geriatric patient. Clin Geriatr Med. 2007; 23(2):371–390, vii

[48] Salahudeen MS, Duffull SB, Nishtala PS. Anticholinergic burden quantified by anticholinergic risk scales and adverse outcomes in older people: a systematic review. BMC Geriatr. 2015; 15:31

[49] Cooper JA, Cadogan CA, Patterson SM, et al. Interventions to improve the appropriate use of polypharmacy in older people: a Cochrane systematic review. BMJ Open. 2015; 5(12):e009235

[50] Garfinkel D, Ilhan B, Bahat G. Routine deprescribing of chronic medications to combat polypharmacy. Ther Adv Drug Saf. 2015; 6(6):212–233

[51] Lavan AH, Gallagher PF, O'Mahony D. Methods to reduce prescribing errors in elderly patients with multimorbidity. Clin Interv Aging. 2016; 11:857–866

[52] By the American Geriatrics Society 2015 Beers Criteria Update Expert Panel. American Geriatrics Society 2015 Updated Beers Criteria for Potentially Inappropriate Medication Use in Older Adults. J Am Geriatr Soc. 2015; 63(11): 2227–2246

[53] Tay L, Tan K, Diener E, Gonzalez E. Social relations, health behaviors, and health outcomes: a survey and synthesis. Appl Psychol Health Well-Being. 2013; 5(1):28–78

[54] Holt-Lunstad J, Smith TB, Layton JB. Social relationships and mortality risk: a meta-analytic review. PLoS Med. 2010; 7(7):e1000316

[55] Seeman TE, Crimmins E. Social environment effects on health and aging: integrating epidemiologic and demographic approaches and perspectives. Ann N Y Acad Sci. 2001; 954:88–117

[56] Courtin E, Knapp M. Social isolation, loneliness and health in old age: a scoping review. Health Soc Care Community. 2017; 25(3):799–812

[57] Mabire C, Dwyer A, Garnier A, Pellet J. Meta-analysis of the effectiveness of nursing discharge planning interventions for older inpatients discharged home. J Adv Nurs. 2018; 74(4):788–799

[58] Gonçalves-Bradley DC, Lannin NA, Clemson LM, Cameron ID, Shepperd S. Discharge planning from hospital. Cochrane Database Syst Rev. 2016(1): CD000313

[59] Eamer G, Taheri A, Chen SS, et al. Comprehensive geriatric assessment for older people admitted to a surgical service. Cochrane Database Syst Rev. 2018; 1:CD012485

[60] Partridge JS, Harari D, Martin FC, Dhesi JK. The impact of pre-operative comprehensive geriatric assessment on postoperative outcomes in older patients undergoing scheduled surgery: a systematic review. Anaesthesia. 2014; 69 Suppl 1:8–16

[61] Chow WB, Rosenthal RA, Merkow RP, Ko CY, Esnaola NF, American College of Surgeons National Surgical Quality Improvement Program, American

Geriatrics Society. Optimal preoperative assessment of the geriatric surgical patient: a best practices guideline from the American College of Surgeons National Surgical Quality Improvement Program and the American Geriatrics Society. J Am Coll Surg. 2012; 215(4):453–466

[62] Morley JE. Rapid Geriatric Assessment: Secondary Prevention to Stop Age-Associated Disability. Clin Geriatr Med. 2017; 33(3):431–440

[63] Elsawy B, Higgins KE. The geriatric assessment. Am Fam Physician. 2011; 83 (1):48–56

[64] Ellis G, Gardner M, Tsiachristas A, et al. Comprehensive geriatric assessment for older adults admitted to hospital. Cochrane Database Syst Rev. 2017; 9: CD006211

[65] Rosen SL, Reuben DB. Geriatric assessment tools. Mt Sinai J Med. 2011; 78(4): 489–497

[66] Kruschinski C, Wiese B, Dierks ML, Hummers-Pradier E, Schneider N, Junius-Walker U. A geriatric assessment in general practice: prevalence, location, impact and doctor-patient perceptions of pain. BMC Fam Pract. 2016; 17:8

[67] Barkhausen T, Junius-Walker U, Hummers-Pradier E, Mueller CA, Theile G. "It's MAGIC"–development of a manageable geriatric assessment for general practice use. BMC Fam Pract. 2015; 16:4

[68] Oresanya LB, Lyons WL, Finlayson E. Preoperative assessment of the older patient: a narrative review. JAMA. 2014; 311(20):2110–2120

[69] Bergert FW, Braun M, Feßler J, et al. Geriatrisches Assessment in der Hausarztpraxis. DEGAM Hausärztliche Leitlinie: Deutschen Gesellschaft für. Allgemein- und Familienmedizin (DEGAM); 2017

[70] Harari D, Hopper A, Dhesi J, Babic-Illman G, Lockwood L, Martin F. Proactive care of older people undergoing surgery ('POPS'): designing, embedding, evaluating and funding a comprehensive geriatric assessment service for older elective surgical patients. Age Ageing. 2007; 36 (2):190–196

[71] Berian JR, Rosenthal RA, Baker TL, et al. Hospital Standards to Promote Optimal Surgical Care of the Older Adult: A Report From the Coalition for Quality in Geriatric Surgery. Ann Surg. 2018; 267(2):280–290

[72] Nielsen PR, Jørgensen LD, Dahl B, Pedersen T, Tønnesen H. Prehabilitation and early rehabilitation after spinal surgery: randomized clinical trial. Clin Rehabil. 2010; 24(2):137–148

[73] Cabilan CJ, Hines S, Munday J. The Impact of Prehabilitation on Postoperative Functional Status, Healthcare Utilization, Pain, and Quality of Life: A Systematic Review. Orthop Nurs. 2016; 35(4):224–237

2 Age-Related Changes in the Spine

Lee S. Hwang and Edward C. Benzel

Abstract

The progressive degenerative changes associated with aging gradually affect all components of the spine and associated structures. The degenerative process begins early, during the first decade of life in the intervertebral disc. This process involves biochemical changes that are followed by macroscopic alterations, including tears and fissures. Ultimately, this may lead to loss of disc height and disc herniation. Facet joint hypertrophy and laxity often follow. Other accompanying changes include osteoporosis of the vertebral bodies, hypertrophy of the ligamentum flavum, and weakening of the paraspinal musculature. The accumulation of these age-related modifications causes narrowing of the spinal canal and collapse of the vertebral body to varying degrees. In addition, the dynamic adaptation of the spine to the forces involved in daily activities also contributes to the alterations. The excessive compensation can sometimes lead to pathological conditions, such as thoracic hyperkyphosis, which contributes to global sagittal imbalance and deformity. Furthermore, the flexibility and range of motion in both cervical and lumbar spines diminish with age. Degenerative changes in the spine are features of the normal aging process. This chapter provides the reader with an understanding of these age-related changes to provide an understanding of the natural history of spine degeneration in order to guide diagnosis of pathological conditions and determine treatment strategies.

Keywords: Aging spine, degenerative changes, stenosis, spondylosis, spinal osteoarthritis

Key Points

- Progressive degenerative changes associated with aging gradually affect all components of the functional spinal unit and adjacent structures
- The intervertebral discs lose water content, facet joints undergo arthritic changes, spinal ligaments hypertrophy, and paraspinal muscles weaken – eventually leading to narrowing of the spinal canal
- Excessive thoracic kyphosis may become pathologic (hyperkyphosis), causing sagittal imbalance and deformity
- Flexibility and range of motion in both cervical and lumbar spines diminish with age
- Understanding age-related changes in the spine may guide diagnosis of pathological conditions and treatment strategies

2.1 Background

As the spine naturally ages and endures physical stressors associated with the activities of daily living, a gradual decrease in strength and range of motion ensues. At the cellular level, the musculoskeletal system undergoes senescence, apoptosis, alterations in the extracellular matrix due to accumulation of posttranslational modifications of matrix proteins as well as an increase in oxidative stress due to the production of reactive oxygen species. Systemically, the body experiences reduced levels of trophic hormones, decreased function of organs, and generalized impairment of mobility. These multifactorial changes may affect any part of the musculoskeletal system, particularly the spine. Among the age-related pathological processes of the spine, *degenerating spondylosis*, or *spinal osteoarthritis*, is the most common. This condition is radiographically associated with narrowed disc spaces and osteophytes, or bone spurs, at the margins of the vertebral body. Autopsy studies have demonstrated spondylosis in 60% of women and 80% of men by age 49, and in 95% of both genders by age 70.[1]

2.2 The Functional Spinal unit

The bony spine is comprised of multiple segmental levels and columns at each level, providing structural stability as well as functional mobility, while protecting the nerve roots and the spinal cord. The functional spinal unit refers to the smallest anatomical unit that includes all the basic functional characteristics of the entire spine, first described by Schmorl and Junghanns.[1] Each segmental level consists of two adjacent vertebrae separated dorsally by facet joints and ventrally by the intervertebral disc. These components collectively constitute the functional spinal unit (▶ Fig. 2.1). The vertebrae are also supported by ligaments, joint capsules, and paraspinal musculature. The spinal ligaments include the interspinous and supraspinous ligaments, the ligamentum flavum, and the anterior and posterior longitudinal ligaments. The muscles spanning over two vertebrae include the splenius, erector spinae, transversospinal, and segmental muscles. The stability and mobility of the spine are primarily achieved via the interplay between the aforementioned structures and the powerful flexor and extensor muscle groups. Normal spinal function also relies on the proper interaction with the *three-joint complex*, which is comprised of the intervertebral disc and the two facet joints (functional spinal unit). Any significant alteration of these components may cause dysfunction, eventually leading to pain, deformity, and neurologic compromise.

2.3 The Intervertebral Disc

Intervertebral discs are located between the vertebral bodies, transmitting the load from body weight and muscle activity and simultaneously facilitating motion. Such motion includes bending, twisting, and cushioning (axial load-related deformation). The intervertebral disc (▶ Fig. 2.2) consists of a gelatinous core (nucleus pulposus) and a fibroblast-like cell matrix with parallel collagen fibers arranged in concentric rings called lamellae (annulus fibrosus).[2,3] Elastin fibers, also within the lamellae, contribute to restoration of the disc morphology after movement of the spine.[4] The nucleus pulposus dissipates the

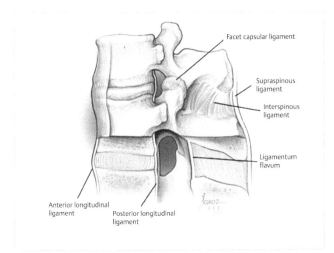

Fig. 2.1 The functional spinal unit is comprised of two adjacent vertebrae with corresponding facet joints, intervertebral disc, and intervening ligaments – acting collectively as a motion segment. Reprinted with permission, Cleveland Clinic Center for Medical Art & Photography © 2017. All Rights Reserved.

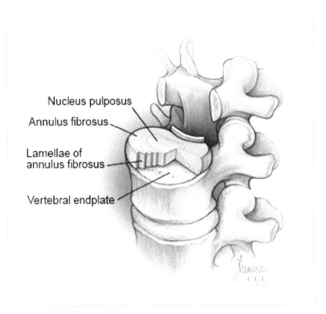

Fig. 2.2 The intervertebral disc consists of a gelatinous core, called nucleus pulposus, and a matrix with parallel collagen fibers arranged in concentric rings called lamellae (annulus fibrosus). The endplate forms a physical barrier to prevent bulging of the nucleus pulposus into the vertebral body and partially absorbs the hydrostatic pressure dissipated by the nucleus pulposus under loading. Reprinted with permission, Cleveland Clinic Center for Medical Art & Photography © 2017. All Rights Reserved.

compressive forces on the disc by exerting hydrostatic pressure on the annulus fibrosus. The nucleus pulposus contains collagen fibers, elastin fibers, and aggrecan-containing proteoglycan gel with interspersed chondrocyte-like cells.[5] Collagen comprises up to 70% of the annulus fibrosus but only 20% of the nucleus pulposus.[6] On the other hand, up to 50% of the nucleus pulposus contains proteoglycans, whereas the annulus fibrosus only contains 20%. Finally, the contents of the disc matrix vary due to continuous turnover by enzymes such as matrix metalloproteases and aggrecanases produced by the disc cells.[7,8]

Degenerative changes can occur as early as 10 years of age, with microscopic tears in the nucleus pulposus, focal disc cell proliferation, and granular matrix transformation, along with an increase in acidic mucopolysaccharides in the disc matrix.[9] These changes progress through young adulthood, and by the third decade of life, the nucleus pulposus begins to lose its gelatinous consistency and develops multiple large clefts with significant granular changes in the matrix. At the molecular level, there is also a loss of proteoglycans and water content, with an increase in collagen. An adult disc, aged 30 to 50 years, has less clear distinction between the nucleus pulposus and the annulus fibrosus. By the fifth decade, the nucleus pulposus is dry, with a solid, rubbery consistency, merging with the inner annulus and containing even more collagen and fewer cells. In individuals older than 70 years, the intervertebral disc becomes more scar-like, with large tissue defects. The progressive alterations in the matrix composition often results in a loss of disc height, which subsequently increases the load on the facet joints and predisposes the bony segment to arthritic changes and the ligamentum flavum to hypertrophy, eventually leading to narrowing of the spinal canal.

Aging and degeneration are also associated with dramatic changes in vascularization and innervation of the disc. A healthy adult disc is avascular. On the other hand, in the setting of degeneration and herniation, blood vessels penetrate through the disc space in response to angiogenesis factors,

metalloproteases, and various cytokines.[10,11,12] In addition, nociceptive nerve fibers expressing substance P have been found in the nucleus pulposus of discs associated with chronic pain.[13]

2.4 The Cartilage Endplate

The thin hyaline cartilage endplate separates the disc from the bony interface of the adjacent vertebral body, providing biomechanical integrity and disc nutrition. At birth, the cartilage endplate is approximately 50% of the intervertebral space, in comparison to approximately 5% in adults.[9] Over time, vascular channels are gradually replaced by the extracellular matrix. The endplate acts as a growth plate for the adjacent vertebral body, similar to the epiphyseal growth plate of long bones. In adulthood, the endplate is approximately 0.6 mm thick with calcification, occupying the central 90% of the interface between the disc and the vertebral body.[9] The endplate forms a physical barrier to prevent bulging of the nucleus pulposus into the spongiosa of the vertebral body, acts as a filter between the disc and vertebral body, and partially absorbs the hydrostatic pressure dissipated by the nucleus pulposus under loading conditions (▶ Fig. 2.2).[14] The endplate is also the main pathway for nutrients to reach the avascular nucleus pulposus by diffusion from the blood supply of the vertebral body.[15]

By the third decade of life, the endplate has sustained various alterations, including fissure and cleft formation, microfractures, and decreased chondrocytes, as well as extensive ossification. The diminished vasculature results in reduced

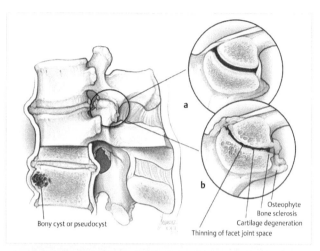

Fig. 2.3 **(a)** Normal facet joint of lumbar spine **(b)** With aging, the facet joint undergoes arthritic changes including complete loss of articular cartilage, vertebral bony cysts and pseudocysts, dense bone sclerosis, and osteophyte formation. Reprinted with permission, Cleveland Clinic Center for Medical Art & Photography © 2017. All Rights Reserved.

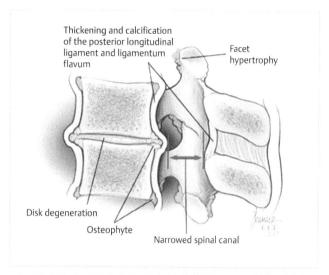

Fig. 2.4 Hypertrophy and calcification of spinal ligaments, along with loss of intervertebral disc height, contribute to the gradual narrowing of the spinal canal. Reprinted with permission, Cleveland Clinic Center for Medical Art & Photography © 2017. All Rights Reserved.

nutritional supply to the intervertebral disc and dense sclerosis of the adjacent vertebral bodies.

2.5 The Facet Joints

The bony articulations between the posterior elements of adjacent vertebrae are called facet, or zygapophyseal, joints. These synovial joints of the spine contain hyaline cartilage overlying subchondral bone. They prevent excessive mobility of the spine and distribute axial load over a broad area, resisting most of the intervertebral shear forces.[16] Furthermore, the posterolateral fibrous capsule, comprised of multilayered fibrous tissue and synovial membrane, is richly innervated with small C-type pain fibers.[17]

Similar to large synovial joints, suboptimal orientation and malalignment of the facet joints increase the risk of arthritic changes, including complete loss of articular cartilage, bony cysts and pseudocysts, dense bone sclerosis, and large osteophyte formation (▶ Fig. 2.3). In late stages, endplate fractures can occur that resemble breaches in the subchondral bone plate, with protruding portions of the articular cartilage into the subarticular bone. These progressive degenerative changes, often with concomitant loss of intervertebral disc height and segmental instability, lead to increased load and subsequent subluxation of the facet joints, then ultimately multilevel spondylosis and stenosis.

2.6 The Vertebral Bodies

The vertebral bodies provide most of the static stability of the spine, and age-related degeneration decreases the structural strength. Over time, the bone undergoes modifications in cytoarchitecture, density, remodeling, and repair. The increasingly fragile bone is then predisposed to osteoporotic fractures, which may ultimately cause disc herniation into the vertebral bodies and spinal deformities.

2.7 The Spinal Ligaments

The ligamentous complex surrounding the spine provides structural support and limits excessive motion in all planes. Copious amounts of well-organized collagen fibers provide tensile strength in all ligaments except the ligamentum flavum, which contains a high percentage of elastin.[18]

The spinal ligaments undergo various age-related changes, including reduced concentration of collagen and water content, decrease in reducible collagen cross-links, and disorganization of collagen fibers.[19] There is also an increase in elastin with age, which decreases the tensile strength and affects the stabilizing function of the longitudinal ligaments. Hypertrophy of the ligamentum flavum, along with loss of intervertebral disc height, contributes to the gradual narrowing of the spinal canal (▶ Fig. 2.4).[20,21]

2.8 The Spinal Muscles

The trunk and pelvic muscles are crucial for maintenance of posture and active movement. During motion, equilibrium and control of stability are maintained by the antagonistic actions of the extensor dorsal musculature and abdominal flexors. The presence of muscles reduces the load and stress on the vertebral body, intradiscal space, and other mechanical components of the spine.

Aging leads to loss of muscle mass, fatty infiltration, and deposits of connective tissue. Starting as early as age 25, the muscle mass decreases 3 to 8% per decade until age 50, when the degeneration rate increases to 10% per decade.[22] During age-related sarcopenia, the reduced number and size of myocytes results in a significant decrease in the strength of the muscle fibers. In women, sarcopenia is affected by levels of estrogen, vitamin D, and IL-6; whereas, in men, testosterone, physical performance, and TNF-α are the most significant contributing factors.[23] The loss of muscle mass compromises spinal stability, and the resulting imbalance may contribute to progressive structural disorganization as well as development of degenerative scoliosis.

2.9 Changes in Spinal Balance

The degenerative changes of the spine accumulate and contribute to the development of progressive kyphosis with aging. In childhood and through the third decade of life, the angle of thoracic kyphosis averages 20 to 29°.[24] After 40 years of age, the mean thoracic kyphosis increases to 53° in individuals aged 60 to 74 and to 66° in those older than 75 years of age.[25] The kyphosis angle increases more rapidly with age in women relative to men.[26]

The age-related thoracic kyphosis may be difficult to distinguish from a pathological condition described as hyperkyphosis – a thoracic kyphosis angle greater than 40°, which represents the 95th percentile of normal for young adults.[24] In older adults, the incidence of hyperkyphosis ranges from 20 to 40% among both men and women.[27] The multifactorial contributing factors include chronic vertebral compression fractures, osteoporosis, and degenerative disc disease, as well as functional changes in muscle strength and posture.[28]

The overall spinal alignment depends on the regional alignment of individual spinal segments as well as the pelvis.[29] The combinatorial effects of various degenerative changes, including thoracic hyperkyphosis and loss of lumbar lordosis, contribute to a global sagittal imbalance.[30] The disequilibrium of forces along the spinal column may eventually lead to deformity as well as adaptive changes in the pelvis, lower limbs, and overall spinal posture.[31,32,33]

2.10 Changes in Spinal Flexibility

Flexibility and range of motion (ROM) rely on the soft tissues of the joints, tendons, ligaments, and muscles and are specific to each joint and level of the spine. The maximal ROM is achieved in the mid- to late 20 s and gradually decreases with age, approximately 20 to 30% between the ages of 30 and 70.[34] The overall ROM in the cervical spine diminishes by 4 to 6° per decade, with the most severe limitation in extension.[35,36,37,38] There is also a significant reduction in lumbar flexion, extension, and lateral flexion in both females and males after 40 years of age.[39] Inadequate ROM and inflexibility throughout the spine may significantly impact functional tasks, activities of daily living, and general mobility.[40] These restrictions can also contribute to gait abnormalities and increase the risk of falls.

2.11 Conclusion

In the aging population, degenerative stenosis and deformities of the spine are prevalent. Age-related changes in the components of the functional spinal unit, as well as the surrounding ligaments and musculature, often lead to progressive microscopic and macroscopic disorganization and disequilibrium. The dynamic adaptation of the spine to the forces involved in daily activities also contributes to the alterations. The excessive compensation can sometimes lead to pathological conditions, such as thoracic hyperkyphosis, which contributes to global sagittal imbalance and deformity. Furthermore, the flexibility and range of motion in both cervical and lumbar spines diminish with age. Degenerative changes in the spine are features of the normal aging process, developing at variable time points in life and with variable severity in each individual. Understanding these specific changes may guide diagnosis of pathological conditions and treatment strategies.

Key References

[1] Ailon T, Shaffrey CI, Lenke LG, Harrop JS, Smith JS. Progressive spinal kyphosis in the aging population. Neurosurgery. 2015; 77 Suppl 4:S164–S172

[2] Boos N, Weissbach S, Rohrbach H, Weiler C, Spratt KF, Nerlich AG. Classification of age-related changes in lumbar intervertebral discs: 2002 Volvo Award in basic science. Spine. 2002; 27(23):2631–2644

[3] Dreischarf M, Albiol L, Rohlmann A, et al. Age-related loss of lumbar spinal lordosis and mobility–a study of 323 asymptomatic volunteers. PLoS One. 2014; 9(12):e116186

[4] Hukins DW, Kirby MC, Sikoryn TA, Aspden RM, Cox AJ. Comparison of structure, mechanical properties, and functions of lumbar spinal ligaments. Spine. 1990; 15(8):787–795

References

[1] Junghanns SA. The human spine in health and disease. New York, NY: Grune and Stratton; 1971

[2] Postacchini F, Bellocci M, Massobrio M. Morphologic changes in annulus fibrosus during aging. An ultrastructural study in rats. Spine. 1984; 9(6):596–603

[3] Roberts S. Disc morphology in health and disease. Biochem Soc Trans. 2002; 30(Pt 6):864–869

[4] Yu J, Winlove PC, Roberts S, Urban JP. Elastic fibre organization in the intervertebral discs of the bovine tail. J Anat. 2002; 201(6):465–475

[5] Marchand F, Ahmed AM. Investigation of the laminate structure of lumbar disc anulus fibrosus. Spine. 1990; 15(5):402–410

[6] Eyre DR, Muir H. Quantitative analysis of types I and II collagens in human intervertebral discs at various ages. Biochim Biophys Acta. 1977; 492(1):29–42

[7] Doita M, Kanatani T, Ozaki T, Matsui N, Kurosaka M, Yoshiya S. Influence of macrophage infiltration of herniated disc tissue on the production of matrix metalloproteinases leading to disc resorption. Spine. 2001; 26(14):1522–1527

[8] Roberts S, Caterson B, Menage J, Evans EH, Jaffray DC, Eisenstein SM. Matrix metalloproteinases and aggrecanase: their role in disorders of the human intervertebral disc. Spine. 2000; 25(23):3005–3013

[9] Boos N, Weissbach S, Rohrbach H, Weiler C, Spratt KF, Nerlich AG. Classification of age-related changes in lumbar intervertebral discs: 2002 Volvo Award in basic science. Spine. 2002; 27(23):2631–2644

[10] Bibby S, Jones DA, Lee RB, Jing YU, Urban J. Biochimie. Biologie et physiologie du disque intervertebral. Rev Rhum. 2001; 68:903–908

[11] Goupille P, Zerkak D, Lemaire V, et al. Role des deteriorations discales dans la survenue d'une lombalgie. Rev Rhum. 2000; 67(Suppl 4):253–260

[12] Rannou F, Corvol M, Revel M, Poiraudeau S. Degenerescence discale et hernie discale: role des metalloproteases et cytokines. Rev Rhum. 2001; 68:913–920

[13] Freemont AJ, Peacock TE, Goupille P, Hoyland JA, O'Brien J, Jayson MI. Nerve ingrowth into diseased intervertebral disc in chronic back pain. Lancet. 1997; 350(9072):178–181

[14] Broberg KB. On the mechanical behaviour of intervertebral discs. Spine. 1983; 8(2):151–165

[15] Roberts S, Urban JPG, Evans H, Eisenstein SM. Transport properties of the human cartilage endplate in relation to its composition and calcification. Spine. 1996; 21(4):415–420

[16] Adams MA, Hutton WC. The effect of posture on the role of the apophysial joints in resisting intervertebral compressive forces. J Bone Joint Surg Br. 1980; 62(3):358–362

[17] Bogduk N. The innervation of the lumbar spine. Spine. 1983; 8(3):286–293

[18] Hukins DW, Kirby MC, Sikoryn TA, Aspden RM, Cox AJ. Comparison of structure, mechanical properties, and functions of lumbar spinal ligaments. Spine. 1990; 15(8):787–795

[19] Okuda T, Baba I, Fujimoto Y, et al. The pathology of ligamentum flavum in degenerative lumbar disease. Spine. 2004; 29(15):1689–1697

[20] Beamer YB, Garner JT, Shelden CH. Hypertrophied ligamentum flavum. Clinical and surgical significance. Arch Surg. 1973; 106(3):289–292

[21] Fukuyama S, Nakamura T, Ikeda T, Takagi K. The effect of mechanical stress on hypertrophy of the lumbar ligamentum flavum. J Spinal Disord. 1995; 8 (2):126–130

[22] Melton LJ, III, Khosla S, Crowson CS, O'Connor MK, O'Fallon WM, Riggs BL. Epidemiology of sarcopenia. J Am Geriatr Soc. 2000; 48(6):625–630

[23] Iannuzzi-Sucich M, Prestwood KM, Kenny AM. Prevalence of sarcopenia and predictors of skeletal muscle mass in healthy, older men and women. J Gerontol A Biol Sci Med Sci. 2002; 57(12):M772–M777

[24] Fon GT, Pitt MJ, Thies AC, Jr. Thoracic kyphosis: range in normal subjects. AJR Am J Roentgenol. 1980; 134(5):979–983

[25] Boyle JJ, Milne N, Singer KP. Influence of age on cervicothoracic spinal curvature: an ex vivo radiographic survey. Clin Biomech (Bristol, Avon). 2002; 17 (5):361–367

[26] Ensrud KE, Black DM, Harris F, Ettinger B, Cummings SR, The Fracture Intervention Trial Research Group. Correlates of kyphosis in older women. J Am Geriatr Soc. 1997; 45(6):682–687

[27] Kado DM, Prenovost K, Crandall C. Narrative review: hyperkyphosis in older persons. Ann Intern Med. 2007; 147(5):330–338

[28] Ailon T, Shaffrey CI, Lenke LG, Harrop JS, Smith JS. Progressive spinal kyphosis in the aging population. Neurosurgery. 2015; 77 Suppl 4:S164–S172

[29] Ames CP, Smith JS, Scheer JK, et al. Impact of spinopelvic alignment on decision making in deformity surgery in adults: A review. J Neurosurg Spine. 2012; 16(6):547–564

[30] Dreischarf M, Albiol L, Rohlmann A, et al. Age-related loss of lumbar spinal lordosis and mobility–a study of 323 asymptomatic volunteers. PLoS One. 2014; 9(12):e116186

[31] Berthonnaud E, Dimnet J, Roussouly P, Labelle H. Analysis of the sagittal balance of the spine and pelvis using shape and orientation parameters. J Spinal Disord Tech. 2005; 18(1):40–47

[32] Farcy JP, Schwab FJ. Management of flatback and related kyphotic decompensation syndromes. Spine. 1997; 22(20):2452–2457

[33] Glassman SD, Bridwell K, Dimar JR, Horton W, Berven S, Schwab F. The impact of positive sagittal balance in adult spinal deformity. Spine. 2005; 30(18): 2024–2029

[34] Bello-Haas VD. Chapter 6: Neuromusculoskeletal and Movement Function. In: Bonder BR, Bello-Haas VD, eds. Functional Performance in Older Adults. 3rd ed. Philadelphia, PA: F.A. Davis Company; 2009:130–167

[35] Chen J, Solinger AB, Poncet JF, Lantz CA. Meta-analysis of normative cervical motion. Spine. 1999; 24(15):1571–1578

[36] Peolsson A, Hedlund R, Ertzgaard S, Oberg B. Intra- and inter-tester reliability and range of motion of the neck. Physiother Can. 2000; 52: 233–242

[37] Salo P, Ylinen J, Kautiainen H, Häkkinen K, Häkkinen A. Neck muscle strength and mobility of the cervical spine as predictors of neck pain: a prospective 6-year study. Spine. 2012; 37(12):1036–1040

[38] Simpson AK, Biswas D, Emerson JW, Lawrence BD, Grauer JN. Quantifying the effects of age, gender, degeneration, and adjacent level degeneration on cervical spine range of motion using multivariate analyses. Spine. 2008; 33(2): 183–186

[39] Intolo P, Milosavljevic S, Baxter DG, Carman AB, Pal P, Munn J. The effect of age on lumbar range of motion: a systematic review. Man Ther. 2009; 14(6): 596–604

[40] Kado DM, Huang MH, Barrett-Connor E, Greendale GA. Hyperkyphotic posture and poor physical functional ability in older community-dwelling men and women: the Rancho Bernardo study. J Gerontol A Biol Sci Med Sci. 2005; 60(5):633–637

3 Diagnosis and Treatment of Osteoporosis in the Aging Spine Patient

Paul A. Anderson and Neil Binkley

Abstract

Low bone mass (osteopenia and osteoporosis) is a common condition that is poorly managed in our current health care system. Poor bone health can increase fragility and fracture risk and also adversely affect outcomes following spinal surgery. The spine practitioner can help patients by taking ownership of bone health. Secondary fracture prevention is aimed at making the first fracture the last fracture by diagnosing and treating poor bone health and intervening to reduce fall risk. Unfortunately, less than 20% of patients who have an osteoporosis-related fracture receive treatment for osteoporosis. Fracture liaison services are becoming increasingly available and provide a comprehensive approach to reduce the risk of subsequent fracture. These programs reduce secondary fractures by 40%. Preoperative bone health optimization is a newer approach aimed at optimizing bone health prior to surgery. Recent investigations show a link between poor surgical outcomes with vitamin D deficiency and osteoporosis. Conversely, as might be expected, treatment with bisphosphonates or bone anabolic medications improves surgical outcomes. The critical components of these programs are assessing the risk of poor bone health, identifying and correcting vitamin D deficiency, eliminating toxins that adversely affect bone (e.g., smoking and excess alcohol intake) recommending fall prevention as required, practicing weight bearing exercises, and maintaining proper nutrition. Dual-energy X-ray absorptiometry (DXA) is an essential part of evaluation, as it classifies bone status and can be ordered and interpreted by all spine practitioners. Advances in DXA testing include vertebral fracture assessment and trabecular bone scoring that may aid in identification of patients with occult fracture and patients with poor quality. Since bone is fundamental to the function of the spine, practitioners should include diagnostic and treatment of bone health when evaluating patients with spinal diseases.

Keywords: Secondary fracture prevention, Osteoporosis, preoperative bone health optimization, osteoporotic-related fracture, Vitamin D

Key Points

- Low bone mass is endemic but poorly managed in our current health care system and negatively affects quality of life and independence.
- Even after fragility fracture, only 20% of patients receive osteoporosis care
- Assessment of bone health can be done by all spine practitioners.
- Secondary fracture prevention programs are effective and reduce secondary fracture risk by ~40%.
- Low bone mass and associated metabolic abnormalities are associated with poorer outcomes after elective spine surgery

- Principles of quality bone health assessment and management include:
  1. All patients with fractures after age 50 need evaluation, including basic laboratory and bone mineral density measurement
  2. This evaluation includes:
     a) Laboratory measurement of calcium, creatinine, alkaline phosphatase, 25-OH vitamin D, CBC
     b) Personal review of the DXA scan image
     c) Consideration of falls, home safety, vision and, if weakness or balance issues are present, physical therapy evaluation.
  3. Calcium intake of 1000 to 1200 mg daily, vitamin D of at least 1,000 IU; consider protein supplementation in older adults.
  4. Treat with pharmaceuticals for 3 to 5 years if fracture risk is high, such as for recent fractures, falls, FRAX risk ≥ 20% for major fracture.

3.1 Background

Low bone mass, (osteopenia and osteoporosis), is an underappreciated health crisis that increases risk for fracture in older adults, with resultant decreased quality of life, morbidity, including loss of independence, and increased mortality. The spine is the most common site of symptoms from osteoporosis due to fracture and deformity. Further, many patients with low bone mass are frequently seeking care for related or unrelated spinal diseases. Spine surgeons need to be aware that poor bone status may adversely influence surgical outcomes and increase the likelihood of complications and revision surgeries (▶ Fig. 3.1). The purpose of this chapter is to review the epidemiology of osteoporosis. Focus will be on the morbidity and mortality associated with spinal fractures, as well as the influence of osteoporosis on spine surgery outcomes. Additionally, current guideline-based diagnoses and overall management approaches will be reviewed. There will be an emphasis on secondary fracture care and on preoperative optimization of spinal patients for surgery.

The occurrence of a low-energy fracture in an older patient is a sentinel event that is a teaching and management opportunity. The goal is to make this fracture the last one. This is done through a systematic approach, including education, assessment, correction of metabolic abnormalities, treatment, rehabilitation, and follow-up. In 2004, the Surgeon General of the United States reported that there is "the gap between what we know and its application," "much of what we know is not always applied in practice" and "primary care and orthopedic surgeons rarely discuss osteoporosis in patients having fractures."[1] Unfortunately, fewer patients are being treated following fractures now than was the case in 2004.[2] Indeed, leaders in the medical osteoporosis community have called this failure to

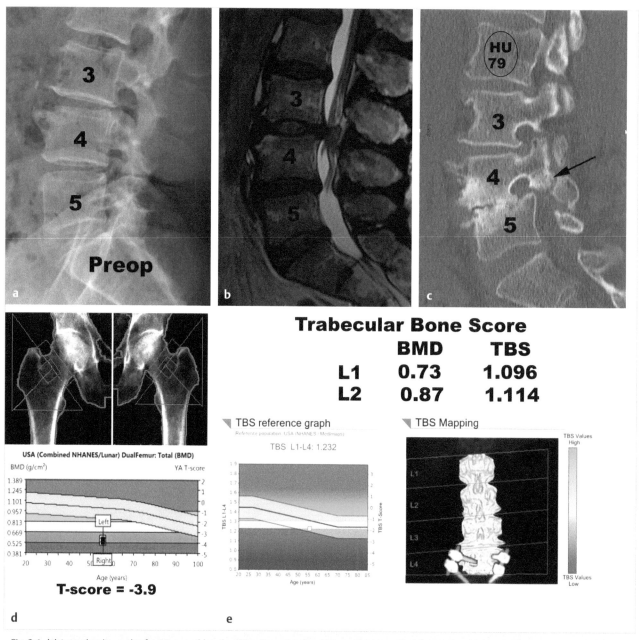

Fig. 3.1 **(a)** Lateral radiograph of a 51-year-old male with a long-standing history of seizure disorders and multiple falls who has developed lumbar spinal stenosis at L3–4 and L4–5. He failed medical management and underwent laminectomy decompression at L3–4 and L4–5. **(b)**T2 weighted MRI scan showing spinal stenosis at L3–4 and L4–5 with normal alignment. **(c)** Six-month postoperative lateral radiograph. The patient has recurrent back and leg pain, was found to have progressive L4–5 disc degeneration and pars fracture with iatrogenic spondylolisthesis at L4–5 (arrow). The Hounsfield units at L2 vertebral body measure 79, indicating probable osteoporosis. This was felt secondary to long-standing medication use to control seizures. **(d)** Bone mineral density was obtained of the hips, showing a T-score of -3.9, indicating severe osteoporosis. **(e)** Trabecular Bone Score (TBS) obtained after revision surgery where a posterior instrumentation at L4–5 was performed. The TBS was 1.096 and 1.114 at L1 and L2 respectively. This indicates a severe qualitative bony defect.

treat a "crisis."[3] This has spurred efforts to improve delivery of secondary fracture care with the goal to prevent further fractures.

3.2 Epidemiology

Low bone density (osteopenia and osteoporosis) is common and is present in an estimated 53 million Americans in 2010.[4]

This is expected to increase to 65 million in 2020 and over 71 million in 2030. Twenty percent of these patients have osteoporosis with dual-energy X-ray absorptiometry (DXA) T-scores below -2.5. Fractures occur in 2.1 million older adults annually, a number greater than that of stroke, heart attack and breast cancer combined.[5] It is estimated that these fractures cost greater than $20 billion per year; an amount expected to significantly increase. In 2011, over 325,000 patients were hospitalized for hip fracture, while 260,000 were hospitalized for spine fracture.[6] However, only one in three spine fractures are clinically appreciated, and many do not require hospitalization. As the population ages, hospitalization for fractures is expected to increase. Approximately 1% of patients in their 50 s are admitted to the hospital because of fragility fractures, while of those over 80 years, approximately 5.5% receive a diagnosis of fragility fracture.[5] This is greater for females than for males. Burge estimated that between the years of 2005 and 2025, there will be a 76% increase in the number of women with fragility fracture and a 24% increase in men.[5] Costs will correspondingly increase by 73% in females and 27% in males. Schousboe has shown that clinical vertebral fractures increase significantly after the age of 65 and are more frequent in the United States than in Northern Europe.[7] For example, the vertebral fracture incidence triples per 100,000 person-years between the ages of 70 and 80 for women in the U.S.

3.3 Morbidity and Mortality of Fractures in Older Adults

Fractures in older adults are life-changing events. The adverse effects of fracture on quality of life and independence have not received adequate attention by the medical community and may be unappreciated by patients. There is a significantly increased chance of loss of independence, higher mortality, chronic pain, loss of function, and reduced health-related quality of life. Tajeu compared 43,000 patients with hip fractures against age-matched comparators at one year follow-up.[8] Mortality was 28.6% at one year compared to 12% for the control group, with a risk ratio of 2.2. Debility, defined as transfer from community living to long-term care, occurred in 20% of those with hip fracture and 5.5% of controls. Destitution, defined as transfer to Medicaid or Medicare supplement, was twice as likely after hip fracture than among controls, occurring in 6.6% compared to 3.1%.

Near-term mortality after vertebral fractures is similar to that of hip fracture. Lau used the Medicare database of 97,300 patients with vertebral fracture and compared mortality to control group.[9] The Hazard ratio ranged 2.2 to 3 compared to no-fracture controls, depending on age at the time of the original fracture. Kaplan Meier analysis shows significant increased mortality over time after vertebral fracture. For instance, at 5 years, only 30% of patients with osteoporotic fracture had survived, compared to 70% of controls. Chen noted that a patient's independence was significantly altered after vertebral fracture. At 2 years, 24% of patients were living at home, with another 15% requiring home health care services.[10] Forty-one percent were transferred to skilled nursing facilities, and 19% to other long-term care facilities.

Although only one-third of vertebral fractures are clinically evident, they may be associated with significant pain. Chen reported that average baseline pain was 7.8, improving significantly to 3.4 over 6 months in conservatively treated patients.[10] This high pain level is notable in that it is significantly greater than those patients enrolled in the SPORT trial for spinal stenosis. Tosteson, using the SF-36, reported long-term, health-related quality of life at 5 years for 215 patients having hip and spine fracture compared to 200 controls.[11] Self-reported limitations and activities of daily living (ADLs) were commonly reported in 25% of those with spine and 58% with hip fractures. If patients had combined hip and spine fractures, over two-thirds reported self-limited ADL limitations. The SF-36 physical components score was a mean of 40 in spine fracture patients, 34 in hip fractures, and 30 if the patient had combined hip and spine fractures, compared to normal age-matched control of 50. Interestingly, the mental health components scores did not vary despite the fractures. Svensson reported patients' perceptions after vertebral compression fractures using a structured narrative technique of 10 community ambulators over the age of 80.[12] Fear concerns were dominant; they particularly struggled to understand a deceiving body and breakthrough pain and reported feelings of fear: of a trajectory into isolation, of dependency, and of an uncertain future.

3.4 Risk of Secondary Fracture

It is well known that "fracture begets fracture." For example, Hodsman calculated the risk of secondary fractures out to 10 years in patients over 65.[13] At 2 years, 11% of hip fracture patients and 12% of spine fracture patients had secondary fractures. This increased to 15 and 16% at 5 years and 25% at 10 years. Center reviewed 2,245 patients at 16-year follow-up.[14] The risk per 1,000-patient years in females was 80 and was even higher in males, at 101. The relative risk compared to those patients without a fracture was 2.5 in females and 6.2 in males. Kanis performed a meta-analysis of drug trials including 60,121 patients, 26% of whom had prior fractures.[15] The risk of a future fracture was doubled in patients who already had a fracture and was greater for males and younger-aged patients. Anderson performed a meta-analysis of nine randomized controlled trials of vertebroplasty compared to nonoperative treatment.[16] Secondary fractures occurred within 12 months in 19% of nonoperatively treated patients, and there was no difference in those having had vertebroplasty. Lindsay noted that with each new fracture, there was a significant and increasing risk of incident fractures.[17] Patients with one fracture had a 12% risk of secondary fractures, while those with 2 or more fractures had a 25% risk. Thus, the presence of a clinical or subclinical fracture in an older patient or from a low-energy mechanism should prompt investigation and consideration of treatment for related osteoporosis.

3.5 Diagnosis of Osteoporosis

3.5.1 Dual-energy X-ray Absorptiometry (DXA)

Dual-energy X-ray absorptiometry (DXA) is the gold standard to determine in vivo bone mineral density (BMD). The technique utilizes high and low energy X-rays which have different, nonlinear X-ray attenuation. As a result, the density which these two X-ray energies pass through tissues can be determined. DXA calculates the areal BMD (gm/cm^2) of a region of interest. Typical regions of interest are the proximal femur, lumbar vertebrae, and distal radius, all three of which are common fracture sites. The bone mineral density (BMD) is then compared to a reference standard, specifically the BMD of 20- to 30-year-old females. The T-score is equal to the BMD of the patient minus the BMD of the reference standard divided by the standard deviation of the reference standard.

$$Tscore = (BMD(subject) - BMD(reference))/SD(reference)$$

The Z-score is calculated using age- and gender-matched controls as a reference standard. A Z-score is used for males and premenopausal females.

One strength of DXA is that larger and therefore stronger bones will have a higher areal BMD and, as such, DXA is a good tool to predict future fracture risk. However, there are many limitations of DXA. Arthritic or degenerative changes, deformity, and the presence of surgical implants prevent accurate measurement of BMD. DXA is only measuring planar bone mineral density and will include cortical trabecular bone. In the spine, trabecular bone is far more significant in preventing fractures than the cortices. Further, variation occurs between scanners and technicians, with different resulting outcomes. Finally, recent investigations suggest that over 25% of scans have incorrect reporting.[18]

3.5.2 Classification of Osteoporosis

The World Health Organization (WHO) classified bone status based on DXA T-score (▶ Table 3.1).[19] However, the WHO classification poorly predicts fracture, with more than 50% occurring in people with low bone mass or normal T-scores. Further, this system provides limited guidance for treatment. The National Osteoporosis Foundation and the National Bone Health Alliance (NBHA) recognized that bone mineral density as defined by the WHO criteria does not explain risk of fracture in half the cases.[20] As such, they recently proposed that the definition of osteoporosis be expanded to include any one of the following: a T-score of less than -.2.5; a fragility spine or hip fracture; low bone mass (-1.0 to -2.5) plus fragility fracture; and low bone mass and high Fracture Risk Assessment Tool (FRAX) probability (▶ Table 3.2).

The Fracture Risk Assessment Tool (FRAX) is a prediction tool that calculates the 10-year hip and 10-year major osteoporotic (spine, hip, wrist and humerus) fracture risk.[21,22] FRAX is standardized for many countries and is based on 12 criteria, including demographics, height and weight, a history of prior fractures, parents with fractures, cigarette use, use of glucocorticoids, having rheumatoid arthritis or secondary osteoporosis, consuming more than 3 alcoholic beverages per day, and femoral neck bone mineral density based on either gm/cm^2 or T score (▶ Table 3.3). The FRAX risk can also be calculated without the use of DXA. The FRAX tool can be accessed at https://www.sheffield.ac.uk/FRAX/index.aspx.

Many guidelines recommend use of FRAX estimated fracture risk to determine the optimum medical treatment, including the therapeutic intervention threshold based on fracture risk. The most commonly used high-risk FRAX thresholds are a 10-year major fracture risk of 20% and a 10-year hip fracture risk of 3%, indicating patients who should be considered for pharmaceutical treatment.

3.5.3 Indications for DXA

The indications for DXA testing are: all women aged 65 + and men aged 70 +; women aged 50 to 64 with a FRAX score greater than 9.3 percent; major osteoporosis-related fracture risk per the United States Preventative Service Task Force (USPSTF); men between the ages of 50 to 69 who exhibit one or more of the following: a prior fracture, glucocorticoid use, or rheumatoid arthritis; and, finally, anyone with a recent fracture (▶ Table 3.4).[23]

3.5.4 Recent Advances in Diagnosis of Osteoporosis

Two recent advancements available in some DXA scanners have improved fracture-risk predictive capabilities. Vertebral Fracture Assessment (VFA) uses a lateral radiographic image of ideally the entire thoracolumbar spine (▶ Fig. 3.2).[24] The Genant visual semiquantitative (VSQ) scale is usually applied to identify

Table 3.1 World Health Organization Criteria for Diagnosis of Osteopenia and Osteoporosis

Classification	T-Score*
Normal	Greater than -1.0
Osteopenia	Between -1.0 and -2.5
Osteoporosis	Less than -2.5

* T-score measured at femoral neck

Table 3.2 National Bone Health Alliance (NBHA) recommendations for diagnosis of osteoporosis

T-score < -2.5 of hip, lumbar spine, or distal third of radius

Low energy spine or hip fracture (independent of bone mineral density)

Low bone mass (T-score -1.0 to -2.5) with fragility fracture of proximal humerus, wrist, pelvis

Low bone mass (T-score -1.0 to -2.5) and high FRAX* risk probability

* Fracture Risk Assessment Tool

Table 3.3 Fracture Risk Assessment Tool (FRAX)

Criteria		Results:
Age	Current smoker	10-year major fracture risk (%)
Gender	Glucocorticoid use	10-year hip fracture risk (%)
Height	Rheumatoid arthritis	
Weight	Secondary osteoporosis	
Prior fracture	Alcohol ≥ 3 units per day	
Parent with hip fracture	Femoral neck BMD (gm/cc) May use T-score	

Table 3.4 Indications for DXA

Females > 65

Males > 70

Females 50–64 and FRAX > 9.3 for major fractures

Males 50–64 with history of prior fracture, glucocorticoid use, or rheumatoid arthritis

Anyone with recent fragility fracture

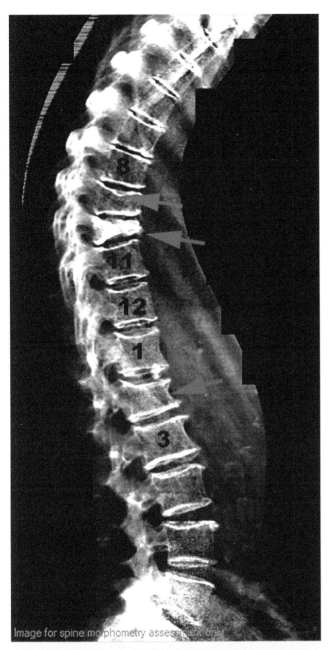

Fig. 3.2 Vertebral fracture assessment (VFA) obtained during routine DXA of a patient with three occult fractures at T9, T10 and T12.

applied to existing lumbar spine DXA data. A region of interest identical to that for DXA is chosen, and each pixel on 2-dimensional imagesis assigned a value based on bone thresholding. The TBS is calculated based on the variation between pixels which are greater in osteoporotic bone than normal trabecular bone when compared to normal. The trabecular bone score can be independent of BMD and have greater predictive value than T-score (► Fig. 3.1e). The TBS can be utilized to improve fracture-risk estimation in FRAX, with high TBS scores reducing risk and vice versa. TBS values > 1.31 are consistent with intact bone microarchitecture, < 1.23 with degraded bone microarchitecture, and a score in between these values with partially degraded bone microarchitecture.

3.5.5 Opportunistic Screening using CT

Computed tomography (CT) is a widely used diagnostic tool. In the U.S. in 2015, there were 240 CT examinations per 1,000 patients.[27] In 2013, over 31 million patients had abdominal or pelvic CTs that examined the lumbar spine and proximal femur, which could provide useful information regarding bone mineral density. CTs obtained for other indications can be used to quantitatively assess bone status; this has been termed "opportunistic osteoporosis screening."[28]

The CT scan uses rotating X-ray emitters and detectors that allow calculation of energy attenuation in each 3-dimensional piece (voxel) of tissue. The X-ray attenuation is normalized and is calculated as the linear attenuation coefficient, known as the Hounsfield unit (HU). Each scanner calculates an HU for each voxel and is displayed on planar images using a grey scale. The X-ray attenuation is proportional to the atomic mass cubed and the number of atoms in each voxel of tissue. Thus, in general for bone, HU is proportional to the BMD.

Several methods to assess bone status using CT have been developed. The simplest is to determine the mean HU in an elliptical region of interest (ROI) using standard PACS software (► Fig. 3.1c).[29] Typically, for the spine this will be drawn in the anterior two thirds of the vertebral body on either axial or sagittal sections. A representative section, usually through mid-body or through the pedicle, is selected, and a region of interest is drawn to include only trabecular bone.[29] It is important to avoid any bony defects, fractures, or bony islands. Standard thresholds to determine the likelihood of osteoporosis are determined for L1, which is also available on both chest and abdomen CTs, making it an ideal vertebra to use if available. The author recommends drawing as large an ellipse as possible. Reliability studies show no difference between averaging multiple small ellipses and drawing one large region of interest.

More accurate quantitative CT scans can be obtained by simultaneously scanning the patient and a phantom containing various concentrations of calcium hydroxyapatite. These are then used to interpolate the bone mineral density of any region of interest. This has been termed synchronous quantitative CT (qCT).[30] This is an excellent research tool but is not widely used clinically. Asynchronous qCT utilizes calibration data obtained daily on CT scanners and does not require the simultaneous scanning of patient and phantom. This approach is as reliable as standard synchronous qCT and may be used to calculate bone mineral density and to determine T-scores similarly to DXA.[30] Phantomless quantitative CT uses water and air density as

individuals with mild, moderate or severe vertebral fractures.[24] In conjunction with this approach, the anterior, middle, and posterior vertebral body height at each level can be measured and compared to controls. With the VSQ system, fractures are classified as mild (20–25% height loss), moderate (25–40% height loss) and severe (> 40% height loss). The VFA allows identification of occult fractures and correlates to functional deficits in BMD. For example, Muszkat reported that 17% of patients having routine DXA had moderate or severe vertebral fractures based on VFA, and of those, 88% were occult.[25]

The trabecular bone score (TBS) provides an index of bone quality by serving as a surrogate of bone microarchitecture.[26] The TBS uses special software to assess bone texture and can be standards to calculate bone mineral density. At present, this is used mainly as a research tool.

There are notable factors that affect X-ray attenuation and thus HU. CT manufacturers and day-to-day fluctuations are minor. Intravenous contrast increases spinal HU by approximately 11.[31] The most important factor is voltage tube energy of the CT scanner.[32] Most CT scans use 120 kV; however, newer scanners allow dual-energy CT scans, and a significant negative correlation exists between higher voltage and lower HU.

Thresholds have been determined to estimate the presence or absence of osteoporosis based on Hounsfield units. Pickard recommends an HU threshold for L1 vertebral body of 135, which optimizes the sensitivity and specificity. An HU greater than 160 will rule out osteoporosis, while a value less than 110 most likely indicates it. Schreiber compared HU to DXA and T-scores. He found that normal bone (T-scores > -1.0) had a mean HU of 133, osteopenic patients (T-score -1.0 to -2.5) had a mean of 101, and osteoporotic patients (T-score < -2.5) had a mean of 78.

Determining Hounsfield units has proven helpful in managing spine patients. A significant linear correlation exists between elastic modulus, apparent yield strain, and pull-out forces and HU, although thresholds have not been determined.[33] Further, Weiser found a linear correlation between bone mineral density obtained from synchronized CT and pedicle screw cycles to failure and load to failure.[34]

Opportunistic CT scans have been evaluated in spine patients. Meredith reported a significant correlation between decreased preoperative HU and proximal junction kyphosis due to fracture in patients having spinal deformity.[35] Patients with fracture had mean HU of 146, compared to 199 in the nonfracture group. Du reported that the incidence of incidental durotomy was twice as high in patients with low HU, although the cause for this phenomenon was not reported.[36] Fusion success was negatively affected by osteoporosis diagnosed by HU. Schreiber evaluated 140 patients and determined that the mean HU for those with successful lumbar fusion was 203, while it was only 140 in patients with nonunion.[37] Okuyama similarly reported that union success was strongly correlated to higher bone mineral density.[38] Nguyen performed a match cohort study and found that in patients with nonunion, the HU value was significantly lower (167 vs. 201) than in those who had union.[39] Wagner found a strong correlation between CT HU and DXA in patients undergoing lumbar fusion. Twelve percent were osteoporotic, of whom two-thirds had never been diagnosed or treated.[40] Mi et al found that patients having cage subsidence after posterior interbody fusion had lower HU than those without subsidence, and at follow-up had less fusion mass. They calculated that an HU threshold in L4 of 132 identified those patients at risk for subsidence.[41]

An important opportunistic use for CT scan is to identify occult fractures. In patients having abdominal CT scans, Graffy determined that 8.2% of patients had occult vertebral fractures, which strongly correlated to decreased HU.[42] Lee noted that DXA poorly predicted fractures in patients having abdominal CT scans.[27] The HU was less than 145 in 97% of patients with occult fracture, while all had DXA T-scores were greater than -2.5. Eighty-two percent of patients with occult fractures on CT were not mentioned in the radiologic reports.

Emohar compared HU in a nonfracture control group to patients with cervical, thoracolumbar, and pelvic fractures.

There was strong correlation with lower HU values in patients with fracture compared to control. In a similar study, authors found that patients with ankylosing spondylitis had markedly lower trabecular HU, suggestive of osteoporosis.[43]

3.5.6 Secondary Osteoporosis

Primary osteoporosis is bone loss due to aging and, in postmenopausal women, the loss of estrogens. Secondary osteoporosis occurs frequently and is due to other medical conditions and medications. It is important that laboratory testing be performed to identify secondary causes of bone loss in patients with a known diagnosis of osteoporosis or prior fragility fracture.[19] In one study, approximately 40% of patients had secondary osteoporosis contributors.[44] Simple laboratory tests include a complete blood count, a comprehensive metabolic panel, 25(OH)D, intact parathyroid hormone, phosphate, and 24-hour urine collection for calcium, sodium and creatinine. Other tests are indicated depending on history and physical findings. In patients with suspicious spine fractures, multiple myeloma should be considered and is assessed by serum and urine protein electrophoresis.

3.5.7 Bone Turnover Markers

Bone turnover markers (BTM) are proteins and peptide molecules used to assess dynamic cellular activity of bone formation and bone resorption. These markers are useful to monitor the effectiveness of treatment but not for the diagnosis of osteoporosis. Current guidelines of the American Association of Clinical Endocrinology (AACE) recommend the use of serum C-terminal telopeptide (s-CTX) to assess bone resorption and serum N-terminal propeptide of type I collagen synthesis (P1NP) to assess bone formation.[19] Patients who respond effectively to antiresorptive therapy should have lower bone turnover and thus lower BTMs. Elevated s-CTX indicates continued high bone turnover and suggests poor treatment compliance, malabsorption, or secondary causes of osteoporosis. In contrast, both formation and resorption BTMs are increased by bone anabolic therapies.

3.6 Treatment of Osteoporosis

3.6.1 General Principles

Universal recommendations for management of patients with osteoporosis are to ensure adequate calcium and vitamin D intake, a high protein diet, treatment of any vitamin D deficiency, regular weight-bearing exercises, fall prevention, cessation of smoking and reduction of excess use of alcohol (▶ Table 3.5). The intervention threshold for use of pharmaceutical medications in many countries is based on fracture risk, as calculated using FRAX. With this approach, patients at high risk (cut points vary by country) should be considered candidates for medical therapy. In other regions of the world, notably the U.S., a hybrid approach of recommending treatment for those with a T-score below -2.5 and for those at elevated fracture risk (> 20 major osteoporosis related fracture or > 3% hip fracture) is utilized. Patients with major fragility fractures are candidates for either antiresorptive or anabolic therapy.

Table 3.5 General Approach to Diagnosis and Management of Osteoporosis

1. Recognition of poor bone health as a problem and a condition that spine practitioners can manage	
2. All patients with fractures after age 50 should have basic laboratory and DXA testing	Basic metabolic panel Complete blood count 25(OH) Vitamin D Personally review DXA
3. Think about falls	Home safety Balance issues Poor vision Generalized weakness
4. Supplements	Calcium 1,000–2,000 mg/day Vitamin D_3 1,000–2,000 U/day Consider protein in older adults
5. Medications (3–5 years) for patients with high fracture risk	FRAX > 20% 10-year major osteoporotic fracture risk Recent fracture Falls Planned fusion in presence of osteopenia or osteoporosis

Table 3.6 Serum 25(OH)D concentration and vitamin D supplementation approaches

	25(OH) Vitamin D (ng/mL)	Supplementation
Normal	> 30	1–2,000 Daily vitamin D_3
Insufficient	20–30	50,000 U vitamin D_2 or D_3 weekly for 8–12 weeks Or 5,000 U vitamin D_2 or vitamin D_3 daily for 10–12 weeks Recheck to determine if adequate 25(OH) vitamin D level has been achieved
Deficient	< 20	50,000 U vitamin D_2 or D_3 weekly for 8–12 weeks Or 5,000 U Vitamin D_2 or Vitamin D_3 daily for 10–12 weeks Recheck to determine if adequate 25(OH) vitamin D has been achieved

*Note: Individuals with low 25(OH)D values very commonly require long-term daily supplementation, not simply one-time correction of vitamin D deficiency.

3.6.2 Supplements

Vitamin D is essential for proper bone physiology since it promotes calcium absorption, osteoblastic differentiation, osteoblastic mediated mineralization, and calcium regulation, and it collagen cross-linking. Clinically, low vitamin D is associated with sarcopenia and increased fall risk. Vitamin D is associated many other disease states such as cardiovascular disease, diabetes, hypertension, and cancer.

Vitamin D is formed in the skin upon exposure to UV radiation where 7-dehydro-cholesterol is converted to cholecalciferol (vitamin D_3). To become active, cholecalciferol requires two hydroxylations. The first occurs in the liver, where vitamin D_3 is converted to 25-hydroxyvitamin D [25(OH)D]. The kidneys subsequently hydroxylate 25(OH)D to the active form 1–25(OH)$_2$ D.

Measurement of serum 25(OH)D is accepted as the best approach to determine an individual's vitamin D status. This metabolite is chosen because it circulates at relatively high concentration and has a long half-life (~3 weeks) and reflects long-term stores. Determination of the optimal level of 25(OH)D has proven difficult because of differences in 25(OH)D assays, which prevents the performance of reasonable meta-analyses. The NIH Vitamin D Standardization Program (VDSP) has developed methodologies allowing use of standardized 25(OH)D data, so progress may be made in this regard. Additionally, but importantly, virtually all previous and ongoing randomized trials of vitamin D supplementation have failed to require volunteers to be low in vitamin D prior to study initiation. It is self-evident that providing more of any nutrient, in this case vitamin D, to individuals that are replete in that nutrient cannot possibly have benefit and could only, potentially, cause harm. In summary, systematic reviews of 25(OH)D status using various assays and also large randomized controlled trials (RCTs) with flawed methodology will not serve to define hypovitaminosis D. In this setting, a common-sense approach to defining vitamin D adequacy was to assume that communities of hunter-gathers in equatorial climates who spend most of their time with high levels of skin exposure represent evolutionary "normal" vitamin D status. In Tanzania, hunter-gather tribes were found to have a mean 25(OH)D of 46 ng/mL. Similarly, surfers in Hawaii had a mean 25(OH)D level (using retrospective assay standardization as recommended by the VDSP) of approximately 36 ng/ml.

Importantly, there is substantial between-individual response in the 25(OH)D increase achieved following initiation of an individual dose of daily vitamin D supplementation. In general, it is recommended to choose larger doses so that as many patients as possible achieve a normal level. Understandably, based on the issues noted above, it is to be expected that expert opinion regarding the optimum 25(OH)D level varies. The 2011 Institute of Medicine report considers a 25(OH)D level of ≥ 20 ng/mL to be adequate, whereas recent AACE guidelines recommend > 30 ng/mL as adequate while calling levels between 20 and 30 ng/mL insufficient and those < 20 ng/mL deficient (▶ Table 3.6).[23,45]

While controversial, many experts believe that the two available forms of vitamin D (D_3, cholecalciferol and D_2, ergocalciferol) vary in potency. Some, though not all, studies find supplementation with vitamin D3 to be more potent at increasing circulating 25(OH)D; as such, it is generally preferred for treatment. Cholecalciferol is widely available as a stand-alone supplement in doses of 1,000, 2,000 and 5,000 IU. Additionally, 50,000 IU D3 supplements are available. Vitamin D_2 is available in similar doses and is the only form available in the U.S. by prescription. The AACE guidelines recommend 1,000 to 2,000 units per day for general population.[19] Patients who are vitamin D insufficient (less than 20 ng/mL) are treated either with 50,000 units of vitamin D_2 or D_3 per week for eight weeks or 5,000 IU of vitamin D_3 daily. At 12 weeks, the 25(OH)D level is checked to assure that it is greater than 30 ng/mL. Note that it is important to wait at least 12 weeks to reach a new 25(OH)D steady state given the ~3 week half-life of 25(OH)D. Subsequent to attaining an optimal 25(OH)D level, and one similar to the normal population, 1,000 to 2,000 units of vitamin D_3 are recommended as a daily maintenance dose. Alternative doses may be required in patients with obesity, malabsorption, or who are taking medications that affect vitamin D metabolism. Indeed, it is not possible to estimate an individual's intake given the difference in 25(OH)D response noted above; as such, in individuals who have sustained fractures, it is prudent to recheck a 25 (OH)D level following initiation of a daily maintenance dose.

Like most issues in the vitamin D literature, the definition of toxicity is controversial. Nonetheless, 25(OH) D levels up to ~150 ng/mL are generally well tolerated without evidence of toxicity. The acute toxicity of vitamin D is elevated serum calcium. Massive doses of vitamin D are unwise, as one study of 500,000 IU found this to increase risk of falls and fractures; the mechanism(s) of these unexpected findings are unknown.

Finally, while controversial, it is widely believed that vitamin D deficiency leads to muscle weakness, with resultant increased fall risk. As such, vitamin D supplementation of older adults with a history of falls or at increased fall risk is recommended by both the American Geriatrics Society and the USPSTF.[23,46] If indeed vitamin D deficiency leads to muscle weakness, it conceivably could contribute to the development of sarcopenia, the age-related reduction in muscle mass and strength. Sarcopenia is increasingly recognized as an important contributor to "osteoporosis-related" fractures due to increased fall risk.

3.6.3 Calcium Supplementation

A calcium-rich diet or supplementation is required for optimum bone health. The recommended dietary allowance for calcium by the AACE is 1,000 mg for adults aged 19 to 50, increasing to 1,200 mg per day in females older than 50.[19] Based largely upon meta-analyses, it has been reported that calcium supplementation may increase cardiovascular disease risk; however, this potential relationship remains contentious. Indeed, a recent meta-analysis did not support the linkage.[47] That a potential relationship of calcium supplementation with nonskeletal disease is controversial could be expected, given the limitations of randomized trials noted earlier. However, increased calcium intake may be associated with nephrolithiasis and therefore should be used with caution in patients with a history of hypercalcemia or nephrolithiasis. A variety of calcium supplements are available: calcium carbonate is low-cost and requires fewer tablets; however, it may cause more gastrointestinal symptoms. Calcium citrate is more expensive and requires a greater number of tablets to achieve a similar amount of calcium. Additionally, calcium citrate does not require acid for absorption and, as such, is preferred in patients with gastrointestinal disorders but may be difficult to swallow. Other supplements such as magnesium, strontium, vitamin A, and vitamin K have not been proven beneficial in management of osteoporosis

3.6.4 Nutrition

Despite the obesity epidemic, undernutrition is common in older adults with fracture. As such, provision of adequate total calories and, importantly, protein is an important component of bone health. Maintaining muscle mass will increase skeletal loading and therefore help preserve bone density in addition to mitigating muscle loss with advancing age (i.e., sarcopenia). As such, adequate protein intake is essential to minimize fracture risk. The AACE recommends 0.8 gm/kg/day based on results

after hip fracture. Other organizations recommend higher protein intake of 1.0 to 1.2 grams/kg body weight daily.[19]

3.6.5 Elimination of Toxins

Excessive alcohol intake is a known risk factor for both fractures due to diminished BMD and an increased propensity to fall. There are a variety of multifactorial mechanisms relating alcohol intake to fracture, and therefore it is recommended that patients with low bone mass consume no more than two drinks per day. Similarly, smoking is a strong risk factor for osteoporosis and increases risk of fractures. All smokers should be counseled for cessation of all tobacco products. Caffeine should be limited to 1 to 2 servings per day, as it may increase urinary calcium excretion and reduce calcium absorption.

3.6.6 Exercise and Physical therapy

Exercise is an important component to maintain and restore bone health and prevent fracture. Disuse, inactivity, and bed rest all contribute to rapid bone loss and an increased risk of fracture. General conditioning should be prescribed in post fracture patients, including weight-bearing exercise once the fracture has healed. Weight-bearing is essential and can include the upper extremity with patients using weights.

Falls are common in the aging population and result from multiple mechanisms. Unfortunately, falls are often iatrogenic. Patients with a history of a fall should have a careful review and adjustment of medications. Elderly patients are more than 10 times likelier to fall when taking benzodiazepines and opioids. A gerontologist may be useful in adjusting medications to reduce fall risk. Treatable neurological diseases, such as cervical and lumbar stenosis, should be identified and treated as required. Further, undiagnosed Parkinsonism is frequent in elderly men presenting with hip fracture.

Other useful interventions are fall prevention, which includes home visits assessing safety, instruction in the use of walking aids, and balance training. In addition, early physical therapy after a fragility fracture can aid the patient in activities of daily living and proper body mechanics. Finally, other modalities, such as tai chi, have shown significant benefit in osteoporotic patients including increasing bone mass. Although there are many forms of tai chi, it appears that all are effective in reducing fall risk and managing osteoporosis.

3.6.7 Pharmaceutical Treatment

Ultimately, osteoporosis results from an imbalance between bone resorption and formation. Bone is constantly being remodeled by activation of preosteoclast to osteoclasts, which resorb bone creating resorption pits. These resorption pits are subsequently filled with new bone by osteoblasts. With decline of estrogens at menopause, an imbalance occurs, with osteoclastic resorption exceeding osteoblastic new bone formation. Additionally, this osteoclastic over-activity leads to trabecular perforation, with resultant reduction in bone strength. There are two general categories of medications used to currently manage osteoporosis: antiresorptive and anabolic agents. The antiresorptive agents include bisphosphonates, calcitonin, denosumab and estrogens. There are two currently approved anabolic agents: teriparatide and abaloparatide.

Antiresorptive Medications

Bisphosphonates are the most widely used antiresorptive agents. They bind to hydroxyapatite on the resorptive surfaces and prevent osteoclastic bone resorption and induce osteoclast apoptosis. Four agents are currently approved in the US: alendronate 70 mg/wk, ibandronate 150 mg/mo, risedronate 35 mg/wk and zoledronate 5 mg/yr via infusion. Multiple studies show consistent fracture reduction in postmenopausal osteoporotic women of approximately 50% with use of bisphosphonates.[19]

Denosumab is a monoclonal antibody that inhibits rank ligand to prevent osteoclast activation and activity. Denosumab (60 mg) is administered subcutaneously every six months and is associated with a 40 to 68% fracture reduction. However, it has similar complications as bisphosphonates (see below).

Calcitonin has been widely used in the past as an antiresorptive agent. It also occasionally will mitigate the pain of compression fractures associated with osteoporosis. However, in meta-analysis, calcitonin has been associated with increased risk of cancer (despite lack of a physiologic rationale for this) and this, combined with little effect upon BMD and a lack of evidence of nonvertebral fracture risk reduction make it rarely used as a first line medication today.

Estrogens and estrogen analogs remain controversial. Because of concerns regarding increased risk of cancer, heart disease and venous thromboembolic disease, estrogen use in postmenopausal women has dramatically declined. As a result, there currently exists a large cohort of women who have not been given any estrogen following menopause; this will almost certainly lead to a much higher rate of osteoporosis in upcoming years. Indeed, recent data document that the historical decline in U.S. hip fracture risk has now plateaued, notably in younger postmenopausal women. One potential explanation for this is the minimal use of estrogen following menopause. The use of estrogens seems likely to increase in the near future; indeed, a recent consensus statement by The North American Menopause Society made strong recommendations regarding the safety and efficacy of estrogens.[48] As such, the use of estrogens following menopause may be increasing, but such use needs to be individualized. Their exact role in the management of metabolic disease is currently in flux.

Anabolic Medications

Two anabolic agents are currently approved by the U.S. FDA: teriparatide, recombinant PTH (134) and abaloparatide, a PTHrP analog. In a seminal RCT study, teriparatide was compared to placebo control in 1,637 postmenopausal females with mean duration of 21 months follow-up.[49] Lumbar spine BMD increased by 9%, spine fracture risk was reduced by 65%, and nonspine fracture by 53%. Abaloparatide has recently been approved for use in primary and secondary osteoporosis treatment. Its properties are similar to those of teriparatide, although it is less likely to produce hypercalcemia. A recent randomized control trial showed that use of abaloparatide resulted in significantly greater fracture reduction and increased bone mass than placebo control.[50]

3.6.8 Complications of Pharmaceuticals

Two complications of bisphosphonates and demosumab are widely reported: atypical femur fractures (AFF) and avascular necrosis of the jaw (ONJ). These complications create fear and confusion which prevent wider appropriate use of these medications. AFFs are stress fractures in the proximal femur, usually at or below the lesser trochanter. Initially, a nonspecific leg/hip/buttock pain often is associated with associated thickening of the lateral femoral cortex, and, subsequently, a complete fracture may develop with minimal or no trauma. AFFs may occur in individuals with no bisphosphonate exposure, but overall they are strongly associated with duration of bisphosphonate treatment. For example at two years, the AFF incidence per 1,000 cases is 0.2, while at 5 years it is 0.5, and at 10 years is 1.2.[51] It is estimated that bisphosphonates prevent between 15 and 100 osteoporotic fractures for every one that may be associated with their use.[51] Thus, at least for a short duration of treatment, e.g., 3 to 5 years, the risk/benefit relationship strongly favors bisphosphonate treatment. The incidence of ONJ in connection with use of bisphosphonates is less than that of AFFs and is strongly associated with dose, particularly with the use of IV zoledronate for treatment of cancer patients. In the cancer patient, higher doses are administered than those used for osteoporosis.

Anabolic agents can increase urinary excretion and calcium and can cause nephrolithiasis. The anabolic agents require daily injection and this, plus their high costs, create barriers to their use. Anabolics are contraindicated in patients with ongoing malignancies or who have had irradiation because of increased risk of osteosarcoma seen in animal models. To this date, no evidence associates anabolic therapy in humans with an increased risk of osteosarcoma.

3.6.9 Drug Holidays

To reduce these complication risks, drug holidays are often prescribed (albeit without a sound base of evidence). It is known that, at 7 years, bisphosphonates continue to reduce fracture risks and that withdrawal of bisphosphonates will result in lowering bone mineral density. However, discontinuing bisphosphonates still has a positive effect on fracture risk. Therefore, drug holidays are felt to be reasonable and are recommended in moderate- and low-risk patients after 3 to 5 years of bisphosphonate treatment.[19] How long these holidays should last and how to best monitor them is not based on evidence. A reasonable approach is to recommend that a DXA scan be performed at intervals during the bisphosphonate holiday to assure that bone mass is being maintained. In higher-risk populations, it is recommended by some organizations to continue bisphosphonates and to avoid a drug holiday.

3.7 Secondary Fracture Prevention

3.7.1 Fragility Fracture as a Teaching Moment

A fracture in older adults can be a seminal event for the patient, and it is an opportunity to help patients maintain independence by preventing future fractures. Thus, while we have the patient's attention (i.e., after they have just sustained a fracture), we must view it as a teaching moment to convey the necessity of preventing subsequent fracture. While it is common for older adults to say "anyone would have fractured if they fell like I did," indeed this is not the case; these individuals are at substantially increased risk and in need of comprehensive evaluation and treatment to reduce their risk for future fracture. Vertebral fractures related to low bone mass are associated with a 5-fold increase in risk of another fragility fracture and a 2.5-fold increase risk of a hip fracture.

Secondary fracture prevention through a comprehensive program aimed at assessment of secondary causes for bone loss, bone density testing, and when appropriate treatment are highly effective. Bawa reviewed the Medicare data base of 31,000 fragility fracture patients, of whom only 10% have any osteoporotic treatment prescribed.[52] Thus, it is becoming widely recognized that osteoporosis treatment is in crisis and that different approaches are needed to optimize care after fracture.[3] Notably, in those 10% receiving treatment after fracture, there was a 40% reduction of secondary fractures. In 2005, the United Kingdom instituted a program that mandated secondary fracture prevention after hip fracture. In the years following institution of this program, there was a 30% reduction in secondary major and hip fractures.[53] In a meta-analysis of 11 studies on the effect of alendronate for primary or secondary prevention of osteoporotic fractures, the risk reduction in patients having a spine and hip fracture treated with alendronate was 45 and 53%, respectively.[54] The number of patients necessary to treat in order to prevent one fracture was 31 and 48 in spine and hip, respectively.

Pelvic and sacral insufficiency fractures frequently present with buttock and sacral pain and/or radiculopathy. In a randomized control trial, 65 patients with pelvic insufficiency fractures were given teriparatide or placebo and were assessed by CT scan, pain level, and functional tasks such as the "get up and go" tests.[55] The study was discontinued early because patients in the treatment group were significantly improved in 4 weeks compared to the placebo group. In all cases, there was lower pain, better function, and better healing in the teriparatide group. Similarly, in a randomized control trial in sacral and sufficiency fractures, the time to ambulate was significantly shorter in the teriparatide group compared to control.[56] Thus, there is high-quality evidence that medical therapy reduces secondary fractures.

3.7.2 Secondary Fracture Prevention Programs

A variety of secondary fracture prevention approaches, or so-called Fracture Liaison Services (FLS), are available. These programs should be easy to implement and flexible for local conditions and should consider a fracture as a teachable moment for the patient. Initiating education and coordination of care between the bone specialist and primary care provider (PCP) is required. Ganda has reviewed the efficacy of four types of secondary fracture preventions.[57] Type A has an embedded FLS coordinator, who is usually a nurse practitioner or physician assistant on the trauma team. This person assumes all care of the bone, including diagnostics and prescribing of medications, and coordinates care with other providers. In the Type B model, a coordinator is again embedded with the trauma team; however, future care for bone health is delegated to the PCP. The Type C model does not include a care coordinator and therefore

has lower cost. The practitioner caring initially for the patient provides education regarding osteoporosis and then refers the patient to primary care for further management. In the Type D model, only education is performed, and it is left to the patient to seek further care from his or her PCP. In a systematic review, Ganda found that in Type A programs, 80% of patients received a DXA, and over half received treatment for osteoporosis.[1] The results for other approaches were poorer, with 59 and 40% in Type B programs, 43 and 23% in Type C programs; only 8% of patients in Type D programs received any pharmaceutical treatment. Thus, the intensity of the initial treatment, particularly having a coordinator embedded with the initial care team, is essential for the success of these programs. Not only is there a reduction of secondary fractures, there may also be less risk of mortality. In a Cochrane review of bisphosphonates there was 55% reduction of the risk of mortality in patients with fragility fractures treated with alendronate.[54] Given the suboptimal results of osteoporosis treatment approaches over the past two decades, the FLS approach is clearly an improvement and should be widely employed.

3.7.3 American Orthopedic Association Own the Bone Program

In response to the U.S. Surgeon General's report identifying a crisis in osteoporosis care, the American Orthopedic Association (AOA) responded by creating the Own the Bone program.[1] Own the Bone focuses on prevention of secondary fractures after low-energy injury. The program is coordinated through the AOA and provides education for practitioners and patients, a robust database, assessment of 10 performance measures, multidisciplinary conferences, and other recognition offerings. The program currently has over 150 sites enrolling patients and is available in all 50 states and Washington DC.[58] The success of the program requires a local practitioner who is designated the "champion." The most successful programs are those of Type A or Type B where there is a midlevel provider embedded in the care team who assumes care for the bone disease.

The Own the Bone database has over 55,000 encounters, with 40,000 new patients enrolled. About a third of them have follow-up visits. Initially, it started with hospitalized patients and therefore included a predominance of hip fractures, but increasingly, more spine fractures and other outpatient fractures are being included. Not surprisingly, about a third of patients who are enrolled in Own the Bone have already had a prior recent fracture, and only 10% had ever received any osteoporosis care. Own the Bone has a nominal initiation cost.

3.8 Presurgical Bone Health Optimization

3.8.1 Introduction to Bone Health Optimization

Recently, with an increased emphasis on safety, patients' overall health is being optimized prior to surgery. Effective measures include diabetic control, maintaining normotension, cardiac risk stratification, use of beta blockers and aspirin where

Table 3.7 Preoperative Bone Health Optimization

1. Diagnostics	Criteria
25(OH)Vitamin D	> 30 ng/ml
DXA	T-score > -1.0
Opportunistic CT	HU > 135
Nutrition	1.0–1.2 gm/kg/da
2. Preoperative Treatment	
All adult patients > 50 years	Correct vitamin D deficiency
	Calcium supplementation
	High FRAX risk – antiresorptive therapy or anabolic
One – two level fusions	Normal T-score – no treatment
	High FRAX or T-score < -1.0 – 3 months antiresorptive or anabolic therapy
	T-score < - 2.5 – Anabolic for 3–6 months
Multilevel fusion	Normal T-score – no treatment
	High FRAX or T-score < -1.0 – 3 months anabolic treatment
	High FRAX or T-score < -2.5 – 6–12 months anabolic treatment

appropriate, and discontinuation of smoking. Given that inadequate bone state is associated with poor outcomes of spine surgery, optimization of bone health is gaining popularity. The goals of bone health optimization are to correct vitamin D deficiency, assure adequate calcium consumption, assess bone mineral density and, if required, improve bone health by antiresorptive and anabolic agents (▶ Table 3.7). The use of anabolic agents for this purpose has the advantages of quickly increasing bone mass and improving osteoblastic activity to aid fusion. Various protocols are being developed, and no consensus has been reached. Many centers modify existing guidelines and delay surgery until it is felt that a restored active skeletal mass is conducive to bone healing and prevention of fracture-related complications.

3.8.2 Vitamin D Deficiency

Vitamin D deficiency is common in patients undergoing spine surgery. Stoker reviewed 260 spinal fusion patients and found only 16% had normal 25(OH)D levels, while 27% were insufficient and 57% deficient.[59] There was a strong correlation to increased Oswestry Disability Index (ODI) and vitamin D deficiency. Ravindra confirmed this observation in 235 elective spine patients from a neurosurgical practice.[60] Thirty percent were deficient and 39% were insufficient. Predictors of vitamin D deficiency were increasing age, female, higher BMI, and diabetes mellitus, whereas patients taking supplements had higher 25(OH)D levels.

However, the effect of vitamin D deficiency on spinal disease and surgical outcomes is less well studied. Kim reviewed 350 patients from an orthopedic practice, each of whom had a diagnosis of lumbar spinal stenosis.[61] Severe back and leg pain occurred 3 to 4 times more likely in vitamin D-deficient patients than those with normal levels. Thus, there was strong negative correlation between vitamin D deficiency and pain, although the exact mechanism is unexplained.

Ravindra correlated outcomes after lumbar spine fusion to preoperative 25(OH)D level in 133 patients.[62] Fusion failure was 3.5 times more likely in vitamin D-deficient patients than in those with normal serum levels. Further, the time to fusion was dependent on 25(OH)D level. Kim correlated postoperative ODI and 25(OH)D and found that no patients preoperatively had a 25(OH)D level greater than 30 ng/mL while two-thirds were deficient at less than 20 ng/mL.[63] There was a strong negative correlation between 25(OH)D level and ODI postoperatively. Unfortunately, at this time it is unknown if delaying surgery and correcting the vitamin D deficiency will change any of these observed clinical or radiographic outcomes. Nonetheless, as vitamin D is inexpensive and essentially side-effect free, optimization of vitamin D status prior to spinal surgery, if feasible, is appropriate.

3.8.3 Bisphosphonates

Antiresorptive therapy is the mainstay for osteoporosis treatment, and thus many patients having spine surgery may be using these medications. There has been concern regarding the effect on bone healing from the use of bisphosphonates and denosumab. In humans, there appears to be either no effect or positive effect from bisphosphonates on fracture healing of the appendicular skeleton.[64] Animal models of spinal fusion confirm these clinical observations and show either no effect or a positive effect from the use of bisphosphonates.[64] In human lumbar interbody spine fusions, Nagahama performed an RCT comparing 35 mg of alendronate weekly postoperatively to a control group.[65] Significantly greater improvement in ODI occurred within 12 months. Spine fusion appeared to occur more consistently and earlier in the alendronate-treated patients. In another RCT, intravenous infusion of zolendronic acid was compared to controls in 79 patients who had posterior fusion for degenerative spondylolisthesis without instrumentation.[66] Similar to alendronate, at 12 months there is a statistically greater improvement in ODI. However, based on CT scan there was no difference in fusion success at 12 months, although fusion appeared to occur earlier, at 3, 6, and 9 months. Ding performed a matched cohort study comparing treatment with 5 mg zoledronate to control in 94 osteoporotic patients having lumbar fusion.[67] The treated group had more rapid healing, improved clinical outcomes, and no hardware loosening or adjacent-segment fractures compared to controls.

3.8.4 Anabolic Treatment

The use of anabolic agents to aid spine fusion in animal studies consistently shows a strong correlation with fusion success.[68] Studies confirm increased preosteoblastic activation and increased callous formation. At this time, use of anabolic agents for preoperative spine optimization is off-label use unless the patient has osteoporosis, i.e., a T-score of ≤ -2.5 or a history of fragility fracture. A weekly injection of N1–84 teriparatide (available in Europe) in patients undergoing lumbar interbody fusion was performed in 75 patients.[69] Bone fusion significantly improved at 4 and 6 months, although there was no difference in clinical outcome. Inoue examined osteoporotic insertional torque of pedicle screws in patients given preoperative teriparatide versus those without and found significantly greater insertional torque of 1.28 Nm compared to 1.08 Nm in the teriparatide group. There was strong correlation with duration of teriparatide and insertional torque out to 120 days.

3.8.5 Current Recommendations for Bone Health Optimization in Spine Patients

Diagnostics

Patients should be evaluated with a DXA scan using indications discussed above and according to AACE guidelines.[19] If a CT scan has been obtained or is available, then assessment of HU at the site of surgery and at L1 should be performed. Mean vertebral body HU less than 135 indicates a high likelihood of osteoporosis and should prompt a DXA scan and potentially treatment before fusion. When using DXA, consider VFA to diagnose occult fractures and TBS to improve understanding of bone microarchitecture.

Supplements

Vitamin D supplementation and calcium optimization through dietary intake, or diet plus supplements if needed to achieve a daily intake of 1,000 to 1,200 mg, should be recommended prior to surgery. Measuring serum 25(OH)D is useful to titrate the supplementation dose and can be repeated to assure that an adequate response occurred. Alternatively, 2,000 – 5,000 U vitamin D_3 daily can be recommended with the recognition that there are substantial differences in 25(OH)D response to any given oral dose.

Suggested Treatment

Patients with normal bone mass (i.e., a T-score better than -1.0) require no further treatment other than optimization of calcium and vitamin D.

Patients with low bone mass are candidates for bone health optimization. Correction of insufficient bone mass as a component of surgery depends upon the surgery procedure planned. Decompression can probably proceed concomitantly with treatment of osteoporosis if required. The surgeon should realize that osteoporotic patients will be more likely to have a pars/pedicle fracture after decompressive laminectomy and that more care to preserve bone integrity is needed.

Patients with short segment fusion likely benefit from improved bone health, which may speed fusion and increase outcomes. We currently recommend 3 months of treatment in patients with low bone mass prior to surgery.

Patients undergoing multilevel fusion and or osteotomy benefit most from preoperative bone health optimization. Patients with osteopenia and osteoporosis who are to undergo such procedures are treated with an anabolic agent for a minimum of 6 months prior to surgery, in addition to vitamin D and calcium supplements. It is likely that further attention to improved nutrition in depleted patients will have an additive benefit. Smoking cessation and reduction of alcohol intake is also important.

3.9 Conclusions

Osteoporosis is epidemic; it is underrecognized and undertreated and is associated with increased fracture risk in older adults. Osteoporosis and vitamin D deficiency negatively affect spinal outcomes, including fusion, and are likely to be associated with greater complications, such as hardware failure, proximal junction kyphosis, and proximal fracture. Osteoporosis and fracture risk are modifiable, however, and new programs to assess the efficacy of preoperative optimization are needed. Secondary fracture prevention should be a critical component of all patients who sustain a fragility fracture.

References

[1] American Orthopaedic Association. Leadership in orthopaedics: taking a stand to own the bone. American Orthopaedic Association position paper. J Bone Joint Surg Am. 2005; 87(6):1389–1391

[2] Balasubramanian A, Tosi LL, Lane JM, Dirschl DR, Ho PR, O'Malley CD. Declining rates of osteoporosis management following fragility fractures in the U.S., 2000 through 2009. J Bone Joint Surg Am. 2014; 96(7):e52

[3] Binkley N, Blank RD, Leslie WD, Lewiecki EM, Eisman JA, Bilezikian JP. Osteoporosis in Crisis: It's Time to Focus on Fracture. J Bone Miner Res. 2017; 32 (7):1391–1394

[4] Wright NC, Looker AC, Saag KG, et al. The recent prevalence of osteoporosis and low bone mass in the United States based on bone mineral density at the femoral neck or lumbar spine. J Bone Miner Res. 2014; 29(11):2520–2526

[5] Burge R, Dawson-Hughes B, Solomon DH, Wong JB, King A, Tosteson A. Incidence and economic burden of osteoporosis-related fractures in the United States, 2005–2025. J Bone Miner Res. 2007; 22(3):465–475

[6] Watkins-Castillo S, Wright N. Prevalence of Fragility Fractures 2014 [Available from: http://www.boneandjointburden.org/2014-report/vb1/prevalence-fragility-fractures

[7] Schousboe JT. Epidemiology of Vertebral Fractures. J Clin Densitom. 2016; 19 (1):8–22

[8] Tajeu GS, Delzell E, Smith W, et al. Death, debility, and destitution following hip fracture. J Gerontol A Biol Sci Med Sci. 2014; 69(3):346–353

[9] Lau E, Ong K, Kurtz S, Schmier J, Edidin A. Mortality following the diagnosis of a vertebral compression fracture in the Medicare population. J Bone Joint Surg Am. 2008; 90(7):1479–1486

[10] Chen AT, Cohen DB, Skolasky RL. Impact of nonoperative treatment, vertebroplasty, and kyphoplasty on survival and morbidity after vertebral compression fracture in the medicare population. J Bone Joint Surg Am. 2013; 95(19): 1729–1736

[11] Tosteson AN, Gabriel SE, Grove MR, Moncur MM, Kneeland TS, Melton LJ, III. Impact of hip and vertebral fractures on quality-adjusted life years. Osteoporos Int. 2001; 12(12):1042–1049

[12] Svensson HK, Olofsson EH, Karlsson J, Hansson T, Olsson LE. A painful, never ending story: older women's experiences of living with an osteoporotic vertebral compression fracture. Osteoporos Int. 2016; 27(5):1729–1736

[13] Hodsman AB, Leslie WD, Tsang JF, Gamble GD. 10-year probability of recurrent fractures following wrist and other osteoporotic fractures in a large clinical cohort: an analysis from the Manitoba Bone Density Program. Arch Intern Med. 2008; 168(20):2261–2267

[14] Center JR, Bliuc D, Nguyen TV, Eisman JA. Risk of subsequent fracture after low-trauma fracture in men and women. JAMA. 2007; 297(4):387–394

[15] Kanis JA, Johnell O, De Laet C, et al. A meta-analysis of previous fracture and subsequent fracture risk. Bone. 2004; 35(2):375–382

[16] Anderson PA, Froyshteter AB, Tontz WL, Jr. Meta-analysis of vertebral augmentation compared with conservative treatment for osteoporotic spinal fractures. J Bone Miner Res. 2013; 28(2):372–382

[17] Lindsay R, Silverman SL, Cooper C, et al. Risk of new vertebral fracture in the year following a fracture. JAMA. 2001; 285(3):320–323

[18] Lewiecki EM, Binkley N, Morgan SL, et al. International Society for Clinical Densitometry. Best Practices for Dual-Energy X-ray Absorptiometry Measurement and Reporting: International Society for Clinical Densitometry Guidance. J Clin Densitom. 2016; 19(2):127–140

[19] Camacho PM, Petak SM, Binkley N, et al. AMERICAN ASSOCIATION OF CLINICAL ENDOCRINOLOGISTS AND AMERICAN COLLEGE OF ENDOCRINOLOGY

CLINICAL PRACTICE GUIDELINES FOR THE DIAGNOSIS AND TREATMENT OF POSTMENOPAUSAL OSTEOPOROSIS - 2016. Endocr Pract. 2016; 22 Suppl 4:1–42

[20] Cosman F, de Beur SJ, LeBoff MS, et al. National Osteoporosis Foundation. Clinician's Guide to Prevention and Treatment of Osteoporosis. Osteoporos Int. 2014; 25(10):2359–2381

[21] Cauley JA, El-Hajj Fuleihan G, Luckey MM, FRAX(®) Position Development Conference Members. FRAX® International Task Force of the 2010 Joint International Society for Clinical Densitometry & International Osteoporosis Foundation Position Development Conference. J Clin Densitom. 2011; 14(3):237–239

[22] Donaldson MG, Palermo L, Schousboe JT, Ensrud KE, Hochberg MC, Cummings SR. FRAX and risk of vertebral fractures: the fracture intervention trial. J Bone Miner Res. 2009; 24(11):1793–1799

[23] U.S. Preventive Services Task Force. Screening for osteoporosis: U.S. preventive services task force recommendation statement. Ann Intern Med. 2011; 154(5):356–364

[24] Fuerst T, Wu C, Genant HK, et al. Evaluation of vertebral fracture assessment by dual X-ray absorptiometry in a multicenter setting. Osteoporos Int. 2009; 20(7):1199–1205

[25] Muszkat P, Camargo MB, Peters BS, Kunii LS, Lazaretti-Castro M. Digital vertebral morphometry performed by DXA: a valuable opportunity for identifying fractures during bone mass assessment. Arch Endocrinol Metab. 2015; 59(2):98–104

[26] Harvey NC, Glüer CC, Binkley N, et al. Trabecular bone score (TBS) as a new complementary approach for osteoporosis evaluation in clinical practice. Bone. 2015; 78:216–224

[27] Lee SJ, Binkley N, Lubner MG, Bruce RJ, Ziemlewicz TJ, Pickhardt PJ. Opportunistic screening for osteoporosis using the sagittal reconstruction from routine abdominal CT for combined assessment of vertebral fractures and density. Osteoporos Int. 2016; 27(3):1131–1136

[28] Pickhardt PJ, Lee LJ, del Rio AM, et al. Simultaneous screening for osteoporosis at CT colonography: bone mineral density assessment using MDCT attenuation techniques compared with the DXA reference standard. J Bone Miner Res. 2011; 26(9):2194–2203

[29] Schreiber JJ, Anderson PA, Rosas HG, Buchholz AL, Au AG. Hounsfield units for assessing bone mineral density and strength: a tool for osteoporosis management. J Bone Joint Surg Am. 2011; 93(11):1057–1063

[30] Pickhardt PJ, Bodeen G, Brett A, Brown JK, Binkley N. Comparison of femoral neck BMD evaluation obtained using Lunar DXA and QCT with asynchronous calibration from CT colonography. J Clin Densitom. 2015; 18(1):5–12

[31] Pickhardt PJ, Lauder T, Pooler BD, et al. Effect of IV contrast on lumbar trabecular attenuation at routine abdominal CT: correlation with DXA and implications for opportunistic osteoporosis screening. Osteoporos Int. 2016; 27(1):147–152

[32] Garner HW, Paturzo MM, Gaudier G, Pickhardt PJ, Wessell DE. Variation in Attenuation in L1 Trabecular Bone at Different Tube Voltages: Caution Is Warranted When Screening for Osteoporosis With the Use of Opportunistic CT. AJR Am J Roentgenol. 2017; 208(1):165–170

[33] Aiyangar AK, Vivanco J, Au AG, Anderson PA, Smith EL, Ploeg HL. Dependence of anisotropy of human lumbar vertebral trabecular bone on quantitative computed tomography-based apparent density. J Biomech Eng. 2014; 136(9):091003

[34] Weiser L, Huber G, Sellenschloh K, et al. Insufficient stability of pedicle screws in osteoporotic vertebrae: biomechanical correlation of bone mineral density and pedicle screw fixation strength. Eur Spine J. 2017; 26(11):2891–2897

[35] Meredith DS, Schreiber JJ, Taher F, Cammisa FP, Jr, Girardi FP. Lower preoperative Hounsfield unit measurements are associated with adjacent segment fracture after spinal fusion. Spine. 2013; 38(5):415–418

[36] Du JY, Aichmair A, Ueda H, Girardi FP, Cammisa FP, Lebl DR. Vertebral body Hounsfield units as a predictor of incidental durotomy in primary lumbar spinal surgery. Spine. 2014; 39(9):E593–E598

[37] Schreiber JJ, Hughes AP, Taher F, Girardi FP. An association can be found between hounsfield units and success of lumbar spine fusion. HSS J. 2014; 10(1):25–29

[38] Okuyama K, Abe E, Suzuki T, Tamura Y, Chiba M, Sato K. Influence of bone mineral density on pedicle screw fixation: a study of pedicle screw fixation augmenting posterior lumbar interbody fusion in elderly patients. Spine J. 2001; 1(6):402–407

[39] Nguyen HS, Shabani S, Patel M, Maiman D. Posterolateral lumbar fusion: Relationship between computed tomography Hounsfield units and symptomatic pseudoarthrosis. Surg Neurol Int. 2015; 6 Suppl 24:S611–S614

[40] Wagner SC, Formby PM, Helgeson MD, Kang DG. Diagnosing the Undiagnosed: Osteoporosis in Patients Undergoing Lumbar Fusion. Spine. 2016; 41(21):E1279–E1283

[41] Mi J, Li K, Zhao X, Zhao CQ, Li H, Zhao J. Vertebral Body Hounsfield Units are Associated With Cage Subsidence After Transforaminal Lumbar Interbody Fusion With Unilateral Pedicle Screw Fixation. Clin Spine Surg. 2017; 30(8):E1130–E1136

[42] Graffy PM, Lee SJ, Ziemlewicz TJ, Pickhardt PJ. Prevalence of Vertebral Compression Fractures on Routine CT Scans According to L1 Trabecular Attenuation: Determining Relevant Thresholds for Opportunistic Osteoporosis Screening. AJR Am J Roentgenol. 2017; 209(3):491–496

[43] Emohare O, Cagan A, Polly DW, Jr, Gertner E. Opportunistic computed tomography screening shows a high incidence of osteoporosis in ankylosing spondylitis patients with acute vertebral fractures. J Clin Densitom. 2015; 18(1):17–21

[44] Barzel US. Recommended testing in patients with low bone density. J Clin Endocrinol Metab. 2003; 88(3):1404–1405, author reply 1405

[45] Institute of Medicine Committee to Review Dietary Reference Intakes for Vitamin D. Calcium. The National Academies Collection: Reports funded by National Institutes of Health. In: Ross AC, Taylor CL, Yaktine AL, Del Valle HB, eds. Dietary Reference Intakes for Calcium and Vitamin D. Washington (DC): National Academies Press (US) National Academy of Sciences; 2011

[46] American Geriatrics Society Workgroup on Vitamin D Supplementation for Older Adults. Recommendations abstracted from the American Geriatrics Society Consensus Statement on vitamin D for Prevention of Falls and Their Consequences. J Am Geriatr Soc. 2014; 62(1):147–152

[47] Kopecky SL, Bauer DC, Gulati M, et al. Lack of Evidence Linking Calcium With or Without Vitamin D Supplementation to Cardiovascular Disease in Generally Healthy Adults: A Clinical Guideline From the National Osteoporosis Foundation and the American Society for Preventive Cardiology. Ann Intern Med. 2016; 165(12):867–868

[48] The NAMS 2017 Hormone Therapy Position Statement Advisory Panel. The 2017 hormone therapy position statement of The North American Menopause Society. Menopause. 2017; 24(7):728–753

[49] Neer RM, Arnaud CD, Zanchetta JR, et al. Effect of parathyroid hormone (1–34) on fractures and bone mineral density in postmenopausal women with osteoporosis. N Engl J Med. 2001; 344(19):1434–1441

[50] Miller PD, Hattersley G, Riis BJ, et al. ACTIVE Study Investigators. Effect of Abaloparatide vs Placebo on New Vertebral Fractures in Postmenopausal Women With Osteoporosis: A Randomized Clinical Trial. JAMA. 2016; 316(7):722–733

[51] Shane E, Burr D, Abrahamsen B, et al. Atypical subtrochanteric and diaphyseal femoral fractures: second report of a task force of the American Society for Bone and Mineral Research. J Bone Miner Res. 2014; 29(1):1–23

[52] Bawa HS, Weick J, Dirschl DR. Anti-Osteoporotic Therapy After Fragility Fracture Lowers Rate of Subsequent Fracture: Analysis of a Large Population Sample. J Bone Joint Surg Am. 2015; 97(19):1555–1562

[53] Hawley S, Leal J, Delmestri A, et al. REFReSH Study Group. Anti-Osteoporosis Medication Prescriptions and Incidence of Subsequent Fracture Among Primary Hip Fracture Patients in England and Wales: An Interrupted Time-Series Analysis. J Bone Miner Res. 2016; 31(11):2008–2015

[54] Wells GA, Cranney A, Peterson J, et al. Alendronate for the primary and secondary prevention of osteoporotic fractures in postmenopausal women. Cochrane Database Syst Rev. 2008(1):CD001155

[55] Peichl P, Holzer LA, Maier R, Holzer G. Parathyroid hormone 1–84 accelerates fracture-healing in pubic bones of elderly osteoporotic women. J Bone Joint Surg Am. 2011; 93(17):1583–1587

[56] Yoo JI, Ha YC, Ryu HJ, et al. Teriparatide Treatment in Elderly Patients With Sacral Insufficiency Fracture. J Clin Endocrinol Metab. 2017; 102(2):560–565

[57] Ganda K, Puech M, Chen JS, et al. Models of care for the secondary prevention of osteoporotic fractures: a systematic review and meta-analysis. Osteoporos Int. 2013; 24(2):393–406

[58] Bunta AD, Edwards BJ, Macaulay WB, Jr, et al. Own the Bone, a System-Based Intervention, Improves Osteoporosis Care After Fragility Fractures. J Bone Joint Surg Am. 2016; 98(24):e109

[59] Stoker GE, Buchowski JM, Bridwell KH, Lenke LG, Riew KD, Zebala LP. Preoperative vitamin D status of adults undergoing surgical spinal fusion. Spine. 2013; 38(6):507–515

[60] Ravindra VM, Godzik J, Guan J, et al. Prevalence of Vitamin D Deficiency in Patients Undergoing Elective Spine Surgery: A Cross-Sectional Analysis. World Neurosurg. 2015; 83(6):1114–1119

[61] Kim TH, Lee BH, Lee HM, et al. Prevalence of vitamin D deficiency in patients with lumbar spinal stenosis and its relationship with pain. Pain Physician. 2013; 16(2):165–176

[62] Ravindra VM, Godzik J, Dailey AT, et al. Vitamin D Levels and 1-Year Fusion Outcomes in Elective Spine Surgery: A Prospective Observational Study. Spine. 2015; 40(19):1536–1541

[63] Kim TH, Yoon JY, Lee BH, et al. Changes in vitamin D status after surgery in female patients with lumbar spinal stenosis and its clinical significance. Spine. 2012; 37(21):E1326–E1330

[64] Hirsch BP, Unnanuntana A, Cunningham ME, Lane JM. The effect of therapies for osteoporosis on spine fusion: a systematic review. Spine J. 2013; 13(2):190–199

[65] Nagahama K, Kanayama M, Togawa D, Hashimoto T, Minami A. Does alendronate disturb the healing process of posterior lumbar interbody fusion? A prospective randomized trial. J Neurosurg Spine. 2011; 14(4):500–507

[66] Chen F, Dai Z, Kang Y, Lv G, Keller ET, Jiang Y. Effects of zoledronic acid on bone fusion in osteoporotic patients after lumbar fusion. Osteoporos Int. 2016; 27(4):1469–1476

[67] Ding Q, Chen J, Fan J, Li Q, Yin G, Yu L. Effect of zoledronic acid on lumbar spinal fusion in osteoporotic patients. Eur Spine J. 2017; 26(11):2969–2977

[68] Lubelski D, Choma TJ, Steinmetz MP, Harrop JS, Mroz TE. Perioperative Medical Management of Spine Surgery Patients With Osteoporosis. Neurosurgery. 2015; 77 Suppl 4:S92–S97

[69] Ebata S, Takahashi J, Hasegawa T, et al. Role of Weekly Teriparatide Administration in Osseous Union Enhancement within Six Months After Posterior or Transforaminal Lumbar Interbody Fusion for Osteoporosis-Associated Lumbar Degenerative Disorders: A Multicenter, Prospective Randomized Study. J Bone Joint Surg Am. 2017; 99(5):365–372

4 Surgical Decision-Making in the Aging Population

Jenny (Jianning) Shao, Thomas E. Mroz, and Samuel C. Overley

Abstract

The number of older adults who require spine surgery has increased significantly in the past decade. Along with this increase in patient population, there is also a corresponding increase in the accompanying comorbidities and deterioration of anatomical integrity of the spine, which in turn necessitate unique considerations in surgical approach, possible complications, and preoperative screening. This chapter provides a comprehensive review of the important effects of aging on surgery, necessary components of the preoperative screening that needs to be implemented for this population, and a discussion on how to tailor spine surgery to the older adult in the context of their overall health and preoperative risk factors. Specifically, the timing and selection of specific surgeries for older adults will be discussed for surgeries of both the cervical and lumbar spine. Risk factors, suboptimal patient responses, and postoperative complications, along with possible changes in surgery to minimize these complications will also be discussed. While a preoperative workup is performed for all patients undergoing spine surgery, older adults require a more comprehensive evaluation that corresponds to their unique constellation of potential complications and comorbidities. In this chapter, we discuss the important preoperative considerations, such as patient frailty, mental status, and social support and advocate for the implementation of a standardized evaluation for these factors before major spine surgery. Ultimately, this chapter seeks to provide a better understanding of the risks and complications that accompany spine surgery in aging patients as well as to suggest possible alterations in surgical approach and preoperative workup to minimize these complications and optimize patient outcome.

Keywords: Preoperative workup, surgical complications in aging patients, age-related comorbidities

4.1 Introduction: The Changing Landscape of Spine Surgery

The population of spine surgery patients has changed significantly during the past two decades; as the proportion of the U.S. population over the age of 62 increases (by 21.1% from 2000 to 2010), the prevalence of spinal conditions is also on the rise.[1] As such, the demand for surgical interventions of the spine to treat disorders ranging from degenerative spinal stenosis to spinal deformities has increased in the aging population throughout the last few decades.[1,2,3,4,5,6,7,8,9] Older adults accounted for the fastest growth in the population of patients undergoing surgeries of the lumbar spine during the past few decades.[2,4] A similar trend is also seen in patients undergoing cervical spine surgeries. For instance, the adjusted rate for older adults undergoing cervical spine fusions rose by 206% from 1992 to 2005.[2,9,10]

This increased demand for spine surgery in the aging population necessitates an understanding of age-related changes in the spine, their effects on patients' responses to surgery, and their impact on surgical decision-making. To this end, we will explore the complications associated with surgeries of both the cervical and lumbar spine in the elderly as well as the preoperative workup recommendations for this patient population. Lastly, we will examine bone mineral density (BMD) workup for spinal fusions and explore the best management strategies prior to elective surgeries. As we progress through this chapter, it will hopefully become evident that the aging patient may go through several important changes and could respond differently to surgical operations than a younger individual, thus necessitating careful consideration of surgical decisions in spine surgeries of the older adult.

4.2 Surgical Complications and Aging

Aging patients, which will henceforth refer to those over 65 years of age, often have both worse outcomes and increased incidence of complications following spine surgery when compared with younger cohorts.[11] As such, it is not surprising that the aging population also has the highest risk of mortality associated with surgeries of the spine.[1] However, this picture is complicated by the increased incidence of comorbidities in older adults, which can confound the impact of age on postoperative surgical complications.[12,13] Furthermore, reports have indicated that withholding surgery from an older adult can actually result in increased morbidity.[9,12] As such, the relative risks and benefits of surgical intervention must be comprehensively assessed for each patient before proceeding. Thus, it is imperative that we explore the relationship between age and postoperative complications associated with surgeries of the cervical and lumbar spine.

Key Points

- Older adults undergoing major spine surgery present a unique constellation of risk factors, comorbidities, and potential complications that must be considered.
- Aging patients manifest rapid deterioration following cervical spondylotic myelopathy (CSM), thereby necessitating prompt surgical intervention for optimal results. Withholding spine surgery from this population of patients may increase morbidity due to rapid disease progression.
- Dysphagia is a major complication of anterior cervical spine surgery in the older adult.
- Minimally invasive spine surgery (MIS) may be a safer alternative for aging populations undergoing surgery of the lumbar spine.
- Preoperative workup in older adults should include a thorough evaluation of the patient's cardiovascular, renal, and pulmonary function, in addition to a comprehensive assessment of the patient's frailty, nutritional status, social support, and mental status.

4.2.1 Cervical Spine

One disorder that exhibits increasing prevalence with age is cervical spondylosis, which can lead to cervical myelopathy, characterized by symptoms such as difficulty in gait and numbness and/or weakness of the hands.[14,15,16] Untreated cervical spondylotic myelopathy (CSM) has a poor natural history and severely impairs both ambulatory functions and quality of life.[1,14,15,16] Although surgical decompression has been shown to improve patient symptoms, several studies have suggested a higher complication rate in patients of advanced age, generally over the age of 65.[1] A 2008 study comparing the surgical outcomes of elderly patients undergoing decompressive surgery for cervical spondylotic myelopathy with those of younger cohorts showed that the older population had a 38% complication rate, compared to a 6% complication rate in the younger group.[8] Similarly, a recent study, which analyzed 5,154 elderly patients and 30,808 nonelderly patients found that elderly age significantly increased the risk of complications following anterior cervical discectomy and fusion (ACDF) and posterior fusion procedures for the treatment of CSM.[14] The elderly group had a 22.26% complication rate after ACDF surgery (compared with a 14.66% complication rate in the nonelderly group, p-value < .001) and a 32.34% complication rate after posterior decompression (compared with a 27.85% complication rate in the nonelderly group, p-value = .0084).[14] Common complications include dysphagia, nerve injury, postoperative pain from paraspinal muscle injury, epidural hematoma, and pulmonary distress.[1,2,3,4,5,7,8] Some severe complications reported for older adults undergoing surgery for CSM include delirium, dementia, and nerve injury.[1,2,3,4,5,7,8] However, it is worth noting that age is not the only factor that increases risks for complications. Medical comorbidities such as diabetes and obesity also increase the risk of adverse outcomes.[1,2,3,4,5,7,8,11,17] Since older patients tend to have a greater number of comorbidities than younger cohorts, it's possible that the comorbidities themselves may account for the increased complication rates, thus serving as a confounder in the relationship between age and postoperative complications.

The literature on this topic, while conflicted, seems to support a role for surgical intervention for CSM in older adults, with several groups reporting no effect of age on postoperative complications for surgical treatment of CSM after adjusting for baseline Japanese Orthopedic Association (JOA) scores.[2,3,4,5,8,9,10] A meta-analysis comprised of 2,868 patients reported no significant difference in the incidence of complications following surgery for CSM between the elderly and nonelderly groups.[9] Similar results have also been reported by other groups, one of which showed that octogenarians had similar rates of postoperative complications as a younger cohort following decompression surgery.[12] However, it was noted that the elderly age group exhibited a rapid deterioration following CSM onset, necessitating prompt surgical intervention for optimal results.[12] Thus, withholding surgery from older adults from fear of possible complications may actually increase morbidity due to the rapid disease progression in this age cohort.[13] While the relative risks and complications of any surgery must be weighed before proceeding, there is clearly a role for surgical intervention for the alleviation of CSM symptoms and improvement in quality of life in the aging population. However, it is important to be cognizant of the possible complications and take measures perioperative to minimize their risks, as will be discussed in a future section.

4.3 Dysphagia in Older Adults and Effect on Cervical Surgery

Another possible complication of cervical surgery is dysphagia, especially in older adults. Older adults are inherently more vulnerable to dysphagia due to the increased comorbidities, such as gastroesophageal reflux disease (GERD).[18,19,20] Of note, the prevalence of dysphagia in persons above the age of 50 in nursing homes is estimated to be anywhere from 40 to 60% in the Midwestern United States.[18] In addition to GERD, other comorbidities that may predispose an individual to developing dysphagia include cerebrovascular accidents, Parkinson's Disease, and Amyotrophic Lateral Sclerosis (ALS), all of which are more prevalent in the aging population.[18,19,20] Since functional dysphagia requires integrity of the oropharynx, anything that compromises that integrity or associated nervous innervation of the oropharynx can lead to dysphagia.[18] As such, dysphagia is a well-established complication of anterior cervical spine surgery. In particular, a recent report demonstrated certain risk factors, such as female gender, the utilization of anterior cervical plates, multiple surgical levels, surgery at C3/4, and using human bone protein rhBMP-2, are associated with an increased risk for developing dysphagia after cervical surgery.[19,20] While more studies are required to establish more comprehensive risk factors in cervical surgery associated with postoperative dysphagia, it is well established that cervical anterior spine surgery is an important contributor to the development of dysphagia. Thus, it is important that a set of guidelines concerning the risk factors for developing dysphagia be developed to guide the instrumentation and approach of cervical spine surgery for older adults.

4.3.1 Lumbar Spine

Lumbar spinal stenosis is the most common degenerative condition of the aged spine, often presenting with symptoms of neurogenic claudication.[1,21,22] Surgical interventions involving lumbar decompression, instrumented lumbar fusion, and minimally invasive methods have been shown to significantly improve patients' quality of life.[1,21,22,23] However, as with decompressive surgeries of the cervical spine, lumbar decompression in older adults is complicated by dissenting opinions concerning associated complications.[1,21,22] Specifically, there is disagreement in the literature concerning whether increased age is significantly correlated with increased complications and worse outcomes.[1,21,22] While some studies have reported increased complications following surgery for degenerative lumbar spinal stenosis (DLSS), the vast majority of literature suggests that confounding factors such as operative time and blood loss were actually more influential than age in predicting surgical outcomes.[1,12,21,22] Indeed, both of these factors were found to be predictive of systemic and wound complications in a retrospective review of 88 elderly patients who underwent DLSS surgery.[14] This result was corroborated by the results from a large European spine registry, which comprised 1,764 elderly patients undergoing DLSS surgery. In this case, aspirin use and blood loss were predictive of the incidence of postoperative complications.[1] Of note, a multicenter cohort study in Switzerland in 2010 indicated that patients who are 80 years or older can expect a clinically meaningful outcome from decompressive surgery for DLSS, with notable improvement in quality of life, as measured by EuroQol-5 Dimension (EQ-5D) quality of life questionnaires.[21] Furthermore, no statistically significant difference in complications were reported between the older and younger cohorts.[14] Even patients aged 90 years and older showed no correlation between DLSS outcomes/complication rates and age.[18] Rather, the odds ratio for comorbidity in this cohort was 9.20 (p = 0.040). A strong correlation with postoperative complications were associated with blood loss, operation time, and days spent in the intensive care unit.[18] Similar results have been reported abundantly, indicating that advanced age in itself is not linked to major complications in DLSS surgeries.[1,12,21,22,24]

Given the clear impact of operation time and blood loss on surgical outcomes and complication rates in older patients, literature suggests that minimally invasive surgery (MIS) may be ideal for patients of advanced age.[11,24] The decreased blood loss, minimal disruption of the anatomy, and reduced pain associated with these procedures render them a viable alternative to conventional decompression surgery for the aging population.[11,24] Recent studies attest to the efficacy of minimally invasive surgeries in DLSS treatment; a study performed on 57 patients over the age of 75 undergoing DLSS MIS showed significant improvement in patient function and quality of life, as measured by Oswestry Disability Index scores and 36-item Short Form Survey scores.[1,24] Furthermore, no major complications were noted in the study. As these results suggest, MIS is a safe and effective alternative to conventional, open decompressive surgeries for the treatment of DLSS in older adults.[1,24]

4.4 Recommendations for Preoperative Workup in Older Adults

Preoperative workup for spine surgery in older adults must include a comprehensive review of systems as well as identification of any condition that may increase the risk of perioperative complications. We will explore here the major elements of the cardiovascular, pulmonary, and renal system workups in the geriatric population. In addition, we will also explore the impact of BMD on the outcomes of spinal fusion procedures. While meticulous preoperative workup is necessary for all patients undergoing major spine surgery, special considerations are necessary for older adults. Specifically, important factors that may affect patient outcome in this population include frailty, nutrition, social support, and mental status.

4.4.1 Cardiovascular

Given that over 50% of patients above 70 years of age have cardiovascular disease upon autopsy, cardiovascular complications and measures to reduce their risk should be considered before any surgery.[11] As such, a preoperative workup in older adults should always include a thorough medical history, surgical

history, cardiac physical examination, and baseline electrocardiogram assessments to evaluate the status of the patient's cardiovascular health and to detect possible cardiovascular risk factors.[12] Specifically, patient reports of dyspnea or syncope should alert the surgeon to possible previous undiagnosed myocardial infarctions or arrhythmias and should be investigated before proceeding with surgery.[11]

To determine a patient's risk for perioperative cardiovascular complications, surgeons can use the Revised Cardiac Risk Index, which was published in 1999 from a study comprised of 2,893 patients and validated in 1,422 patients who underwent major noncardiac surgery.[12,25] Specifically, six risk factors were identified which had significant correlation with postoperative cardiovascular complications, namely, histories of ischemic heart disease, congestive heart failure, cerebrovascular disease, diabetic insulin therapy, chronic kidney disease (as defined by a preoperative creatinine level of 2 mg/dL or higher), and high-risk surgeries.[12,25] The predictive power of these risk factors can be appreciated by examining the risk for major cardiovascular complications in the context of the number of predictors present.[13] A patient with zero of the six risk factors only has a 0.4% risk of having a significant cardiovascular complication, where as a patient with three or more risk factors has over an 11% risk of having a major cardiovascular complication.[12]

4.4.2 Pulmonary System

Aging is often accompanied by a decline in respiratory function and reserve capacity, which can often give way to chronic obstructive diseases.[12] Indeed, airway obstruction has been noted to complicate spine surgery in the older adult patient. In a case series of 100 patients aged over 70 years, almost 40% exhibited abnormal pulmonary function.[13] Thus, as part of preoperative workup for older adults, pulmonary function tests such as the one-second forced expiratory volume (FEV1) should be performed.[12] Furthermore, arterial blood gas concentrations should also be determined to detect possible loss of pulmonary reserve capacity.[12] A preoperative PCO2 concentration of greater than 45 mm Hg has been associated with an increased occurrence of postoperative pulmonary complications.[12] This is especially important if a ventral surgical approach is being considered or if the patient manifests symptoms of pulmonary compromise, such as dyspnea, orthopnea, or poor exercise tolerance.[12] If clear pulmonary impairment is present, however, operations that require thoracotomy should be avoided.[12] While there is no clearly defined guidelines of ideal pulmonary function prior to spine surgery, it is widely agreed that optimal preoperative respiratory function is associated with better patient outcomes and reduced rates of postoperative complications.[12]

4.4.3 Renal System

Older adults have been shown to have reduced renal function compared to younger patients. Indeed, renal decline in aging patients is more established than that of any other organ system.[12] Thus, a preoperative workup for older adults should include a thorough interrogation of the integrity of the patient's renal function.[12] Specifically, serum creatinine levels, the gold standard for assaying kidney function, should be determined, especially if the patient has symptoms of chronic renal failure.[12] Furthermore, the patients' medications should also be considered when assaying renal functions, since drugs such as nonsteroidal anti-inflammatory drugs (NSAIDs) can reduce renal blood flow and even cause renal ischemia if taken in high enough doses.[12] Combined with an already age-related decreased filtration rate, continued use of NSAIDs prior to surgery can lead to dangerous renal complications.[12] Thus, patients scheduled for spine surgery should discontinue NSAID usage as prescribed by the surgeon.[12]

4.4.4 Bone Mineral Density

Osteoporosis is a significant medical problem in the older patient population, affecting 26% of women over 65 years of age and 50% of women over 85 years of age.[12] This is clinically relevant in spine surgery, as osteoporosis leads to decreased BMD and is associated with poor bone remodeling characteristics.[12,26] As such, the pullout strength of pedicle screws can be reduced and both rates of and time to fusions may be negatively impacted.[12,26] Thus, in preoperative workup of older adults with decreased BMD, measures should be taken to increase bone density secondarily, improving screw purchase and promoting positive bone remodeling and healing.[12,26] This is often achieved via pharmacologic agents.[12]

4.4.5 Patient Frailty

To appreciate the effect that frailty has on patient outcomes, it is important to first establish what constitutes frailty. While some subjectivity is inherent in the definition, it is broadly agreed upon that frailty is characterized as a reduction in physiological function and reserve throughout multiple organ systems, as manifested by clinical symptoms and presentation.[27,28] Several indices have been proposed to quantify frailty, including the modified Frailty Index (mFI) and the Canadian Study for Health and Aging Frailty Index (CSHA-FI).[27] Utilizing these indices, several studies have reported that frailty is a significant predictor of patient outcomes and postoperative complications in major spine surgery.[27,28] Importantly, a recent study reported that frailty was directly associated with increased reoperation rates, higher mortality, and increased complications (including pneumonia, deep vein thrombosis, shock, cardiac arrest, pulmonary embolism, etc.) after surgery in a statistically significant manner.[3] There is also a direct correlation between increasing mFI and mortality in the first 30 days.[3] In the aforementioned study, an increase in mFI from 0 to 0.27 was mirrored by an increase in mortality from 0.3% to 10%.[27] Thus, it is evident that frailty is a significant predictor of patient outcomes and complications in major spine surgery. As such, preoperative evaluation of patient frailty with indices such as the mFI, along with appropriate patient counseling with explicit communication of the risks associated with the patient's frailty index, is crucial for optimal patient outcomes in major spine surgery.[27,28]

4.4.6 Nutrition

The nutritional status of a patient has also been established as an important predictor of postoperative complications, morality, and patient outcomes. While this is true for patients of all ages, it is especially important in patients in the elderly population.[29,30] Indeed, a recent study on the impact of nutrition status and patient outcomes in patients undergoing lumbar spine fusion surgery showed that malnutrition was significantly correlated with increased 1-year mortality rates, with an adjusted odds ratio (OR) of 6.16, as well as increased rates of major complications over 90 days (OR 4.24), such as infection (OR 2.27) and wound dehiscence (OR: 2.52).[29] In addition, patients with poor nutritional status also had an increased length of stay in comparison to well-nourished patients, thereby increased their risk of contracting nosocomial infections.[29] Several reports have indicated that malnutrition serves as a significant contributor to comorbidities and complications in aging patients and leads to decreased resilience and resistance to "physical stressors" postoperatively.[29,30] Thus, given the importance of nutritional status on patient outcomes and complications, it is important to implement nutritional screening as part of the preoperative workup routine, the results of which should inform the future steps of the patient's treatment.[29,30] For instance, a recent study indicated that patients with severe malnutrition could be administered parenteral nutrition preoperatively to boost their nutritional status.[30] In particular, efforts should be made to reduce hyperglycemia and curtail insulin resistance via a preoperative nutritional regimen, as this may lead to improved would healing and expedite the recovery of bowel function following surgery.[30] Furthermore, "immune-modulating formulas" consisting of arginine, omega-3 fatty acids, and other nutrients have been demonstrated to improve patient outcomes.[30] These ingredients serve as important components of metabolic pathways that are involved in wound healing and immune function.[38] Therefore, we propose the implementation of nutritional screening as part of the preoperative evaluation for older adults undergoing major spine surgery, with appropriate follow-up nutritional treatments.[29,30]

4.4.7 Social Support

The presence of social support is crucial in the optimal recovery of older adults, as evidenced by several reports on the effects of social support (or lack thereof) on patient mortality.[31] Broadly, social isolation is characterized by living alone and having few friends and family members in their immediate contacts.[31] Indeed, the English Longitudinal Study of Aging identified loneliness and social isolation as key risk factors in postoperative mortality in the aging population.[31] Furthermore, this study found that a lack of social support was also correlated with an increased progression of frailty, the adverse effects of which have been discussed earlier in this section.[31] Specifically, patients who reported high levels of loneliness demonstrated an increased risk of becoming physically frail over four years with a relative risk ratio of 1.74 (CI: 95%)[31] It is important to note, however, that this increase in physical frailty was not associated with a change in the frailty index.[31] Thus, while the evidence for social support's importance in postoperative patient outcomes is less quantitative, it is nevertheless important to determine the patient's level of social support prior to major spine surgery.[31] If preoperative screening reveals that the patient is socially isolated, then it may be important to assign a social worker or external support system to the patient to ensure optimal adjustment during the postoperative period.

4.4.8 Mental Status

There is an increased prevalence of mental status disturbances in older adults that predispose them to increased rates of postoperative complications and mortality rates.[32] Common disruptions in mental status in older adults can broadly be categorized into cognitive impairment and mood changes, most prominently depression.[32] In 2002, approximately 13.9% of the elderly had dementia, and 22.3% of the elderly had some type of cognitive impairment.[40] Given this significant proportion of the older population who suffer from cognitive impairment, it is crucial to determine the effect of preoperative mental status on postoperative outcomes.[32] Several studies have shown that there is a strong correlation between cognitive impairment and postoperative complications, most prominently postoperative delirium, which has an incidence of 32 to 42% in the older adult population.[32] Even more troubling, the presence of postoperative delirium is associated with major complications, including increased length of hospital stay and mortality.[32] Specifically, studies have shown the preoperative cognitive impairment is predictive of postoperative pulmonary complications.[32] In one particular cohort study, patients with mild cognitive impairment, as defined by a Montreal Cognitive Assessment (MoCA) test score of 19 to 25, demonstrated significant deterioration in respiratory function as assayed by spirometry, rates of atelectasis, and requirement for mechanical ventilation.[32] Given the significant impact of cognitive function on postoperative outcomes and complications, it is imperative to implement cognitive testing as part of the preoperative evaluation prior to major spine surgery.[32] This can be accomplished with cognitive tests such as the MoCA and the Mini-Mental Status Exam (MMSE), both of which have been well-validated in the assessment of baseline cognitive function.[32]

In addition to cognitive function, the patient's mood before surgery is also an important predictor of patient outcomes.[32] A significant proportion of older adults, approximately 15% to 20%, suffer from depression.[32] This statistic is even higher among older patients in the preoperative period. Unfortunately, preoperative depression and anxiety are correlated with worse postoperative outcomes.[32] Indeed, even after controlling for sex, previous myocardial infarctions, and comorbidities like diabetes, patients with depression had a higher mortality rate after 6 months. In addition, depression has also been correlated with major complications during the postoperative period.[32] Thus, given the adverse effect of depression on patient outcome, it may be important to conduct a mood screening before major spine surgery and to take appropriate measures during the preoperative period. This may include ensuring proper treatment for depression, periodic therapy sessions, and maximizing social support for the patient.

4.5 Matching Patient and Surgeon Expectations

The ability to match patient and surgeon expectations is integral to obtaining a successful outcome in spine surgery. This becomes even more important (and complicated) when considering spine surgery in the aging population. Expectations regarding aging (ERA) are clinically defined as the expected ability of an elderly patient to maintain both their physical and cognitive health. ERA are typically based on both a physical activity level and cognitive function in the preoperative state to help better define goals of potential surgery and help the patient to better understand their expected recovery course and final outcome following any planned intervention. Much research has gone into helping predict which aging patients will have a positive outcome versus those who have a poor outcome. A positive ERA does seem to be one of the most important factors in patients with a good outcome. Of the many factors used in determining ERA, physical activity level remains among the highest impact variables. Patients with a higher preoperative activity level tend to have a higher ERA, which in turn predicts a better outcome.

Furthermore, substantial literature suggests that a higher level of physical activity when examined as an independent variable correlates with a significantly decreased rate of chronic debilitating diseases such as cardiovascular disease, diabetes, cancer, hypertension, obesity, depression, and osteoporosis. The most important correlate however, is the apparent power of one's *expectations* to influence tangible metrics of physical activity, which in turn increase the odds of a successful outcome after spine surgery. For these reasons, ERA is possibly the most powerful modifiable preoperative variable when discussing spine surgery in the aging population.

As surgeons, it is our duty to educate patients on all of the potential treatment options and utilize a shared decision-making process tailored to our patients' goals. When discussing spinal surgery with an aging patient, this becomes even more important. Additionally, as part of the education process, determining an older adult patient's expectations as they relate to aging (ERA) is vital. Gauging ERA as a global sense of "positive vs. negative" gives the surgeon the ability to more accurately educate the patient on the relative odds of having a successful outcome. Simply put, patients with a negative ERA, regardless of the spinal pathology or proposed procedure, will have a harder time obtaining a positive outcome and vice versa. However, ERA is a "modifiable" variable, meaning that it is not always necessary to refuse offering surgery to those with a negative ERA. Surgeons can educate their patients about modifying their expectations, encouraging physical activity and a positive cognitive outlook to improve one's ERA. This, in conjunction with a thorough medical preoperative evaluation and optimization, provides the best possible chance for a successful outcome following spine surgery in the older adult population.

4.6 Tailor Surgery to the Patient

As with any patient with spinal pathology, a tailored surgical approach (once surgery has been decided upon via a shared decision-making process) is vital to a successful outcome. In older adults, several factors may be influenced not only by the age of the patient, but also by their "physiological age," functional capacity, and ERA (as discussed previously). Physiological age refers to a patient's overall health status and physical activity level. For instance, an 85-year-old who plays tennis 5 days a week at a competitive level may be viewed more as a 65-year-old for treatment purposes. Whereas a 65-year-old with multiple comorbidities with a sedentary lifestyle and a negative ERA may be viewed more as a physiological 85-year-old. The importance of this delineation in addition to a patient's current and expected functional capacity and goals often influences surgical treatment strategy.

The evaluation of an older adult with spinal pathology first starts with a detailed history and physical. Determining exactly where a patient's pain lies is integral. Is the pain consistent with neurogenic claudication, a unilateral specific dermatomal radiculopathy, low back pain from sagittal imbalance, or mechanical axial low back pain, or any combination of the aforementioned? The secondary goal of interviewing the aging patient with these chief complaints is determining their level of physical activity and level of impairment from what ails them. After making these assessments, the surgeon should critically evaluate the imaging studies. This is where the mindset of the surgeon must shift when treating an elderly patient with spine disease. The goal in this demographic is often to do the most minimally invasive procedure that will address the greatest percentage of their pain in the least invasive way possible in the particular surgeon's hands.

A few common pathologies in this cohort that are frequently over-treated by spine surgeons are degenerative spondylolistheses and perceived positive sagittal balance due to lumbar stenosis. Recent literature supports decompression alone in patients with low-grade spondylolisthesis. While the discussion remains very polarized amongst surgeons, there is certainly a duty to discuss this option with older adults with a low-grade spondylolisthesis. The discussion should not be too dissimilar to that had with younger patients: there is a chance the slip may progress, and additional surgery may be required if this happens. However, for older adults with a high degree of spondylosis and less dynamic instability, this risk may be more nominal.

Additionally, many older adults with moderate to severe central, lateral recess, and foraminal stenosis will compensate with relative loss of lumbar lordosis and a forward flexed posture to relieve neural compression. This may manifest as an apparent sagittal imbalance and fool the surgeon into offering a deformity correction when the patient may in fact only require a decompression to address their disease. This is where (transforaminal) epidural steroid injections (ESI) become paramount in distinguishing pathology. The senior surgeon's preferred algorithm to distinguish whether a patient's low back pain is a product of compensatory forward flexion to relieve compression due to stenosis versus a true flexible deformity that has resulted in pathologic positive sagittal imbalance is to inject the most compressive levels and follow the patient for improvement in symptoms. If the patient reports even short-term relief in their low back pain after injection, it is likely that they will benefit from a decompressive procedure alone. Conversely, if the injections do not help the symptoms, further discussion regarding a larger deformity correction may ensue. However, these discussions must be tailored to the patient's overall health status and ERA, and the culmination of these discussions may not always end in the offering of such a corrective procedure.

The same outlook must be taken with older adults with a degenerative scoliosis. Often, global coronal and sagittal balance is maintained. The treating surgeon must scrutinize radiographs within the context of the patient's overall health status, functional capacity, and ERA as previously discussed. A slightly positive sagittal balance is often acceptable in this cohort of patients, and when correction is indicated, it is almost never advised to correct to zero, as literature suggests this may predispose for proximal junctional kyphosis. Scrutiny of the posterior-anterior radiograph is critical to assess for rotatory subluxation and lateral subluxation that is often not apparent in the sagittal films. These pathologies are often the culprits for unilateral radicular symptoms, which may be present on the side of slip (compressive radiculopathy) or the contralateral side (tension radiculopathy). Additionally, the fractional curve, frequently at L4–5 or L5–S1, is another often radiographically subtle finding that may be the true pain generator. Again, targeted ESI is helpful to tease out the source of a patient's pain. When confirmed, a limited focal decompression/fusion is often successful, despite a multilevel degenerative scoliosis.

4.7 Conclusion

Surgical decision-making in aging patients can be difficult, but with appropriate recognition and modification of comorbidities, surgery can be considered. If comorbidities exist that cannot be modified, careful education of the patient and family of potential risks should be discussed. When possible, the least invasive operative intervention to treat the patient's dominate symptoms and restore function should be offered. Surgical options and outcomes should be discussed with the patient and, if needed, the patient's social support to provide enough information for shared decision-making to occur between the patient and the surgeon. Critically, every effort should be made to match the expectations of surgical outcome of the patient and the surgeon.

Key References

[1] Deyo RA, Mirza SK, Martin BI, Kreuter W, Goodman DC, Jarvik JG. Trends, major medical complications, and charges associated with surgery for lumbar spinal stenosis in older adults. JAMA. 2010; 303(13):1259–1265

[2] Kim S, Brooks AK, Groban L. Preoperative assessment of the older surgical patient: honing in on geriatric syndromes. Clin Interv Aging. 2014; 10:13–27

[3] Sobottke R, Aghayev E, Röder C, Eysel P, Delank SK, Zweig T. Predictors of surgical, general and follow-up complications in lumbar spinal stenosis relative to patient age as emerged from the Spine Tango Registry. Eur Spine J. 2012; 21(3):411–417

[4] Wang MC, Chan L, Maiman DJ, Kreuter W, Deyo RA. Complications and mortality associated with cervical spine surgery for degenerative disease in the United States. Spine. 2007; 32(3):342–347

[5] Madhavan K, Chieng LO, Foong H, Wang MY. Surgical outcomes of elderly patients with cervical spondylotic myelopathy: a meta-analysis of studies reporting on 2868 patients. Neurosurg Focus. 2016; 40(6):E13

References

[1] O'Lynnger TM, Zuckerman SL, Morone PJ, Dewan MC, Vasquez-Castellanos RA, Cheng JS. Trends for spine surgery for the elderly: implications for access to healthcare in North America. Neurosurgery. 2015; 77 Suppl 4:S136–S141

[2] Baird EO, Egorova NN, McAnany SJ, Qureshi SA, Hecht AC, Cho SK. National trends in outpatient surgical treatment of degenerative cervical spine disease. Global Spine J. 2014; 4(3):143–150

[3] Ciol MA, Deyo RA, Howell E, Kreif S. An assessment of surgery for spinal stenosis: time trends, geographic variations, complications, and reoperations. J Am Geriatr Soc. 1996; 44(3):285–290

[4] Deyo RA, Mirza SK, Martin BI, Kreuter W, Goodman DC, Jarvik JG. Trends, major medical complications, and charges associated with surgery for lumbar spinal stenosis in older adults. JAMA. 2010; 303(13):1259–1265

[5] Galbraith JG, Butler JS, Dolan AM, O'Byrne JM. Operative outcomes for cervical myelopathy and radiculopathy. Adv Orthop. 2011; •••:2012

[6] Goldman L. Cardiac risks and complications of noncardiac surgery. Ann Intern Med. 1983; 98(4):504–513

[7] Harbrecht PJ, Garrison RN, Fry DE. Surgery in elderly patients. South Med J. 1981; 74(5):594–598

[8] Holly LT, Moftakhar P, Khoo LT, Shamie AN, Wang JC. Surgical outcomes of elderly patients with cervical spondylotic myelopathy. Surg Neurol. 2008; 69 (3):233–240

[9] Madhavan K, Chieng LO, Foong H, Wang MY. Surgical outcomes of elderly patients with cervical spondylotic myelopathy: a meta-analysis of studies reporting on 2868 patients. Neurosurg Focus. 2016; 40(6):E13

[10] Nagashima H, Dokai T, Hashiguchi H, et al. Clinical features and surgical outcomes of cervical spondylotic myelopathy in patients aged 80 years or older: a multi-center retrospective study. Eur Spine J. 2011; 20(2): 240–246

[11] Steinmetz MP, Benzel EC. Benzel's Spine Surgery E-Book: Techniques, Complication Avoidance, and Management. Elsevier Health Sciences; 2016

[12] Ulrich NH, Kleinstück F, Woernle CM, et al. LumbSten Research Collaboration. Clinical outcome in lumbar decompression surgery for spinal canal stenosis in the aged population: a prospective Swiss multicenter cohort study. Spine. 2015; 40(6):415–422

[13] Wang MY, Green BA, Shah S, Vanni S, Levi AD. Complications associated with lumbar stenosis surgery in patients older than 75 years of age. Neurosurg Focus. 2003; 14(2):e7

[14] Veeravagu A, Connolly ID, Lamsam L, et al. Surgical outcomes of cervical spondylotic myelopathy: an analysis of a national, administrative, longitudinal database. Neurosurg Focus. 2016; 40(6):E11

[15] Wang MC, Chan L, Maiman DJ, Kreuter W, Deyo RA. Complications and mortality associated with cervical spine surgery for degenerative disease in the United States. Spine. 2007; 32(3):342–347

[16] Wang MC, Kreuter W, Wolfla CE, Maiman DJ, Deyo RA. Trends and variations in cervical spine surgery in the United States: Medicare beneficiaries, 1992 to 2005. Spine. 2009; 34(9):955–961, discussion 962–963

[17] Raffo CS, Lauerman WC. Predicting morbidity and mortality of lumbar spine arthrodesis in patients in their ninth decade. Spine. 2006; 31(1): 99–103

[18] Aslam M, Vaezi MF. Dysphagia in the elderly. Gastroenterol Hepatol (N Y). 2013; 9(12):784–795

[19] Liu F-Y, Yang D-L, Huang W-Z, et al. Risk factors for dysphagia after anterior cervical spine surgery: A meta-analysis. Medicine (Baltimore). 2017; 96(10):e6267

[20] Anderson KK, Arnold PM. Oropharyngeal Dysphagia after anterior cervical spine surgery: a review. Global Spine J. 2013; 3(4):273–286

[21] Ragab AA, Fye MA, Bohlman HH. Surgery of the lumbar spine for spinal stenosis in 118 patients 70 years of age or older. Spine. 2003; 28(4):348–353

[22] Sobottke R, Aghayev E, Röder C, Eysel P, Delank SK, Zweig T. Predictors of surgical, general and follow-up complications in lumbar spinal stenosis relative to patient age as emerged from the Spine Tango Registry. Eur Spine J. 2012; 21(3):411–417

[23] Avila MJ, Walter CM, Baaj AA. Outcomes and Complications of Minimally Invasive Surgery of the Lumbar Spine in the Elderly. Muacevic A, Adler JR, eds. Cureus. 2016;8(3):e519. doi:10.7759/cureus.519

[24] Wang MC, Shivakoti M, Sparapani RA, Guo C, Laud PW, Nattinger AB. Thirty-day readmissions after elective spine surgery for degenerative conditions among US Medicare beneficiaries. Spine J. 2012; 12(10):902–911

[25] Lee TH, Marcantonio ER, Mangione CM, et al. Derivation and prospective validation of a simple index for prediction of cardiac risk of major noncardiac surgery. Circulation. 1999; 100(10):1043–1049

[26] Thomsen K, Christensen FB, Eiskjasr SP, et al. The effect of pedicle screw instrumentation on functional outcome and fusion rates in posterolateral lumbar spine fusion: a prospective, randomized clinical study. Spine. 1997; 22:2813–2822

[27] Leven DM, Lee NJ, Kothari P, et al. Frailty index is a significant predictor of complications and mortality after surgery for adult spinal deformity. Spine. 2016; 41(23):E1394–E1401

[28] Flexman AM, Charest-Morin R, Stobart L, Street J, Ryerson CJ. Frailty and postoperative outcomes in patients undergoing surgery for degenerative spine disease. Spine J. 2016; 16(11):1315–1323

[29] Puvanesarajah V, Jain A, Kebaish K, et al. Poor nutrition status and lumbar spine fusion surgery in the elderly: readmissions, complications, and mortality. Spine. 2017; 42(13):979–983

[30] Evans DC, Martindale RG, Kiraly LN, Jones CM. Nutrition optimization prior to surgery. Nutr Clin Pract. 2014; 29(1):10–21

[31] Gale CR, Westbury L, Cooper C. Social isolation and loneliness as risk factors for the progression of frailty: the English Longitudinal Study of Ageing. Age Ageing. 2017

[32] Kim S, Brooks AK, Groban L. Preoperative assessment of the older surgical patient: honing in on geriatric syndromes. Clin Interv Aging. 2014; 10:13–27

5 Perioperative Optimization in the Aging Population

Ade Olasunkanmi

Abstract

The aging patient is more likely to have a higher burden of comorbidities/multiorgan system disease, thereby presenting a unique challenge in achieving balance with therapies and intervention while maintaining functional independence. As a result, there is growing utilization of health care resources by this segment of the population, challenging the health care delivery system. While there is a higher morbidity in elderly patients, there is no proven significant difference in postoperative mortality or long-term survival between the aging patient and the other surgical groups. Important are new approaches to management, such as comprehensive preoperative assessment and optimization. This allows for maintenance of functional status (less likelihood of loss of functional independence), quality of life (less time in the hospital), and reduction of medical and surgical complications in older adults.[2]

Keywords: Aging population, perioperative optimization, complications, spine surgery, enhanced recovery

Key Points

- Surgery can be safely performed in the aging patient
- Comprehensive preoperative assessment is important for morbidity and mortality counseling
- Frailty does not equal age, although it is common with aging
- There are no strict criteria for withholding surgery in the aging patient
- Modifiable risk factors can be anticipated and managed perioperatively to decrease perioperative complications

5.1 Background

People over 65 years of age are the fastest growing segment of the population due to increased life expectancy and decreased birth rates1, and there is a corresponding increase in the number of surgical procedures in this population of adults.[2,3,4] Older adults comprise over 40% of all surgical patients in the United States and account for a large proportion of health care costs.[5] Despite advances in surgical, anesthetic and medical management, the effects of aging places the older adult at risk of adverse postoperative outcomes[6] and prolonged recovery.[3] The high prevalence of comorbidities and decreased physiologic reserve have been implicated in poor postoperative outcomes. As a result, healthcare for older adults is a prominent concern as the aging population grows in number and complexity. Aging is associated with overall decline in reserves, making it more difficult to recover from a major stress. A poor functional recovery following a successful surgery may be even more devastating to an older patient. The propensity toward complications in the aging surgical population, coupled with the continued growth of the aging population requiring surgery has led to

greater attention to perioperative identification of pre-existing comorbidities and other risk factors.[1,5]

The aging patient is more likely to have a higher burden of comorbidities/multiorgan system disease, thereby presenting a unique challenge in achieving balance with therapies and intervention while maintaining functional independence.[1] Age bias is still evident in clinical practice because of the presumed higher mortality and morbidity rates associated with the older adult. However, several studies have suggested that medical comorbidities, which are more prevalent with age, are primarily responsible for the observed perioperative complications seen in this population. In addition, while there is a higher morbidity in aging patients, there is no proven significant difference in postoperative mortality or long-term survival between the population and the other surgical groups.[1,7,8,9,10,11] Emerging data increasingly suggests that preoperative comprehensive assessment and optimization reduce medical and surgical complications in older adults, such as reduction in the length of hospital stay and the likelihood of a loss of functional independence.[2] The following chapter will discuss elements of the comprehensive perioperative assessment of the aging patient and provide thresholds and interventions to consider for optimization.

5.2 Frailty

Frailty is a decrease in physiological reserves, resulting in diminished resiliency, loss of adaptive capacity, and increased vulnerability to stressors.[12,13] Frailty is the consequence of age-related defects that have accumulated in different physiological systems.[14] The concept of frailty denotes gradual loss of physical and mental function as well as vitality, regardless of coexisting disease.[13] It has been identified as an independent risk factor for mortality, morbidity, and increased length of stay and discharge to institutions other than the home in different surgical populations.[6,13] The prevalence of frailty in older adults is estimated at 9.9% and the prevalence of prefrailty of 44.2%. Frailty is also more common in women compared to men and increases with age. In aging patients undergoing surgery, the prevalence of frailty is higher, at 25 to 56%.[5]

While there are competing models of frailty, its role as a predictor of postoperative adverse events following surgery is being recognized.[6,12,13] The two most accepted models of frailty are the frailty phenotype and frailty index (FI) (► Table 5.1).[6] In the frailty phenotype model, frailty is measured across a set of five criteria or domains; unintentional weight loss (> 10 pounds in the past year), self-reported exhaustion, gait speed, low physical activity level and grip strength.[6,12] A point is awarded for each criterion met by the patient and the total is computed. Patients identified as frail (3 or more points) should be considered for possible geriatric consult for further assessment and identification of needed interventions. The FI or deficit accumulation model is based on the number of accumulated deficits a patient accrues across a number of different domains: current illnesses/comorbidities, cognitive status, emotional, motivation,

Table 5.1 Frailty measurement according to the "Fried" criteria (Adapted from Alvarez-Nebreda et. al.[12])

Characteristic of fragility	Measurement
Shrinking	> 10 pounds unintentional weight loss in last year
Weakness	Grip strength: lowest 20% By gender/BMI, using a hand dynamometer
Exhaustion	Self-report exhaustion during last week Identified by two questions from the CES-D scale
Slowness	Walking time for 15 feet: slowest 20% By gender/height
Low activity	Kcal/week: lowest 20% By gender: men < 383 kcal/week; women < 270 kcal/week, using the Minnesota Leisure Time Physical Activity Questionnaire

BMI: Body Mass Index
CES-D: Center for Epidemiological Studies- Depression scale
Scoring: ≥ 3 criteria = **positive for fragility** phenotype; 1–2 criteria = **intermediate or prefrail**

Fatigue	Are you fatigued? (yes = 1 point)
Resistance	Can you walk up one flight of stairs? (no = 1 point)
Aerobic	Can you walk more than a block? (no = 1 point)
Illnesses	Do you have more than five illnesses? (yes = 1 point)
Loss of weight	Have you lost more than 5% of your weight in the past 6 months? (yes= 1 point)

Scoring ≥ 3 points = **frail**, 1–2 points = **prefrail**, 0 points= **robust**

communication, strength, mobility, balance, elimination, nutrition, activities of daily living, sleep and social.[6,12] The index is the ratio of the number of deficits divided by the number of variables measured. The derived index can be compared to the frailty phenotype classification to determine frailty: FI < /= 0.10 is considered "non-frail", 0.1 < FI < /= 0.2 is considered "vulnerable", 0.21 < FI < /= 0.45 is frail and FI > 0.45 is "most frail".[15] While the frailty index allows for the identification of domains needing intervention during the perioperative period, the process can be very time-consuming and often requires a geriatric consult.[12]

Frailty screening should be undertaken only if it will influence the management of the patient, with the goal of preoperative risk stratification and identifying potentially modifiable factors that can be optimized prior to surgery. There are several tools that can be used for the measurement of frailty. The FRAIL scale, proposed by The Geriatric Advisory Panel of the International Academy of Nutrition and Aging,[16] is used for the screening of frailty; it is based on the frailty phenotype model and includes five features, each worth one point (described above). Other tools include the Risk Analysis Index (RAI), the Edmonton Frail Scale, the modified Frailty Index, and the Clinical Frailty Scale, all based on the FI model. The choice of tool selected for screening should take into consideration the clinical/health care setting, the demands and limitations of the institution, the composition of the multidisciplinary team, the patient population seen, and the goal of the intervention.[12]

5.3 Diabetes

Diabetes mellitus (DM) is a very common chronic disease with a long course and serious systemic implications.[17] The incidence of DM has been increasing rapidly, and it is estimated that over 29 million Americans have a confirmed diagnosis of DM.[18] There are many factors contributing to the rise of this epidemic, including a high prevalence of obesity, unhealthy diet, a sedentary lifestyle, improved or changes to diagnostic criteria, and increase in life expectancy resulting in an aging population.[17] Diabetes is a significant risk factor for complications following surgery, including pneumonia, surgical site infection, 30-day postoperative mortality and morbidity, cardiovascular adverse events, delayed discharge, and hospital readmission.[17,18,19,20] The long-term mortality and high incidence of surgical site infections and cardiovascular complications in the diabetic population represent an increasing medical and socioeconomic burden on the health delivery system and society.[21] The poorer outcomes observed in patients with DM are partly due to the higher rates of comorbidities, such as silent ischemic heart disease, renal impairment, and hypertension.[19] The risk of mortality in diabetic patients is related to the length of time the patient has had DM, optimal glycemic control at the time of hospital admission, and the glycosylated hemoglobin (HbA1c). The presence of poorly controlled diabetes and elevated levels of HbA1c have been implicated in the risk of worse perioperative outcomes.[22] The negative consequence of poor glycemic control is due to the production of advanced glycation end products (AGEs), which results from glycosylation of proteins. Higher levels of AGEs have been linked to development of both fatal and nonfatal cardiovascular disease from rapidly progressive atherosclerosis, resulting from accumulation of glycosylated proteins in the vessel walls. Dysglycemia, encompassing hypoglycemia, hyperglycemia, stress-induced hyperglycemia, and excessive glucose variability (all of which can be associated with poorly controlled blood glucose) has been associated with even poorer postoperative outcomes.[19] Several studies have linked poor glycemic control to impaired function of lymphocytes, decreased phagocytosis, impaired bacterial killing, and impaired chemotaxis, leading to the observed increased risk of postoperative surgical site infection seen in diabetics.[22] Furthermore, surgery and anesthetics have profound effects on glucose level and in the setting of pre-existing poorly controlled diabetes can lead to postoperative complications. Surgery and anesthetics lead to the release of a host of hormones, such as glucagon, growth hormone, adrenaline and noradrenaline. The combination of cytokine release and increased counter-regulatory hormones raises glucose levels and increases insulin resistance. This combination can lead to dangerous and significant hyperglycemia in diabetic patients with poorly controlled glucose, contributing to poor postoperative outcomes.[19]

Long-term glycemic control is monitored using HbA1c. HbA1c reflects an individual's mean blood glucose level over the previous 2 to 3 months and represents the amount of glucose that sticks to the red blood cells. The International Expert Committee Report recommends glycemic control with a goal of HbA1c < 7.0%, and this has been associated with reduced micro- and macrovascular risk. However, it is very difficult to apply the same goal to a broad group of patients.[22] In the 2008 study by

Walid et. al[17], HbA1c greater than 6.1% was associated with increased length of stay and overall cost, from health care resource utilization perspective, among patients undergoing anterior cervical discectomy and fusion and lumbar decompression and fusion. Hikata et. al[23] evaluated postoperative surgical site infection in diabetic patients following posterior thoracolumbar surgery and reported increased or high risk, with HbA1c > 7.0%. They recommended lowering HbA1c to < 7.0% prior to surgery to decrease the risk of postoperative surgical site infection. However, the study was insufficiently powered to support the conclusion. A subsequent study by Canciennne et. al[24] looked at 5,000 patients undergoing single-level lumbar decompression with the goal of identifying the HbA1c threshold level above which the postoperative risk of infection increased significantly. Patients were divided into groups based on their HbA1c level by increments of 0.5 mg/dL. The risk of deep postoperative surgical site infection increased with increase in perioperative HbA1c level. Using a receiver operating characteristic (ROC) curve and multivariate analyses, it determined that perioperative HbA1c above 7.5 mg/dL could serve as the threshold correlating with significantly increased risk of surgical site infection following surgery, with odds ratio 2.9, compared to patients with HbA1c < 7.5 mg/dL (95% CI, $p < 0.0001$).[8]

5.4 Osteoporosis

Osteoporosis presents a unique challenge because it may be associated with fusion failure, iatrogenic instability and fracture following surgery. It is more common with advancing age due to progressive bone loss throughout the adult life. The prevalence of osteoporosis is expected to increase with increasing life expectancy.[25] Older adults are rarely assessed and treated for osteoporosis and low bone mineral density (BMD) despite the high prevalence of this chronic disease and the serious consequences.[26,27] Osteoporosis leads to reduced bone mass and deterioration in the bone microarchitecture, predisposing older adults to fragility fractures and debilitating spinal deformities.[27] The yearly incidence of osteoporotic fractures in the United States exceeds that of new-onset diabetes, coronary artery disease, stroke, heart failure, and breast cancer.[26] Fractures among older adults have been linked to greater mortality, increased requirement for long-term care and significant deterioration in quality of life. Given the high prevalence of osteoporosis in older adults, the clinical problem it presents and the significant impact it has on the quality of life and mortality, it is essential to identify osteoporosis (or osteopenia) prior to elective surgery and to initiate treatment to reduce the risk of postoperative complications and to ensure successful surgical outcome.[26,27] According to the World Health Organization (WHO), all perimenopausal and postmenopausal women as well as patients with known metabolic bone disease or a high number of risk factors should undergo BMD screening with dual-energy X-ray absorptiometry (DEXA) and metabolic laboratory evaluation.[27] The FRAX fracture-risk assessment tool, developed by the WHO, can help identify patients who would benefit from therapy despite not being classified as having osteoporosis.[27,28] FRAX weighs the influence of several risk factors to quantify fracture risk. Measurement of Hounsfield units (HU) on CT of the lumbar spine has been shown to correlate with BMD and can therefore be used as a screening and diagnostic tool for osteoporosis.[29] Using the neck of the femur for the measurement of HU is more reliable than using a degenerative segment in the lumbar spine, which could yield a false negative measurement. Identification or recognition of osteoporosis or risk factors is important so that appropriate referral for preventative strategies can be undertaken. Medical therapy can include pharmacologic agents such as antiresorptive agents that reduce bone loss or anabolic agents that increase bone formation. FDA approved antiresorptive agents include bisphosphonate (alendronate, risedronate, ibandronate and zoledronic acid), calcitonin, and raloxifene. Teriparatide is the only anabolic agent that is FDA approved for the treatment of osteoporosis. It is effective in treating vertebral fractures and is well tolerated. Ohtori et. al[30] in 2013 compared teriparatide and bisphosphonate for treatment of osteoporosis in postmenopausal women undergoing spinal fusion and reported both faster and greater rates of fusion in the teriparatide group. Inoue et. al[31] reported increase in the insertional torque of pedicle screws during spinal fusion with at least 1 month of treatment prior to surgery. Ohtori et al(2015)[32] reported a more effective bony fusion with more than 6 months of treatment with teriparatide, compared to shorter duration of teriparatide or treatment with bisphosphonate.

5.5 Cardiovascular

Cardiovascular disease in older Americans represents a huge burden in terms of health care costs, functional decline, functional disability and morbidity and mortality.[33] High-risk surgical procedures in patients with active cardiac conditions, who have poor exercise tolerance, are associated with very poor perioperative outcomes. It is therefore critical to identify pre-existing cardiac disease, and if present, have it evaluated and treated prior to nonemergent noncardiac procedures.[25]

Perioperative mortality and morbidity from coronary artery disease are common complications following noncardiac surgery, especially in the aging patient. The incidence of cardiac morbidity after surgery depends on the definition and ranges used to measure the morbidity; this can range from elevated cardiac biomarkers (e.g., troponin) to more serious complications such as myocardial infarction, cardiac arrest/serious arrhythmias, and acute heart failure.[34,35] Devereaux et. al[36] reported a 1.9% 30-day mortality in a cohort of patients >= 50 years of age who underwent noncardiac surgery and had elevated troponin levels. In addition to the mortality risk, postoperative cardiac complications lead to prolonged hospital stay, increase in illness burden, and reduction in long-term survival.[34] Age is an important consideration in the risk of major adverse cardiac event after a noncardiac surgery, due to the growing prevalence of cardiovascular disease in adults age 55 or older.[33,37]

The American College of Cardiology/American Heart Association (ACC/AHA) Practice Guidelines[38] recommend the use of a validated risk-prediction tool to predict the risk of perioperative major adverse cardiac event in patients undergoing nonemergent noncardiac surgery. Risk assessment of patients should include integration of clinical risk factors, functional capacity assessment, and the type of surgery. More complex patients may need a formal detailed assessment by a cardiologist or hospitalist.[34] The American Society of Anaesthesiologists (ASA) and the American College of Surgeons National Surgical Quality Improvement Program (ACS-NSQIP) Surgical Risk Calculator (described below) are useful tools for preoperative assessment and risk stratification. The Revised Cardiac Risk Index (RCRI) is a simple, validated and accepted multivariate predictive tool for assessing perioperative risk of major cardiac complications, such as myocardial infarction, pulmonary edema, ventricular fibrillation, or primary cardiac arrest or complete heart block.[34,38] Each of the clinical variables contributes 1 point, with scores of 0, 1, 2 and >= 3 points, corresponding to estimated risks of major cardiac complications of 0.4%, 0.9%, 7%, and 11%, respectively. An RCRI score of 0 implies the patient is low risk, a score of 1 or 2 suggests intermediate risk, and high-risk patients have a score of 3 or higher. The RCRI discriminates well between high- and low-risk patients, but it does not account for age or hypertension, both of which are important factors in perioperative risk assessment.[34] Exercise tolerance or functional status is another important factor that can be an important predictor of perioperative outcome. Poor or low exercise tolerance is associated with poor perioperative outcomes.[25,39] Older adults with poor exercise intolerance have been shown to have more cardiovascular and pulmonary complications.[39] A useful tool for assessing exercise tolerance is the Duke Activity Status Index (DASI). It is a structured questionnaire that grades exercise ability on the basis of questions that are related to exercise equivalences.[25] The 12-item scale was developed to correlate with peak oxygen uptake, and the response to each question in the questionnaire is weighted, with higher scores indicating higher functional status (Max score 58.2).[40] The ACC/AHA guidelines recommend using the metabolic equivalent of task (MET), which is a derivative of the DASI questionnaire, with 4 METs given as the cut-off value for acceptable functional capacity (▶ Table 5.2).[25,38]

Table 5.2 Metabolic Equivalent of Task (MET) (Adapted from Fleisher LA et. al[38])

Physical activity

Light intensity activities (< 3 METs)

Sleeping

Watching television

Writing, desk work, typing

Walking, level ground, strolling, very slow

Moderate intensity activities (3–6 METs)

Bicycling, stationary, very light effort

Walking, briskly

Mowing lawn

Sexual activity

Vigorous intensity activities (> 6 METs)

Jogging (6 mph), hiking

Soccer, basketball game

Running, in place

Rope jumping

Swimming

5.6 Pulmonary

Postoperative pulmonary complications due to pulmonary disease, such as obstructive sleep apnea (OSA) and chronic obstructive pulmonary disease (COPD), are increasingly being recognized as important causes of medical morbidity and mortality. Both OSA and COPD are independent risk factors for major cardiopulmonary events that can complicate functional capacity. The reported incidence of postoperative pulmonary complications varies widely in the literature, from 2% to 19%, and approximately 10% to 30% of patients who undergo general anesthesia experience postoperative pulmonary event, ranging from minor to major complications. In addition, up to 90% of patients experience some degree of atelectasis during anesthesia due to positioning and loss of functional residual capacity.[41] OSA is a common chronic condition characterized by frequent episodes of upper airway collapse during sleep. It can lead to derangements in gas exchange and can affect nocturnal sleep quality and lead to daytime fatigue. OSA is being recognized as an independent risk factor for the development of systemic hypertension, cardiovascular disease, stroke and abnormal glucose metabolism.[42,43] The prevalence of OSA is estimated at between 3% to 7%, variably affecting the population with some subgroups at higher risk. Age (>= 60), among several other factors, increase the vulnerability for the disorder and postoperative pulmonary complication.[41] The majority of people affected remain undiagnosed, despite the increasingly apparent clinical consequences.[42] OSA and COPD are primarily diseases of middle- and older aged adults, who are the most likely to require surgical procedures. Due to the potentially serious complications associated with untreated OSA, it is important to screen for and recognize the disorder and plan appropriate therapy prior to nonemergent/elective surgery to reduce postoperative cardiorespiratory events, which can be twice as common in this population.[34] Smoking cessation and pulmonary rehabilitation are important preoperative strategies that can help improve both short- and long-term outcomes.[41]

A number of screening tests have been developed to identify high risk patients, but the STOP and STOP-Bang questionnaires are convenient and easy to use and can be helpful in this regard. These questionnaires are acronyms: the **s**noring, **t**iredness, **o**bserved apnea, high B**P** (STOP) and **s**noring, **t**iredness, **o**bserved apnea, high B**P**-**B**MI, **a**ge, **n**eck circumference and **g**ender (STOP-Bang) are concise, user-friendly screening tools for OSA that can be used in the outpatient setting.[41,43] The STOP questionnaire has moderate sensitivity (65.6%) and specificity (60%) in detecting OSA. It has a higher sensitivity but lower specificity in detecting moderate and severe OSA (74% and 53%; 80% and 49%, respectively).[43] Because of the relative ease of use, efficiency and high sensitivity, the STOP-Bang questionnaire is currently widely used and has been well validated. It has additional four questions (body mass index – BMI > 35, age > 50, neck circumference > 40 cm, gender = male) in addition to the STOP questions. Each question counts for one point with a "yes" response, for a possible total score of 8 points. The STOP-Bang questionnaire has very high sensitivity (100% for detecting severe OSA and 93% for moderate OSA).[41,43] Patients with a score of 0 to 2 on the questionnaire are considered to be at low risk of OSA. Several studies have shown that patients identified as being at high risk of OSA have higher rates of postoperative complications, such as unplanned reintubation and myocardial infarction.[43] Patients at high risk for OSA on the STOP or STOP-Bang questionnaire should be considered for further evaluation for OSA and interventions such as CPAP prior to proceeding with elective surgical interventions.

5.7 Kidney Disease

Kidney disease is a spectrum of diseases, including acute kidney disease (AKI, chronic kidney disease (CKD) and end-stage renal disease (ESRD), and is a chronic and progressive process with far-ranging consequences on postoperative outcome.[44,45] CKD is a public health problem, with a rising incidence and prevalence of kidney failure.[46] The U.S. Renal Data System estimates that a patient with CKD is 3 times more likely to be hospitalized.[44] The life expectancy of patients with kidney disease has been increasing, with an increasing number undergoing spine surgery[47] and there has been several studies evaluating the impact of the disease on the postoperative outcome. Patients with CKD have higher rates of myocardial infarction, pneumonia, bleeding, septicemia, morbidity, and mortality[44,45,48] as well as a higher rate of 30-day readmission.[49,50] Also, CKD is important to the spine surgeon because of the osseous manifestations of severe renal dysfunction, such as bone loss, anemia, hypertension, and atherosclerotic disease.[44,46] In addition, CKD patients have poorer quality of life, with a higher burden of pre-existing comorbidities, including diabetes, hypertension, dyslipidemia, bone loss, neuropathy cardiovascular disease, and poor quality of life.[44] The goal of preoperative evaluation is to reduce the morbidity and mortality in renal disease patients undergoing surgery. Renal function is assessed by the glomerular filtration rate (GFR) or serum creatinine levels, and several studies have shown an increase in 30-day complications as the GFR decreases below 80 ml/min/1.73 m². Consistent with the recommendation from the National Kidney Foundation, Purvis et. al[46] noted an estimated GFR of 60 ml/min/1.73 m² to be the threshold value of a significant increase in morbidity. Serum creatinine levels can also be used as a complimentary test to assess preoperative kidney function and predict perioperative complications.[46] A creatinine level of greater than 1 ml/dL has been identified as an independent risk factor for postoperative myocardial infarction,[51] while levels greater than 2.0 mg/dL are associated with development of deep venous thrombosis.[52] Although preoperative kidney disease cannot be alleviated prior to surgery, understanding the increased postoperative complication risks and increased morbidity and mortality can inform the surgeon's conversation with the patient.[46] Importantly, in order to decrease the postoperative complications, intraoperative and postoperative management strategies can be developed to manage fluid status/fluid shifts and blood pressure.[44,45,46]

5.8 Nutrition

Nutritional deficiency in older adults can be due to a decrease in appetite, nutritional intake, and/or decreased gut absorption.[53] Malnutrition leads to lower immune response. Muscle atrophy and decreased wound healing then occurs[54]; therefore, optimization of nutritional status in older adults undergoing surgery is important to decrease complications and improve surgical outcomes.[53] Poor nutritional status has an adverse effect on postoperative outcome and is very prevalent with many disease processes as well as other comorbidities. It is an independent risk factor for postoperative complications and increased hospital stay and cost.[53,55] Elective spine surgery is risky in the older adult, given the overall burden of comorbid diseases, and the presence of nutritional deficiency/malnutrition greatly increases overall adverse outcomes. Patients should be screened with adequate history of weight loss/weight gain, muscle gain or loss, oral intake, and BMI, as well as for chronic or acute disease states.[53]

Various scoring and assessment tools exist for screening for nutritional deficiency. The Mini Nutritional Assessment (MNA) tool is the most widely used validated tool for nutritional screening and assessment because of how easy it is to use and its feasibility in a clinical setting.[56] The MNA has four parts: anthropometric measurements, general status, diet information, and subjective assessment, with a maximum score of 30 points. A score of < 17 points is regarded as an indication of malnutrition, 17 to 23.5 points indicate a risk for malnutrition, and a score > 23.5 points indicates that the patient is well nourished.[56] Albumin could be used to determine a patient's nutritional health status prior to surgery, and the role of prealbumin is still being evaluated as a predictor of surgical outcome. Normal values of prealbumin are in the range 16 to 40 mg/dL, and values less than 16 mg/dL are considered to indicate malnutrition.[53] Laboratory tests, such as a lymphocyte count, serum albumin, and prealbumin could offer a high predictive value when combined with a nutrition screening tool such as the MNA. A total lymphocyte count of less than 1,500 cells/mm³, transferring levels less than 200 mg/dL, body mass index (BMI) less than 18.5 Kg/m², and albumin levels less than 3.5 g/dL are all indicators of malnutrition.[53,57]

In malnourished patients, a referral to a nutritionist prior to proceeding with elective surgery should be considered. Various Enhanced Recovery After Surgery (ERAS) pathways have also proposed several steps aimed at reducing postoperative complications related to malnutrition, including permitting solid intake up to 6 hours before surgery and clear intake up to 2 hours before surgery; oral carbohydrate loading to reduce the body's catabolic effect from the stress response to surgery; early postoperative nutrition/feeding; and optimizing social circumstances.[53,55,58]

5.9 Body Mass Index (BMI)

The worldwide population is gaining weight. This trend is expected to grow, with four out of 10 adults already classified as overweight or obese in 2013.[59] Obesity is particularly prevalent in the United States, with 31.7% of adult men and 33.9% of adult women classified as obese. It is an independent risk factor for comorbidities such as hypertension, diabetes and cardiovascular disease, as well as a contributor to the development of low back pain and increased rates of degenerative spine pathologies.[60] Complications correlated to obesity include longer incision, increased blood loss, increased surgery duration, SSI, and venous/pulmonary thromboembolisms.[59,61,62,63] Adult spinal deformity is very common, and the incidence increases with age, with reported prevalence of up to 68% in patients over the age of 65 years. Surgery for the treatment of adult spinal deformity to relieve pain and disability is complicated by the high rates of postoperative complications due to several factors, including obesity.[59,60,61] Several studies have investigated the role of obesity on postoperative complications following surgery with varying findings, partly due to the discrepancy in inclusion criteria, type of procedure and the obesity threshold used.[59,61] Primarily, the disparities arise from nonstratification of the patients based on obesity class.[60] The Centers for Disease Control defined obesity as BMI greater than or equal to 30 Kg/m[2].[64] Based on several studies, when all other covariates are held constant and healthy weight patients (BMI < 25 Kg/m[2]) are compared to other BMI groupings (overweight - 25–29, class 1 obese - 30–34, class 2 obese - 35–39 and class 3 obese - 40+), the BMI threshold for significantly increased risk of postoperative complications was found to be BMI > 40 Kg/m[2]. The patients with BMI > 40 Kg/m2, were found to be at significantly higher risk for longer operative time, increased blood loss, higher risk of readmission/reoperation, higher rates of SSI, and greater odds of DVT,[60,61,62,63] suggesting that this subgroup of obese patients may bear the burden of the increased medical costs and poor outcomes following surgery.[61]

5.10 Morbidity and Mortality Prediction

Aging has been traditionally assessed with chronological age, but chronological age does not offer an adequate assessment of a patient's health or functional status.[1,12] The processes of aging, or frailty,[1,2,12] which leads to a reduction in functional reserve, vary from one individual to another and affect an individual's ability to withstand the stress from an operation or anesthesia.[1] The absence of an overt evidence of organ system dysfunction in an elderly patient does not preclude reduced function or reserve. It is therefore important to assess for and manage pre-existing illnesses or dysfunction that may affect postoperative morbidity and mortality or worse functional outcome.[65,66,67] Medical conditions such as undiagnosed or poorly controlled DM, kidney disease, hypertension, cardiopulmonary disease, cerebrovascular disease, osteoporosis, smoking and poor nutrition status have all been associated with postoperative complications and worse functional outcomes.[1,66,68] Preoperative identification of these risk factors is important to reducing the incidence of perioperative complications.

Various risk modelling systems are available for assessment of complication risk in surgical patients. The American Society of Anesthesiologists (ASA) Physical Status Classification System is used by the anesthesiologists for risk stratification. The ASA score is a subjective assessment of a patient's health that is comprised of five classes, based on the presence and severity of systemic diseases.[1,69,70] The biggest drawback of the ASA system is that it is highly subjective and susceptible to inter-observer disagreement. It also has poor sensitivity to differentiating between the two largest groups, ASA II and III categories.[1] Another frequently used tool is the ACS-NSQIP Surgical Risk Calculator.[71] It was developed from a multi-institutional database of surgical procedures across all surgical specialties and draws on a model utilizing 21 preoperative factors to predict postoperative outcomes in individual patients. It estimates a patient's risk of an unfavorable outcome, such as a complication or death, following surgery. The risk, calculated using data from a large number of patients undergoing similar procedure, is estimated based on the patient's history as provided by the surgeon. Veeravagu et. al[70] found that the ACS-NSQIP consistently predicted complication rates that underestimated the actual complication occurrence. However, it does accurately predict the occurrence of an adverse event after surgery. Another assessment tool that has been well studied and validated is the Charlson Comorbidity Index (CCI).[70] It categorizes patients' comorbidities based on the International Classification of Diseases (ICD) diagnosis codes. Each comorbidity category is assigned a weight based on adjusted risk or mortality, and the sum of all the weights results in a single score for the patient. A higher score predicts a higher risk or increased resource utilization. Arrigo et. al found that the CCI is a significant predictor of 30-day complications following surgery while Whitmore et. al found the tool to be a useful but incomplete predictor of postoperative complications.[70] Another scoring or predictive tool is the Preoperative Score to Predict Postoperative Mortality (POS-POM). It incorporates objective markers such as diabetes, dialysis dependence, dementia, and heart failure to determine perioperative and postoperative risk of mortality. However, it does not include the risk of postoperative morbidity and poor postoperative quality of life or loss of independence.[72]

5.11 Social Support

Social support refers to a network of relations providing emotional and financial support and practical guidance, assistance, and advice. It is important to decrease stress and improve coping mechanisms with many different health conditions. It is critical to do so during hospitalization and is even more important following discharge from the hospital.[73] The recovery following spine surgery is a complex process, and availability of social support may be associated with positive short- and long-term recovery and surgical outcomes.[74] It is important to assess the patient's social support and need for home health prior to hospitalization and before discharge.[3] If the patient's family or social support is inadequate or insufficient, preoperative referral to a social worker for postdischarge planning should be considered.

5.12 Delirium/Dementia Assessment

There is a high prevalence of dementia and cognitive impairment without dementia in the aging population in the United States, and dementia is a known risk factor for morbidity and mortality in this population. Postoperative delirium is a very common complication following surgery in the aging population, and there is a strong correlation between preoperative cognitive impairment and postoperative delirium.[75] Postoperative delirium has been associated with death, increased length of stay, and discharge to long-term care or rehabilitation facilities. Preoperative cognitive impairment is also predictive of postoperative pulmonary complications such as atelectasis and

Table 5.3 Summary Recommendation

Domain	Assessment	Optimization strategies/recommendation
Frailty	Evaluate for indicators	Preoperative strength training; physical therapy before surgery
Diabetes	HbA1c	Delay surgery for levels > 7.5 mg/dL; endocrine consult
Cardiovascular	Cardiac evaluation; DASI; METs	Avoid surgery in patients with METs < 4; Cardiology consult
Pulmonary	Pulmonary evaluation; STOP and STOP-Bang	Pulmonology consult for OSA; consider interventions such as CPAP or BiPAP prior to surgery; Hospitalist consult as in-patient
Osteoporosis	Evaluate risk factors; BMD; FRAX	Vitamin D and calcium; consider pharmacologic agents
Kidney disease	Creatine and GFR	Preoperative optimization; risk counselling; hospitalist consult in-patient; perioperative fluid management
Nutrition	Mini Nutritional Assessment; albumin and prealbumin levels	Nutritional supplementation; dietitian/nutrition consult
Body mass index	Calculate BMI	Avoid surgery with BMI > 40 Kg/m^2; weight loss; bariatric consult
Social support	Evaluate postoperative needs	Social work referral; preoperative SNF/in-patient rehabilitation planning prior to surgery
Delirium/Dementia	Evaluate cognitive ability and capacity; Mini-Cog test	Limit sedating psychotropic medications; Geriatric consult
Mortality and Morbidity	ASA; ACS-NSQIP surgical risk calculator	Appropriate counselling and assessment of risks and benefits

a longer need for mechanical ventilation.[75] Identification is important preoperatively to mitigate these postoperative complications. The Mini-Mental State Exam is a well-validated method for assessment of cognitive function. It is a 30-point questionnaire that is useful in measuring cognitive impairment and easily administered in the clinical setting. The ACS/AGS guideline recommends the use of Mini-Cog test for preoperative assessment of cognitive impairment. The Mini-Cog assesses numerous cognitive domains, such as cognitive function, memory, language comprehension, visual-motor skills, and executive function.[76]

5.13 Applying Perioperative Assessment

The perioperative parameters described above are collected to allow the surgeon and patient to determine the risk vs. benefit of a surgical intervention. As patients age, these risk-benefit conversations should be more deliberate and take into consideration health, functional, and social factors. It is important to know that there are not many strict criteria to withhold surgery and that some of the risk factors cannot be corrected (e.g., pre-existing cardiac or renal disease) but can be anticipated and managed. However, some general guidelines should be considered. First, if a patient has a modifiable risk factor that can be corrected for an elective procedure, then delaying the procedure until the correction has been made should be strongly considered. Second, surgery should not be delayed if the delay to correct a risk factor puts the patient at more risk in the short term. Third, if the existing risk factors place the patient at more risk than the proposed benefit of the surgery, then surgery should not be performed.

5.14 Conclusion

Given the association between aging and overall decline in functional reserves, care deliberation is necessary when considering surgery in the aging patient. It is important to define goals, priorities and life expectancy as well as nonsurgical management.[1,77] While surgery can be performed safely, a comprehensive evaluation and operative risk assessment should be part of the perioperative counseling of the older adult undergoing surgery (▶ Table 5.3).

Key References

[1] Cheng S-P, Yang T-L, Jeng K-S, Lee J-J, Liu T-P, Liu C-L. Perioperative Care of the Elderly. Int J Gerontol. 2007; 1(2):89–97

[2] Alvarez-Nebreda ML, Bentov N, Urman RD, et al. Recommendations for Pre-operative Management of Frailty from the Society for Perioperative Assessment and Quality Improvement (SPAQI). J Clin Anesth. 2018; 47:33–42

[3] Ali R, Schwalb JM, Nerenz DR, Antoine HJ, Rubinfeld I. Use of the modified frailty index to predict 30-day morbidity and mortality from spine surgery. J Neurosurg Spine. 2016; 25(4):537–541

[4] Buckinx F, Rolland Y, Reginster J-Y, Ricour C, Petermans J, Bruyère O. Burden of frailty in the elderly population: perspectives for a public health challenge. Arch Public Health. 2015; 73(1):19

[5] Rollins KE, Varadhan KK, Dhatariya K, Lobo DN. Systematic review of the impact of HbA1c on outcomes following surgery in patients with diabetes mellitus. Clin Nutr. 2016; 35(2):308–316

[6] Curtis JR, Safford MM. Management of osteoporosis among the elderly with other chronic medical conditions. Drugs Aging. 2012; 29(7):549–564

[7] Yazdanyar A, Newman AB. The burden of cardiovascular disease in the elderly: morbidity, mortality, and costs. Clin Geriatr Med. 2009; 25(4):563–577, vii

[8] Epstein NE. More risks and complications for elective spine surgery in morbidly obese patients. Surg Neurol Int. 2017; 8(1):66

References

[1] Cheng S-P, Yang T-L, Jeng K-S, Lee J-J, Liu T-P, Liu C-L. Perioperative Care of the Elderly. Int J Gerontol. 2007; 1(2):89–97

[2] Wick EC, Finlayson E. Frailty-Going From Measurement to Action. JAMA Surg. 2017; 152(8):757–758

[3] Mohanty S, Rosenthal RA, Russell MM, Neuman MD, Ko CY, Esnaola NF. Optimal Perioperative Management of the Geriatric Patient: A Best Practices Guideline from the American College of Surgeons NSQIP and the American Geriatrics Society. J Am Coll Surg. 2016; 222(5):930–947

[4] Pearce L, Bunni J, McCarthy K, Hewitt J. Surgery in the older person: Training needs for the provision of multidisciplinary care. Ann R Coll Surg Engl. 2016; 98(6):367–370

[5] Amrock LG, Deiner S. Perioperative frailty. Int Anesthesiol Clin. 2014; 52(4):26–41

[6] Partridge JSL, Harari D, Dhesi JK. Frailty in the older surgical patient: a review. Age Ageing. 2012; 41(2):142–147

[7] Seymour DG, Pringle R. Post-operative complications in the elderly surgical patient. Gerontology. 1983; 29(4):262–270

[8] Vaz FG, Seymour DG. A prospective study of elderly general surgical patients: I. Pre-operative medical problems. Age Ageing. 1989; 18(5):309–315

[9] Polanczyk CA, Marcantonio E, Goldman L, et al. Impact of age on perioperative complications and length of stay in patients undergoing noncardiac surgery. Ann Intern Med. 2001; 134(8):637–643

[10] Lubin MF. Is age a risk factor for surgery? Med Clin North Am. 1993; 77(2):327–333

[11] Audisio RA, Bozzetti F, Gennari R, et al. The surgical management of elderly cancer patients; recommendations of the SIOG surgical task force. Eur J Cancer. 2004; 40(7):926–938

[12] Alvarez-Nebreda ML, Bentov N, Urman RD, et al. Recommendations for Preoperative Management of Frailty from the Society for Perioperative Assessment and Quality Improvement (SPAQI). J Clin Anesth. 2018; 47:33–42

[13] Ali R, Schwalb JM, Nerenz DR, Antoine HJ, Rubinfeld I. Use of the modified frailty index to predict 30-day morbidity and mortality from spine surgery. J Neurosurg Spine. 2016; 25(4):537–541

[14] Buckinx F, Rolland Y, Reginster J-Y, Ricour C, Petermans J, Bruyère O. Burden of frailty in the elderly population: perspectives for a public health challenge. Arch Public Health. 2015; 73(1):19

[15] Blodgett J, Theou O, Kirkland S, Andreou P, Rockwood K. Frailty in NHANES: Comparing the frailty index and phenotype. Arch Gerontol Geriatr. 2015; 60 (3):464–470

[16] Susanto M, Hubbard RE, Gardiner PA. Validity and Responsiveness of the FRAIL Scale in Middle-Aged Women. J Am Med Dir Assoc. 2018; 19(1):65–69

[17] Walid MS, Newman BF, Yelverton JC, Nutter JP, Ajjan M, Robinson JS. Prevalence of previously unknown elevation of glycosylated hemoglobin (HbA1c) in spine surgery patients and impact on length of stay and total cost. J Hosp Med. 2009; •••. DOI: 10.1002/jhm.541

[18] Boreland L, Scott-Hudson M, Hetherington K, Frussinetty A, Slyer JT. The effectiveness of tight glycemic control on decreasing surgical site infections and readmission rates in adult patients with diabetes undergoing cardiac surgery: A systematic review. Heart Lung. 2015; 44(5):430–440

[19] Akiboye F, Rayman G. Management of Hyperglycemia and Diabetes in Orthopedic Surgery. Curr Diab Rep. 2017; 17(2):13

[20] Rollins KE, Varadhan KK, Dhatariya K, Lobo DN. Systematic review of the impact of HbA1c on outcomes following surgery in patients with diabetes mellitus. Clin Nutr. 2016; 35(2):308–316

[21] Bock M, Johansson T, Fritsch G, et al. The impact of preoperative testing for blood glucose concentration and haemoglobin A1c on mortality, changes in management and complications in noncardiac elective surgery: a systematic review. Eur J Anaesthesiol. 2015; 32(3):152–159

[22] Shaw P, Saleem T, Gahtan V. Correlation of hemoglobin A1C level with surgical outcomes: Can tight perioperative glucose control reduce infection and cardiac events? Semin Vasc Surg. 2014; 27(3):156–161

[23] Hikata T, Iwanami A, Hosogane N, et al. High preoperative hemoglobin A1c is a risk factor for surgical site infection after posterior thoracic and lumbar spinal instrumentation surgery. J Orthop Sci. 2014; 19(2):223–228

[24] Cancienne JM, Werner BC, Chen DQ, Hassanzadeh H, Shimer AL. Perioperative hemoglobin A1c as a predictor of deep infection following single-level lumbar decompression in patients with diabetes. Spine J. 2017; 17(8):1100–1105

[25] Priebe H-J. Preoperative cardiac management of the patient for non-cardiac surgery: an individualized and evidence-based approach. Br J Anaesth. 2011; 107(1):83–96

[26] Curtis JR, Safford MM. Management of osteoporosis among the elderly with other chronic medical conditions. Drugs Aging. 2012; 29(7):549–564

[27] Lehman RA, Jr, Kang DG, Wagner SC. Management of osteoporosis in spine surgery. J Am Acad Orthop Surg. 2015; 23(4):253–263

[28] Unnanuntana A, Gladnick BP, Donnelly E, Lane JM. The assessment of fracture risk. J Bone Joint Surg Am. 2010; 92(3):743–753

[29] Schreiber JJ, Anderson PA, Rosas HG, Buchholz AL, Au AG. Hounsfield units for assessing bone mineral density and strength: a tool for osteoporosis management. J Bone Joint Surg Am. 2011; 93(11):1057–1063

[30] Ohtori S, Inoue G, Orita S, et al. Comparison of teriparatide and bisphosphonate treatment to reduce pedicle screw loosening after lumbar spinal fusion surgery in postmenopausal women with osteoporosis from a bone quality perspective. Spine. 2013; 38(8):E487–E492

[31] Inoue G, Ueno M, Nakazawa T, et al. Teriparatide increases the insertional torque of pedicle screws during fusion surgery in patients with postmenopausal osteoporosis. J Neurosurg Spine. 2014; 21(3):425–431

[32] Ohtori S, Orita S, Yamauchi K, et al. More than 6 Months of Teriparatide Treatment Was More Effective for Bone Union than Shorter Treatment Following Lumbar Posterolateral Fusion Surgery. Asian Spine J. 2015; 9(4):573–580

[33] Yazdanyar A, Newman AB. The burden of cardiovascular disease in the elderly: morbidity, mortality, and costs. Clin Geriatr Med. 2009; 25(4):563–577, vii

[34] Scott IA, Shohag HA, Kam PCA, Jelinek MV, Khadem GM. Preoperative cardiac evaluation and management of patients undergoing elective non-cardiac surgery. Med J Aust. 2013; 199(10):667–673

[35] Botto F, Alonso-Coello P, Chan MT, et al. Vascular events In noncardiac Surgery patIents cOhort evaluatioN (VISION) Writing Group, on behalf of The Vascular events In noncardiac Surgery patIents cOhort evaluatioN (VISION) Investigators, Appendix 1. The Vascular events In noncardiac Surgery patIents cOhort evaluatioN (VISION) Study Investigators Writing Group, Appendix 2. The Vascular events In noncardiac Surgery patIents cOhort evaluatioN Operations Committee, Vascular events In noncardiac Surgery patIents cOhort evaluatioN VISION Study Investigators. Myocardial injury after noncardiac surgery: a large, international, prospective cohort study establishing diagnostic criteria, characteristics, predictors, and 30-day outcomes. Anesthesiology. 2014; 120(3):564–578

[36] Devereaux PJ, Chan MT, Alonso-Coello P, et al. Vascular Events In Noncardiac Surgery Patients Cohort Evaluation (VISION) Study Investigators. Association between postoperative troponin levels and 30-day mortality among patients undergoing noncardiac surgery. JAMA. 2012; 307(21):2295–2304

[37] Schoenborn CA, Heyman KM. Health characteristics of adults aged 55 years and over: United States, 2004–2007. Natl Health Stat Rep. 2009(16):1–31

[38] Fleisher LA, Fleischmann KE, Auerbach AD, et al. ACC/AHA Guideline on Perioperative Cardiovascular Evaluation and Management of Patients Undergoing Noncardiac Surgery: A Report of the American College of Cardiology/American Heart Association Task Force on Practice Guidelines. Circulation. 2014; 2014:130

[39] Reilly DF, McNeely MJ, Doerner D, et al. Self-reported exercise tolerance and the risk of serious perioperative complications. Arch Intern Med. 1999; 159 (18):2185–2192

[40] Hlatky MA, Boineau RE, Higginbotham MB, et al. A brief self-administered questionnaire to determine functional capacity (the Duke Activity Status Index). Am J Cardiol. 1989; 64(10):651–654

[41] Diaz-Fuentes G, Hashmi HRT, Venkatram S. Perioperative Evaluation of Patients with Pulmonary Conditions Undergoing Non-Cardiothoracic Surgery. Health Serv Insights. 2016; 9 Suppl 1:9–23

[42] Punjabi NM. The epidemiology of adult obstructive sleep apnea. Proc Am Thorac Soc. 2008; 5(2):136–143

[43] Chung F, Abdullah HR, Liao P. STOP-Bang Questionnaire: A Practical Approach to Screen for Obstructive Sleep Apnea. Chest. 2016; 149(3):631–638

[44] Jones DR, Lee HT. Surgery in the patient with renal dysfunction. Anesthesiol Clin. 2009; 27(4):739–749

[45] Cherng Y-G, Liao C-C, Chen T-H, Xiao D, Wu C-H, Chen T-L. Are non-cardiac surgeries safe for dialysis patients? - A population-based retrospective cohort study. PLoS One. 2013; 8(3):e58942

[46] Purvis TE, Kessler RA, Boone C, Elder BD, Goodwin CR, Sciubba DM. The effect of renal dysfunction on short-term outcomes after lumbar fusion. Clin Neurol Neurosurg. 2017; 153:8–13

[47] Bains RS, Kardile M, Mitsunaga L, et al. Does chronic kidney disease affect the mortality rate in patients undergoing spine surgery? J Clin Neurosci. 2017; 43:208–213

[48] De la Garza Ramos R, Jain A, Nakhla J, et al. Postoperative Morbidity and Mortality After Elective Anterior Cervical Fusion in Patients with Chronic and End-Stage Renal Disease. World Neurosurg. 2016; 95:480–485

[49] Adogwa O, Elsamadicy AA, Sergesketter A, et al. The Impact of Chronic Kidney Disease on Postoperative Outcomes in Patients Undergoing Lumbar Decompression and Fusion. World Neurosurg. 2018; 110:e266–e270

[50] Choy W, Lam SK, Smith ZA, Dahdaleh NS. Predictors of 30-Day Hospital Readmission After Posterior Cervical Fusion in 3401 Patients. Spine. 2018; 43(5):356–363

[51] Wang TY, Martin JR, Loriaux DB, et al. Risk Assessment and Characterization of 30-Day Perioperative Myocardial Infarction Following Spine Surgery: A Retrospective Analysis of 1346 Consecutive Adult Patients. Spine. 2016; 41 (5):438–444

[52] Wang TY, Sakamoto JT, Nayar G, et al. Independent Predictors of 30-Day Perioperative Deep Vein Thrombosis in 1346 Consecutive Patients After Spine Surgery. World Neurosurg. 2015; 84(6):1605–1612

[53] Qureshi R, Rasool M, Puvanesarajah V, Hassanzadeh H. Perioperative Nutritional Optimization in Spine Surgery. Clin Spine Surg. 2018; 31(3):103–107

[54] de Souza Menezes F, Leite HP, Koch Nogueira PC. Malnutrition as an independent predictor of clinical outcome in critically ill children. Nutrition. 2012; 28(3):267–270

[55] Melnyk M, Casey RG, Black P, Koupparis AJ. Enhanced recovery after surgery (ERAS) protocols: Time to change practice? Can Urol Assoc J. 2011; 5(5):342–348

[56] Guigoz Y, Vellas B. The Mini Nutritional Assessment (MNA) for Grading the Nutritional State of Elderly Patients: Presentation of the MNA, History and Validation. Nestlé Nutrition Workshop Series: Clinical & Performance Program Mini Nutritional Assessment (MNA): Research and Practice in the Elderly. 1999:3–12. doi:10.1159/000062967

[57] Bailey KV, Ferro-Luzzi A. Use of body mass index of adults in assessing individual and community nutritional status. Bull World Health Organ. 1995; 73 (5):673–680

[58] Nelson G, Altman AD, Nick A, et al. Guidelines for pre- and intra-operative care in gynecologic/oncology surgery: Enhanced Recovery After Surgery (ERAS®) Society recommendations–Part I. Gynecol Oncol. 2016; 140(2):313–322

[59] Soroceanu A, Burton DC, Diebo BG, et al. International Spine Study Group. Impact of obesity on complications, infection, and patient-reported outcomes in adult spinal deformity surgery. J Neurosurg Spine. 2015; 23(5):656–664

[60] Bono OJ, Poorman GW, Foster N, et al. Body mass index predicts risk of complications in lumbar spine surgery based on surgical invasiveness. Spine J. 2018; 18(7):1204–1210

[61] Flippin M, Harris J, Paxton EW, et al. Effect of body mass index on patient outcomes of surgical intervention for the lumbar spine. J Spine Surg. 2017; 3(3):349–357

[62] Seicean A, Alan N, Seicean S, et al. Impact of increased body mass index on outcomes of elective spinal surgery. Spine. 2014; 39(18):1520–1530

[63] Epstein NE. More risks and complications for elective spine surgery in morbidly obese patients. Surg Neurol Int. 2017; 8(1):66

[64] Defining Adult Overweight and Obesity. Centers for Disease Control and Prevention. https://www.cdc.gov/obesity/adult/defining.html. Published June 16, 2016. Accessed July 27, 2018

[65] Prough DS. Anesthetic pitfalls in the elderly patient. J Am Coll Surg. 2005; 200(5):784–794

[66] Wang L, van Belle G, Kukull WB, Larson EB. Predictors of functional change: a longitudinal study of nondemented people aged 65 and older. J Am Geriatr Soc. 2002; 50(9):1525–1534

[67] Reuben DB, Rubenstein LV, Hirsch SH, Hays RD. Value of functional status as a predictor of mortality: results of a prospective study. Am J Med. 1992; 93(6):663–669

[68] Rosenthal RA. Nutritional concerns in the older surgical patient. J Am Coll Surg. 2004; 199(5):785–791

[69] Whitmore RG, Stephen JH, Vernick C, et al. ASA grade and Charlson Comorbidity Index of spinal surgery patients: correlation with complications and societal costs. Spine J. 2014; 14(1):31–38

[70] Veeravagu A, Li A, Swinney C, et al. Predicting complication risk in spine surgery: a prospective analysis of a novel risk assessment tool. J Neurosurg Spine. 2017; 27(1):81–91

[71] ACS Risk Calculator - Home Page. https://riskcalculator.facs.org/RiskCalculator/. Accessed July 19, 2018

[72] Mistry PK, Gaunay GS, Hoenig DM. Prediction of surgical complications in the elderly: Can we improve outcomes? Asian J Urol. 2017; 4(1):44–49

[73] Laxton AW, Perrin RG. The relations between social support, life stress, and quality of life following spinal decompression surgery. Spinal Cord. 2003; 41 (10):553–558

[74] Adogwa O, Elsamadicy AA, Vuong VD, et al. Effect of Social Support and Marital Status on Perceived Surgical Effectiveness and 30-Day Hospital Readmission. Global Spine J. 2017; 7(8):774–779

[75] Kim S, Brooks AK, Groban L. Preoperative assessment of the older surgical patient: honing in on geriatric syndromes. Clin Interv Aging. 2014; 10:13–27

[76] Chow WB, Rosenthal RA, Merkow RP, Ko CY, Esnaola NF, American College of Surgeons National Surgical Quality Improvement Program, American Geriatrics Society. Optimal preoperative assessment of the geriatric surgical patient: a best practices guideline from the American College of Surgeons National Surgical Quality Improvement Program and the American Geriatrics Society. J Am Coll Surg. 2012; 215(4):453–466

[77] Oresanya LB, Lyons WL, Finlayson E. Preoperative assessment of the older patient: a narrative review. JAMA. 2014; 311(20):2110–2120

6 Value-Based Care in the Aging Spine

Paul Page, Daniel Burkett, Clayton L. Haldeman, and Daniel K. Resnick

Abstract

Treatment of spinal disorders in a fiscally responsible manner is becoming increasingly important as the cost of healthcare is more closely scrutinized. As healthcare reform continues to shift toward a value-based approach, an objective framework must be utilized when considering whether the cost of an intervention is worth the potential benefit for the patient. In order to quantify the overall value of interventions objectively, a variety of methods have been introduced, including the cost per quality-adjusted life years, minimal clinically important difference, and substantial clinical benefit. In addition to these methods, numerous health-related quality of life surveys have also been developed to identify and objectively track the clinical progress and outcomes of patients in a more focused and clinically relevant fashion. This chapter provides an overview of strategies to evaluate patient-specific treatment value, focusing on treatment decision-making for the older adult spine patient.

Keywords: Value, aging spine, minimal clinically important difference, quality adjusted life years

Key Points

- As the average life expectancy in the United States continues to increase, the need for cost-efficient care of the spine for both degenerative and nondegenerative disorders has become increasingly necessary.
- A variety of health-related quality of life outcome surveys (HRQOL) attempt to quantify often highly subjective postoperative results.
- Characterization of a minimal clinically important difference (MCID) and substantial clinical benefit (SCB) allow for identification of the HRQOL survey results that demonstrate a significant change in patients' perception of their condition.
- Cost per quality-adjusted life years (QALY) is an important measure to assess the value of a treatment.
- In general, spinal surgery in the aging population has demonstrated a comparable cost per QALY in a variety of degenerative conditions.

6.1 Background

Low back pain is ranked as the leading cause of disability worldwide in the latest Global Burden of Disease Study. In 2010 alone, low back pain resulted in 83 million years of life lived with disability. Perhaps not unexpectedly, estimates of prevalence of back pain and spinal disorders in the United States and Canada showed higher rates for the older adult. Martin estimated the cost of treating low back and neck pain at $86 billion dollars in 2005, an increase of 65% from just eight years prior. This trend is predicted to continue. The "silver tsunami" has been termed the growing proportion of the U.S. population over 65, which is expected to increase to 20% by 2040, from 13% in 2010. Complicating all this is the vast array of treatment options and strategies for spinal disorders. Given the cost, prevalence, and wide range of treatment strategies available for spinal disorders, there is a strong need to define value in spine care, especially in the aging population.

6.2 Measures of Outcomes in Spinal Surgery

The concept of a quality-adjusted life year (QALY) is a tool to help in decisions regarding resource allocation. It quantifies health using life years weighted by their quality. One QALY is equal to one year in perfect health. To be dead is to have 0 QALYs. Time spent in less than optimal health is a QALY ranging from 0 to 1, with greater value associated with greater health. Acknowledging that there are states worse than death, negative QALYs are possible as well. More compactly, QALY = quality of life x quantity of life. Cost-effectiveness (CE), therefore, is defined as CE = cost/QALY. The World Health Organization has defined a cost-effective intervention as three times the per-person average income per quality adjusted life (QALY) year gained. In the United States, where the average per-person income is about $40k, any intervention that costs less than $120k per QALY gained, is said to be cost effective.[1]

Various organizations, including the Panel on Cost-Effectiveness in Health and Medicine, have recommended that QALY be used to compare the economic impact of alternative health care interventions. This can be done using the incremental cost-effectiveness ratio (ICER) and has the advantage that it can be used across health care domains, to compare the value of a certain hip replacement to heart surgery, for example. ICER is defined as the change in cost divided by the change in effectiveness, $ICER = [(cost_a - cost_b)/(QALY_a - QALY_b)]$.

For any intervention to be cost-effective, however, it must first be efficacious. Qualitative measures of patient function, such as reduction in painful symptoms, do not fully describe the functionality of the patient and his/her ability to return to gainful employment or have a fulfilling life. As a result, multiple scales have been developed to evaluate health-related quality of life (HRQOL) with more validity. These surveys are administered in the clinical setting in the preoperative and postoperative settings. The most commonly utilized surveys are the Short Form-36 (SF-36) and the Oswestry Disability Index (ODI). They are reviewed briefly below.

6.3 Short Form – 36

SF-36 consists of eight scaled sections relating to vitality, physical functioning, bodily pain, perceptions of health, physical role functioning, emotional role functioning, social role functioning, and mental health. The scoring system ranges from 0 to 100 with a lower score representing worse health and higher grades representing better health. This survey is unique because it combines both physical and mental components into its scoring. Given its broad range of questions, it is frequently utilized in a variety of conditions, including acute coronary syndrome, total knee arthroplasty, and a variety of spine topics.[2,3]

6.4 Oswestry Disability Index

Originally derived from the Oswestry Low Back Pain Questionnaire, the most recent version of the ODI was published in 2000.[4] This validated questionnaire contains 10 topics: pain, lifting, the ability to care for oneself, the ability to walk, the ability to sit, sexual function, the ability to stand, social life, sleep quality, and traveling ability. The scores for these topics are summed and multiplied by two in order to reach a maximum score of 100, which represents complete disability.

6.5 Clinically Important Differences in Outcomes

While the creation of HRQOL surveys have made it easier to quantitatively evaluate the factors that significantly improve the lives of patients, minor changes in these factors may cause a significant clinical difference. The purpose of the minimum clinically importance difference (MCID) measurement is to establish a threshold in which improvement is identified as significant, regardless of what health-related quality of life survey is utilized. It can be considered as the smallest amount of improvement that a patient would identify as being important in their life. By condensing health-related quality of life surveys into a more simplistic result, clearly defined thresholds can be created.

Several methods are used to identify the MCID: distribution-based, anchor-based, and the delphi method. The anchor-based method is currently the most utilized method. This method provides a standard or "anchor" question that is general in nature in order to determine whether the patient feels that he/she is better, worse, or about the same since his/her intervention. These results are then cross-referenced with their post-treatment survey results. In addition to the HRQOL survey, the patient is also asked to decide whether overall their symptoms are "about the same," "somewhat better," or "much better". The MCID is then identified as the difference between those who respond "somewhat better" vs. those who respond "about the same."

Similar to the MCID is the substantial clinical benefit (SCB). SCB is the change in the healthy-related quality of life survey that the patient perceives as substantially better or markedly improved. This value denotes the difference between those who report themselves as "much better" vs. "about the same." While the MCID may be the minimum amount of improvement necessary to be found, the SCB is considered to be the ultimate goal of any therapy.

A study conducted in 2008 by Carreon et al. utilized 454 patients from the Lumbar Spine Study Group and demonstrated a MCID value of 12.8 for ODI and 4.9 points for SF-36.[5,6] A similar study conducted in 2010 by Anderson et al demonstrated that for degenerative cervical spine conditions the MCID was 4.1 on SF-36, and the SCB was found to be 6.5.[7] While a variety of other scales exist to determine outcomes, many are not consistently used to evaluate for value of care. When using these outcome measures to assess value measures, it is important to note that the efficacy of MCID and SCB have been validated by multiple studies.

6.6 Healthcare Economics and Spine Surgery

When considering economics in healthcare, limitations exist as to what treatments are considered to be cost- and value-efficient. Value is defined as the benefit received compared to the cost of the surgical or medical intervention. The most important factor used to evaluate how much benefit is gained from the treatment is consistently assessed by the quality-adjusted life years (QALY). The goal of the QALY is to condense the treatment options into a single common score, for which a variety of disease states and interventions can be assessed by their effect on minimizing morbidity and mortality. The QALY is calculated by measuring the number of years until death with and without treatment in conjunction with the health-related quality of life survey (HRQOL) of the patient. After obtaining a value for this treatment, the cost per QALY can be calculated. The cost-effectiveness of the treatment can then be compared with other commonly implemented therapies.

There has been much debate over what is considered an acceptable cost per QALY. The most commonly used threshold cutoff for therapy efficiency is $50,000 per QALY. The rationale for this value is not based on science, but is rooted in the initial cost-effectiveness literature of end-stage renal disease.[8] The first introduction of a $50,000 QALY threshold was in an article from 1992 regarding HIV interventions.[9] While most authors in the 1990s openly acknowledged that this was an arbitrary choice, it slowly became common practice. One of the most highly cited articles was from 1998,; it ultimately concluded that no true cost-per-QALY threshold could ever be completely agreed upon due to the variability between decision makers, what their values are, and what the available resources are.[10] In addition to these limitations, comparisons between surgical and nonsurgical interventions are not clear.

Due to the limitations of a cost-per-QALY analysis when considering surgical and nonsurgical management, another commonly used measure is the incremental cost-effectiveness ratio (ICER). The ICER is defined as the overall difference in cost between two potential treatment options for a specific pathology. This value can be calculated by taking the cost-per-QALY gained from the procedure in question subtracted by the cost-per-QALY gained by the conservative/nonoperative therapy choice.

6.7 Effects of Advanced Age On Value

While numerous studies have been conducted evaluating the cost-effectiveness of adult spinal surgery, significantly less research has been conducted that specifically highlights the aging population. Spinal surgery in younger, healthy populations has demonstrated cost-effectiveness and good results, but questions have been raised as to whether this same cost-effectiveness holds true in an older adult and medically-complicated population.

An important component when considering surgical intervention in an older adult age group is the presence of confounding comorbidities and a relatively higher risk for postoperative complications. These factors lead to increased potential financial burdens on health networks and patients. A recent study evaluating 21,853 patients undergoing anterior cervical fusion evaluated the Medicare reimbursement from the full inpatient stay and analyzed how pertinent comorbidities affected the overall financial cost. Results demonstrated that average reimbursements were similar between the elderly group (age 65–84) and the younger patient population. The average cost in the elderly population was $13,648 +/- $7,306 compared to $14,234 +/- $8,838 in the younger population. Their results did find that comorbid conditions were found to alter the final reimbursement. Multivariate analysis demonstrated that factors such as advanced age ($1,083), myelopathy diagnosis ($2,150), obesity ($651), congestive heart failure ($1,523), and chronic kidney disease ($1,962) were all factors that increased the cost.[11]

In addition to the above findings regarding degenerative cervical conditions, a significant amount of data has also been gathered regarding the value of lumbar spine surgery. One recent study conducted in 2015 compared the outcomes and cost-effectiveness in the elderly with nonelderly patients for lumbar decompression surgery with and without fusion. In total, 221 patients were evaluated and found to demonstrate statistically similar outcomes in 2-year QALY means for both decompression alone and decompression with fusion. Additionally, the mean 2-year cost-per-QALY gained was similar between the elderly and younger patients with or without fusion. Cost-per-QALY with decompression alone was $23,364 in the younger population and $31,750 in the elderly population. The cost of lumbar decompression with fusion was significantly higher, with the cost-per-QALY being $64,228 compared to $60,183 for the elderly and younger groups.[12] These results demonstrate that decompression alone is highly cost-effective even in an elderly population. This cost-per-QALY is comparable to the treatment of hypertension, which has demonstrated a $22,000 cost-per-QALY for inpatients without diabetes or chronic kidney disease.[13]

Advancements in the technology of constructs and surgical techniques have made the occurrence of revision lumbar surgery less common. Despite the decreased incidence of revision surgeries, these still occur in aging patients and are often more costly than the initial operation. Despite the increased expenses, data has shown that these revision surgeries are still associated with a reasonable cost-per-QALY. A recent study published in 2013 evaluated 69 older adult patients who had undergone revision lumbar surgeries for adjacent segment disease, pseudarthrosis, or recurrent-level stenosis.[14] The mean total 2-year cost-per-QALY was $28,256 +/- $3,000. More specifically, the cost-per-QALY for revisions was $28,829 for adjacent segment disease, $28,069 for pseudoarthrosis, and $27,871 for same-level recurrent stenosis. The cost of decompression revision and extension of the fusion was much higher, with a mean 2-year cost-per-QALY of $80,594.

6.8 Actionable Items

For the surgeon in clinical practice, issues of health care policy and economics can be daunting. Involvement in the political conversation may be a daunting task to a single individual. Given this challenge, the involvement of local and national organizations provides the opportunity for lobbying for the spine provider's interest. Key interest groups such as the American Association of Neurologic Surgeons (AANS), the Congress of Neurologic Surgeons, (CNS), and the North American Spine Society (NASS) offer opportunities for the individual provider to have a voice when approaching larger governing bodies such as the Centers for Medicare and Medicaid Services (CMS). These larger organizations additionally allow for the surgeon to interact with politicians in an organized fashion.

In addition to participating in these organizations, involvement in registries allow the individual surgeon the opportunity to be involved in larger studies that permit the input of data into results that may change value-based care at a greater level. Currently, a wide variety of registries exist that include a variety of spinal pathologies. The chief goal of these registries is to compile information across a multitude of centers to create the most accurate data possible regarding patient outcomes and value-based care. Several national registries are active today, including the AO Spine Non Fusion Registry, NASS Registry, the Vanderbilt Prospective Spine Registry, and the Scoliosis Outcomes Database Registry.

6.9 Conclusion

The evaluation of value in health care is a continually-evolving and imperfect field. Advances such as quality of life surveys and calculations like the QALY and ICER attempt to establish a clearly-defined value for what is considered an acceptable cost for therapies. While these goals are noble, these are limited by the variability in who the final decision maker is, what resources are available, and what their ultimate values and goals are. Despite the additional risk for complications in the elderly population, literature has shown that surgical intervention for this patient population is reasonable and that cost-per-QALY results are comparable to younger patient populations.

References

[1] World Health Organization. Macroeconomics and Health: investing in health for economic development. Geneva, Switzerland: World Health Organization: Report of the WHO Commission on Macroeconomics and Health. 2001

[2] Lim JBT, Chong HC, Pang HN, et al. Revision total knee arthroplasty for failed high tibial osteotomy and unicompartmental knee arthroplasty have similar patient-reported outcome measures in a two-year follow-up study. Bone Joint J. 2017; 99-B(10):1329–1334

[3] Tegn N, Abdelnoor M, Aaberge L, et al. Health-related quality of life in older patients with acute coronary syndrome randomised to an invasive or conservative strategy. The After Eighty randomised controlled trial. Age Ageing. 2017; •••:1–7

[4] Fairbank JC, Pynsent PB. The Oswestry Disability Index. Spine. 2000; 25(22): 2940–2952, discussion 2952

[5] Nayak NR, Coats JM, Abdullah KG, Stein SC, Malhotra NR. Tracking patient-reported outcomes in spinal disorders. Surg Neurol Int. 2015; 6 Suppl 19: S490–S499

[6] Copay AG, Glassman SD, Subach BR, Berven S, Schuler TC, Carreon LY. Minimum clinically important difference in lumbar spine surgery patients: a choice of

methods using the Oswestry Disability Index, Medical Outcomes Study questionnaire Short Form 36, and pain scales. Spine J. 2008; 8(6):968–974

[7] Carreon LY, Glassman SD, Campbell MJ, Anderson PA. Neck Disability Index, short form-36 physical component summary, and pain scales for neck and arm pain: the minimum clinically important difference and substantial clinical benefit after cervical spine fusion. Spine J. 2010; 10(6):469–474

[8] Grosse SD. Assessing cost-effectiveness in healthcare: history of the $50,000 per QALY threshold. Expert Rev Pharmacoecon Outcomes Res. 2008; 8(2): 165–178

[9] Freedberg KA, Tosteson AN, Cotton DJ, Goldman L. Optimal management strategies for HIV-infected patients who present with cough or dyspnea: a cost-effective analysis. J Gen Intern Med. 1992; 7(3):261–272

[10] Owens DK. Interpretation of cost-effectiveness analyses. J Gen Intern Med. 1998; 13(10):716–717

[11] Puvanesarajah V, Kirby DJ, Jain A, Werner BC, Hassanzadeh H. Cost Variation of Anterior Cervical Fusions in Elderly Medicare Beneficiaries. Spine. 2017; 42(17):E1010–E1015

[12] Devin CJ, Chotai S, Parker SL, Tetreault L, Fehlings MG, McGirt MJ. A Cost-Utility Analysis of Lumbar Decompression With and Without Fusion for Degenerative Spine Disease in the Elderly. Neurosurgery. 2015; 77 Suppl 4:S116–S124

[13] Moran AE, Odden MC, Thanataveerat A, et al. Cost-effectiveness of hypertension therapy according to 2014 guidelines. N Engl J Med. 2015; 372(5):447–455

[14] Adogwa O, Owens R, Karikari I, et al. Revision lumbar surgery in elderly patients with symptomatic pseudarthrosis, adjacent-segment disease, or same-level recurrent stenosis. Part 2. A cost-effectiveness analysis: clinical article. J Neurosurg Spine. 2013; 18(2):147–153

7 Cervical Fractures

Alexander B. Dru, Ken M. Porche, and Daniel J. Hoh

Abstract

The aging population is growing rapidly in industrialized countries. It is expected that there will be a concomitant expansion of age-related health issues that parallels this growth. Due to decrease in bone quality, combined with an increased tendency for ground-level falls among the aging population, there is predicted a potential 50% increase in age-related fractures by 2025. Progressive age-related positive sagittal imbalance in this population may further contribute to changes in cervical spinal alignment that may increase risk for cervical spine fractures. Treatment options for cervical fractures, specifically Type II odontoid fractures, has been controversial in this population due to inherent risks related to age and medical comorbidities. Airway complications are of particular concern, with conservative management involving external immobilization. Comparison between various nonoperative and surgical treatment options are reviewed further. In general, survival outcomes from geriatric cervical fractures are impacted by age, injury, severity, and neurological deficit. For Type II odontoid fractures, surgical treatment has generally been shown to have better fusion rates than nonoperative treatment, while being cost-effective for those 65 to 80 years old. Further research is necessary to determine if this benefit extends to those > 80 years.

Keywords: Cervical fracture, odontoid fracture, geriatric fracture, fragility fracture, cervical spine injury, spinal cord injury

Key Points

- Cervical fractures are anticipated to be an increasing problem due to rapid population growth among the aging population, issues related to poor bone mineral density, global spinal sagittal malalignment, and gait instability
- Cervical fractures in the aging population have unique characteristics and challenges compared to those occurring in younger individuals
- For the type II odontoid fracture, operative treatment has been shown to have improved fusion rates compared to nonoperative treatment in patients age 65–80 years old
- For type II odontoid fractures, it remains unclear whether surgical treatment confers any advantage over nonsurgical treatment in patients > 80 years old.
- Halo vest immobilization carries a significant complication rate in the aging population. Rigid cervical collars should be considered as a treatment option when pursuing non-operative management of type II odontoid fractures in the aging population.

7.1 Epidemiology

The aging population is expected to grow exponentially in industrialized countries. The U.S. population age > 65 years was roughly 15% in 2014; it is expected to double after 6 years and reach 25% of the population by 2030.[1,2]

One expected rising medical need is skeletal fractures of the aging spine because of the relationship of advanced age to poor bone mineral density and the propensity for falls. Ground level falls (GLF) are particularly high risk in this population and correlate with increased age. The frequency of GLFs increases with age, ranging from an annual incidence of 30% in those over 65 to an incidence of 50% in those over 80 years of age.[3] This age-related GLF risk in combination with the growing aging population contributes to a predicted increase in the annual fracture rate by 50% from 2005 to 2025.[4] When compared to their younger counterparts, aging patients suffer a disproportionate number of cervical spine fractures,[5] with a high predisposition for C1 and C2 fractures (See ▸ Fig. 7.1).[6,7] The propensity for cervical fractures in this population may be related to multiple factors, including the more common presentation of a GLF with hyper-extension injury to the head and neck in combination with progressive overall kyphotic spinal alignment.

As aging spine fracture incidence increases, the associated costs of treating these fractures will also grow. At present, the annual cost for fracture treatment in the U.S. for this demographic is reported to be $14 billion.[4,8] Management of C2 fractures alone resulted in hospital charges in the U.S. of more than $1.5 billion in 2010.[9] Due to distinct challenges. such as compounding medical comorbidities, decreased physiological reserve, increased frailty, and unique psychosocial needs, the aging population represents an increasing demand on the health care system.[1]

7.2 Biomechanical Considerations

The most common cause of cervical spine fractures in aging patients is from low-energy GLFs as compared to high-energy injuries seen in younger individuals.[6,7,10] One reason for this difference in injury pattern among demographics may be related to global postural changes that occur with age.[1] Increasing age is correlated with progressive cranio-pelvic kyphosis, which becomes most significant by the eighth decade of life.[6] As degenerative spinal changes lead to multilevel loss of disc height, the spine tends to straighten leading to cervical kyphosis, with an unbalanced shifting of the center of gravity anteriorly.[7] This subaxial cervical kyphosis may additionally lead to compensatory mechanisms such as hyperlordotic angulation at the cranio-cervical junction. Additionally, osteoporotic and arthritic changes throughout the vertebral column in aging patients lead to weak bone from decreased bone mineral density and decreased flexibility of the spine from bridging osteophytes that predispose a patient to fractures from low-velocity trauma.[10] Approximately 40% of patients > 65 years old with type II odontoid fractures have positive sagittal malalignment, of which 60% have posterior fracture displacement.[11]

Additional risk factors for cervical fracture in this population include progressive poor bone mineral density with age, particularly in postmenopausal women.[12] Decreased reaction time, increasing impaired balance, ataxia, and gait instability further increase the risk of fall.[1] The combination of these

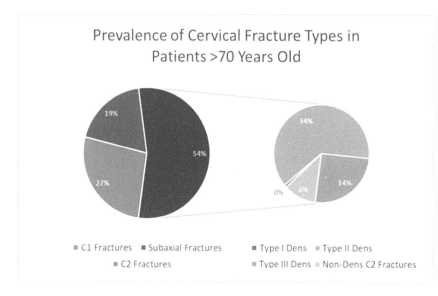

Prevalence of Cervical Fracture Types in Patients >70 Years Old

19% · 54% · 27% · 34% · 14% · 6% · 0%

■ C1 Fractures ■ Subaxial Fractures ■ Type I Dens ■ Type II Dens
■ C2 Fractures ■ Type III Dens ■ Non-Dens C2 Fractures

Fig. 7.1 Breakdown of cervical fracture types by prevalence in patients over 70.

factors–global kyphosis with an unbalanced center of gravity; hyperlordotic angulation at the cranio-cervical junction; impaired gait, balance and reaction time; and poor bone mineral density–culminate in a high susceptibility for upper cervical spine fractures with GLF.

7.3 Common Injury Types

C1 fractures account for 27% of cervical spine fractures in those > 65 years of age.[13] They are classified as those involving a single arch (Type I), those with burst fracture (Type II; aka Jefferson), or lateral mass fractures (Type III). Jefferson fractures generally occur from axial loading, and were classically described as four-point fractures. Now, more commonly Jefferson fractures include two- or three-point fractures as well. C1 fractures may lead to transverse ligament disruption, resulting in atlanto-axial instability.

C2 fractures account for 54% of geriatric cervical spine fractures.[13] Hangman's fractures are defined as bilateral fractures through the pars interarticularis and/or the pedicle of C2. These fractures are often due to hyperextension and axial loading in high-energy mechanisms of injury, and as a result are more commonly observed in younger individuals.

C2 odontoid process (dens) fractures are the most common upper cervical spine fracture in adults > 70 years of age (~89% of cervical fractures, see ▶ Fig. 7.1).[14,15] Hyperflexion is the most common mechanism of injury, with subsequent anterior atlanto-axial displacement. Anderson and D'Alonzi classified these fractures through the apical portion (Type I), through the base of the neck (Type II), and through the body of C2 (Type III).[16] Shallow Type III fractures can be further differentiated from Type II fractures by determining whether the fracture line involves the C2 superior facets.[17] Grauer et al proposed a subtyping of Type II fractures into nondisplaced/horizontal (IIA), antero-superior to postero-inferior/anteriorly displaced (IIB), and antero-inferior to postero-superior/posteriorly displaced (IIC) fractures, which can be utilized in surgical planning.[17] Type II fractures are most common; they increase in frequency with age and additionally have been increasing in proportion each

year.[15] Type II fractures generally demonstrate poor healing rates with conservative management,[15,17] whereas, Type I and Type III fractures can often be successfully treated with nonoperative immobilization. One caveat to that generalization is Type I fractures which significantly disrupt the apical and/or alar ligamentous attachment to the occiput may result in atlanto-occipital instability.[18] ▶ Fig. 7.2 shows the Grauer classification of odontoid fractures. A cervical CT demonstrating a displaced Type II odontoid fracture is depicted in▶ Fig. 7.3. ▶ Fig. 7.2 lists the general guidelines for management of each type.

Isolated subaxial (C3-C7) cervical fractures without a concomitant C1 or C2 fracture account for only 19% of geriatric cervical spine fractures.[13] These injuries include simple axial loading burst or compression fractures or more complex fracture and/or facet dislocations. Less common injury patterns include clay-shoveler's fracture (avulsion of a spinous process) and teardrop fractures (severe hyperflexion with antero-inferior vertebral body fracture and posterior ligamentous disruption).

7.4 Treatment Options

A complete review of the breadth of treatment options of cervical fractures is beyond the scope of this chapter. We will limit the described options to general principles of treatment and those specific to odontoid fractures, which represent the most common injury type. Conservative management includes a variety of external immobilization devices, including cervical collars and the halo vest. Cervical collars can be soft or rigid and strap around the neck to facilitate application and removal. Typically, soft collars do not immobilize the cervical spine, while rigid collars generally are best at stabilizing the lower cervical spine. The halo-vest externally immobilizes the cervical spine by external pin fixation of the skull connected by four rod posts to a rigid torso vest. The halo-vest is best at immobilizing the upper and lower cervical spine. It can be used to reduce flexion, extension, bending, and rotation; however, it is unable to provide distraction once the patient is upright. For certain fractures with significant displacement or angulation,

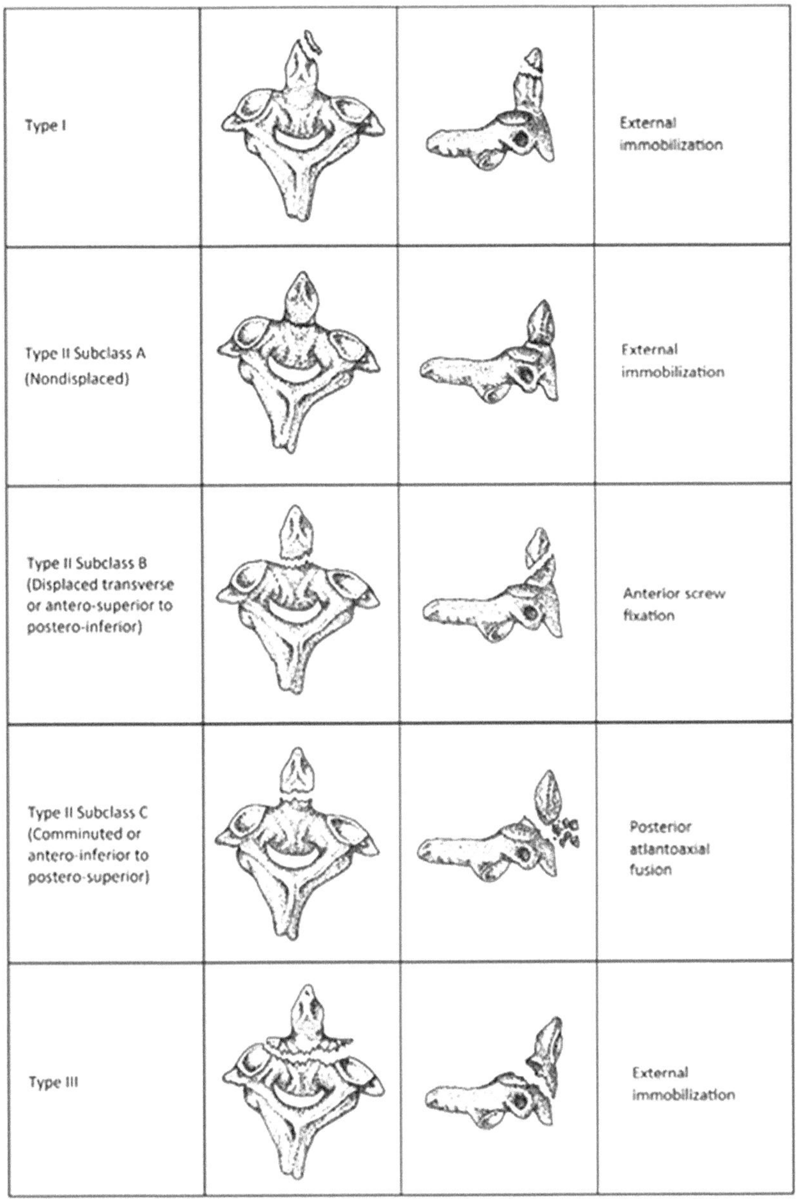

Type I			External immobilization
Type II Subclass A (Nondisplaced)			External immobilization
Type II Subclass B (Displaced transverse or antero-superior to postero-inferior)			Anterior screw fixation
Type II Subclass C (Comminuted or antero-inferior to postero-superior)			Posterior atlantoaxial fusion
Type III			External immobilization

Fig. 7.2 Grauer subclassification of Type II odontoid fractures and treatment algorithm.[18]

closed reduction with traction may be necessary prior to immobilization.[19]

Surgical treatment provides the potential benefit of enhanced immediate fracture immobilization by applying internal fixation directly to the spinal elements, via screw–rod, screw–plate, or wiring techniques. Additionally, spinal fixation devices and graft materials can be used to provide intraoperative reduction maneuvers for improved spinal alignment and bony healing. When necessary, spinal cord decompression can also be performed at the time of surgical stabilization via either anterior and/or posterior approaches (e.g., laminectomy, discectomy/corpectomy).

Odontoid fractures represent the most common cervical injury type in the elderly population, and typically result in atlanto-axial instability with abnormal translational motion through the fractured portion of the dens. Types I and III odontoid fractures demonstrate high fracture healing rates with nonoperative external immobilization, whereas Type II fractures are associated with significant failure rates with the same approach.[9,15] Therefore, there is extensive clinical experience describing various surgical treatment options for specifically Type II odontoid fractures.

In general, surgical fixation of odontoid fractures is via either a posterior or an anterior approach. Posterior spinal fixation with C1–C2 fusion is performed by either C1–C2 wiring, C1–C2 transarticular screw fixation, or by a C1–C2 screw–rod construct. There have been several previously described posterior wiring methods. The Brooks method uses a double-wire loop passed from cranial to caudal beneath the lamina of C1 and C2, which is used to secure a structural iliac crest graft.[20] The Gallie method uses an "H" graft that fits over the posterior arches of C1 and C2 with a wire passed underneath the lamina of C1, over

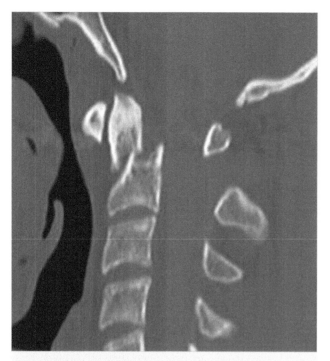

Fig. 7.3 Sagittal CT of displaced Type II odontoid fracture.

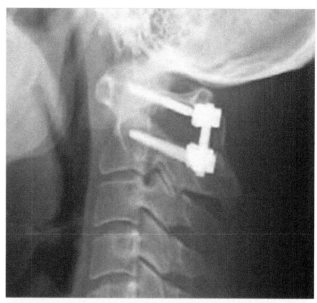

Fig. 7.4 Cervical X-ray of C1–C2 fusion in Type II nondisplaced odontoid fracture.

the spinous process of C2, and tightened to secure the graft in place.[20] The Sonntag method is similar to the Gallie in that the wire is passed underneath only the C1 lamina and is looped around the C2 spinous process. Both the Gallie and the Sonntag approaches only require passing the wire underneath the C1 lamina, as opposed to the Brooks technique, which involves passing the wire under the lamina of both C1 and C2. Posterior wiring fixation alone is associated with a relatively high nonunion rate and has since been supplanted by C1–C2 transarticular screw and C1–C2 screw–rod construct techniques. Posterior wiring, however, remains an important approach, as it provides added supplemental rigidity to primary posterior screw fixation and is an effective method for incorporating structural bone graft into the fusion construct.

C1-C2 transarticular screw fixation results in superior biomechanical immobilization and is associated with high bony healing rates.[18] In this procedure, bilateral posterior screws are placed through the isthmus of C2, crossing the C1-C2 articulation, and into the lateral mass of C1.[17] While this technique provides immediate rigid fixation of C1 and C2, it is associated with a potentially significant risk of injury to the vertebral artery, as it courses adjacent to the C2 foramen transversarium. In the presence of a high-riding, torturous or hyperplastic vertebral artery, modified trajectories may be necessary, or may simply not be technically feasible.[19] Preoperative planning with multiplanar CT reformatted images is necessary to assess an adequate screw path before considering C1–C2 transarticular screw fixation. Additionally, intraoperative navigation is a potentially useful adjunct for particularly challenging screw trajectories.

C1–C2 screw–rod fixation is an alternate approach for posterior spinal stabilization with equivalent biomechanical immobilization as C1–C2 transarticular screws (▸ Fig. 7.4).[19] C1 lateral mass screws can be combined with C2 pedicle, pars or intralaminar screws via a connecting rod to provide internal fixation.

C2 pedicle screws cross the C2 pedicle into the vertebral body, providing rigid fixation of C2 via a long bicortical screw. Because C2 pedicle screws traverse the isthmus, they are subject to the same potential risk of vertebral artery injury as C1–C2 transarticular screws. Alternatively, C2 pars screws enter the C2 isthmus; however, they do not pass the transverse foramen, thereby obviating the risk of potential vertebral artery violation. C2 intralaminar screws involve placement of crossing screws directly through the cancellous channel of the lamina. Intralaminar screws decrease the risk of vertebral artery injury; however, they require an intact C2 lamina (i.e., cannot be performed in the setting of a laminectomy for decompression).

Posterior surgical treatment of odontoid fractures requires stabilization across the C1–C2 motion segment, which ultimately results in significant loss of axial head rotation. An alternative anterior approach allows for direct surgical fixation across the odontoid fracture line, thereby preserving C1–C2 motion.[19] In this approach, a pilot hole is drilled through C2 and coaxially through the dens to its apex. The hole is then tapped and a lag screw is placed to secure the fragment to the body (▸ Fig. 7.5).[18] A second adjacent screw may be placed to prevent rotation around the single screw, which may be increasingly considered for the elderly population.[18,21] The anterior odontoid screw approach relies on eventual bony healing across the fracture line, and, as such, chronic fractures > 6 months after injury may fail secondary to the formation of fibrous nonunion across the fracture gap. Additionally, anterior odontoid screw fixation requires a nondisplaced, well-aligned fracture with specific anatomic limitations with respect to fracture morphology and patient thoracic chest size. Finally, osteoporotic patients have an additional risk of poor bone healing and screw purchase. Therefore, careful preoperative patient assessment is necessary before considering potential anterior odontoid screw fixation.

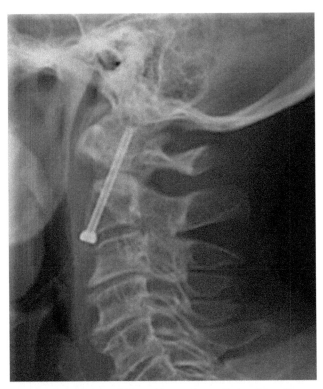

Fig. 7.5 Cervical X-ray of Odontoid screw in nondisplaced Type II odontoid fracture.

7.5 Benefits and Risks

In aging patients, halo vest immobilization is associated with impaired swallowing, respiratory function, and mobilization due to restriction of normal thoracic chest-wall motion. Complications from halo-vests include aspiration, pneumonia, cranial pin-site infection, dural violation, pressure sores, and, rarely, intracranial abscess.[9,22] These risks are countered by the perceived benefit of achieving better rigid upper cervical immobilization compared to cervical collars. Additionally, a halo vest may be preferred in patients suspected of poor compliance with removable or adjustable cervical collars. These risks may be reduced by close interval follow-up of patients in a halo vest to avoid common complications. Cervical collars also carry risk of complications, albeit less than observed with halo vests. Primarily, cervical collars without diligent hygiene and routine surveillance of pressure points can lead to skin breakdown and ulcers.

Surgical treatment carries general risk of bleeding, infection, anesthetic complications, neural or vascular injury, spinal implant malfunction (e.g. screw breakage or loosening), and pseudo-arthrosis. Various surgical approaches carry additional specific risks unique to aspects of the technique. Passing sublaminar wires may injure neural elements, particularly in the setting of spinal canal narrowing (e.g., posteriorly displaced dens fracture).[18] As previously mentioned, C1-C2 transarticular screws can cause vertebral artery injury, with a small incidence of potentially devastating brainstem stroke.[18,19] Excessively long or misplaced lateral mass or pedicle screws risk injury to the internal carotid or vertebral arteries, hypoglossal nerve, and

spinal cord. With anterior odontoid screw fixation, esophageal or pharyngeal perforation and/or airway complications are potential risks from the surgical exposure.[21] In addition, elderly patients are at increased risk of dysphagia and aspiration pneumonia from anterior neck dissection and soft tissue retraction.[21] The surgical risk profile for a given patient should take into account– such individual factors as medical comorbidities, baseline frailty, and functional status–and should be weighed against the benefit of immediate fracture stabilization and neural decompression.

7.6 Pitfalls, Complications and Avoidance

Clinical decision-making in the elderly population, whether nonoperative or operative, is often confronted with the challenge of multiple compounding factors, including lower physiological reserve, increased susceptibility to prolonged bed rest, poor bone mineral density, reduced recovery capacity and medical comorbidities. For surgical patients, preoperative optimization of comorbidities is essential to reduce risk of perioperative complications. Improving preoperative mobility status, nutrition, glucose control and bone mineral density may decrease the likelihood of negative outcomes. Careful attention to screw placement and trajectory is critical to increase bony purchase in patients with osteoporosis. Further, intraoperative use of osteobiologic adjuncts may be necessary to enhance early fusion before spinal implants fixated in osteoporotic bone may loosen. After surgery or external immobilization, diligent management of patient mobilization, adequate oral nutrition intake, and bowel and bladder regimen are essential to minimize risk of pneumonia, urinary tract infections, deep venous thrombosis, and pulmonary embolism. Close follow-up after discharge is necessary to identify potential persistent atlantoaxial instability, fracture nonunion, spinal implant, cervical collar or halo vest-related complications.

An additional consideration in traumatic injuries in the elderly is to cautiously align reasonable expectations for overall clinical and functional outcomes with the patient and caregivers. Patients with chronic life-threatening illnesses, dependent living status, advance directives and clearly defined preferences for end-of-life care may choose to limit aggressive surgical treatment and/or life-supporting technologies.[23] In select cases, appropriate care of elderly trauma patients may be directed at palliation rather than striving for a curative endpoint and/or prolongation of life.

7.7 Outcomes/Evidence

Overall, predicted individual survival from a GLF is strongly negatively correlated with increasing age.[1] Presumably, higher mortality from a GLF with advanced age is linked to increased medical comorbidities, frailty, and limited functional reserve. Additionally, there is also a significant decrease in disposition to home after hospital discharge with increasing age. More elderly patients are being discharged to inpatient rehabilitation or assisted living facilities after hospitalization.

With regard to cervical fractures in the elderly, the most significant factors that impact survival are injury severity and neurologic deficit.[23] Mortality rates in patients with spinal cord injuries are much higher in those with more severe spinal cord injuries and for those > 60 years of age.[24] The most common cause of death, especially with upper cervical fractures, is respiratory failure.[23] With impaired neurologic function and decreased respiratory drive, prolonged immobilization, and potentially respiratory compromise related to general anesthesia and pain medications, one can expect that elderly patients with cervical fractures are particularly vulnerable to inability to mobilize secretions and aspiration.[23,24]

Given the disproportionate predilection for Type II odontoid fractures in the aging population, there have been a number of studies that assessed factors that impact overall survival after injury. A recent prospective study and subsequent systematic review of geriatric Type II odontoid fractures determined that surgical treatment demonstrates an overall survival advantage compared to nonoperative care.[25,26] Further, those treated nonoperatively had a significant worsening in neck disability index (NDI) score as opposed to those who underwent surgery.[27] Overall, there was no significant difference in complication rates between patients managed surgically or conservatively,[25, 27] and no difference in mortality or complication rate was observed between anterior versus posterior surgery.[25] It should be noted, however, that there was likely selection bias in these studies in terms of which patients were determined to be better suited for surgical treatment. In addition, there was a lack of benefit with surgical treatment in those patients > 80 years of age, as morbidity and mortality increase 2- and 3-fold, likely due to increased age-related complications (i.e. airway difficulties).[28,29]

When assessing overall cost-effectiveness, surgical treatment for Type II odontoid fractures was shown to be associated with a $12K and $40K increase in quality-adjusted life years (QALY) compared to non-surgical treatment in those 65 to 74 years and 75 to 84 years old, respectively.[30] A decline in QALY was shown for those > 84 years old with surgery, however, making it not cost-effective.[30] Therefore, at present, surgical management is demonstrated to be cost-effective up until 84 years of age.

With respect to fracture healing, nonoperative treatment has been shown to have a relatively high rate of nonunion, ranging from 22 to 65%.[27,31,32] Factors impacting fracture nonhealing include age > 60 years, posterior fracture displacement, fracture angulation > 10°, delay in diagnosis/treatment > 3 weeks, and fracture comminution.[17,19] When comparing halo vest versus cervical collars, there does not appear to be a difference in overall fracture healing rate.[9] Halo vests as compared to non-halo vest treatment (i.e., rigid collar or surgery), however, are associated with a significant increase in mortality (51% vs. 31%) and complication rate (66% vs. 36%).[33] Nonhealing has been described by 4 types: Type 1, stable anatomic nonunion; Type 2, stable displaced nonunion; Type 3, unstable displaced nonunion; and Type 4, posttraumatic os odontoideum[34] Treatment for anatomically stable nonunion consists of continued conservative management with external immobilization and medication to promote bone healing. Treatment options for symptomatic nonunion dens fractures include prolonged external immobilization or surgical therapy. In a series of 48 elderly nonhealing odontoid fractures, 16 symptomatic patients underwent C1–C2 arthrodesis, and 28 asymptomatic patients underwent nonoperative management with posttreatment follow-up of 5 years.

All patients with surgical intervention achieved fusion. Only 2 of the 28 nonoperative patients achieved radiographic fusion, but all 28 patients reported satisfactory outcomes.[35] Recently, case reports have suggested teriparatide therapy may represent a pharmacologic option for nonhealing patients who cannot undergo surgery and who failed external immobilization alone.[36]

7.8 Conclusion

Moving forward, one can expect further increases in the average life expectancy and expansion of the aging population. With this growth, there will be a concomitant increase in medical illnesses specific to this demographic, of which cervical fractures will likely become even more prevalent. Given the reduced physiologic reserve and chronic medical comorbidities of this population, defining best treatment strategies remains challenging. Current evidence suggests that surgical treatment for Type II odontoid fractures results in better improvement in disability and stabilization of fractures compared to conservative treatment. Further, surgical treatment appears to be more cost-effective than nonoperative treatment, although these benefits appear to extend to only those individuals less than 80 years old. Conservative treatment with a rigid cervical collar is also a reasonable treatment option, although it is less likely to achieve a solid bony fusion of the dens fracture.

When considering management in the aging patient, special attention must be made to identify the specific needs of this population. Diligent follow-up for posttreatment complications is essential. Plan of care, advanced directives, alignment of patient and caregiver expectations, and palliation when appropriate should be considered.

Key References

[1] Hlubek RJ, Nakaji P. Nonoperative Management of Odontoid Fractures: Is Halo Vest Immobilization Warranted? World Neurosurg. 2017; 98:839–840

[2] Bhattacharya B, Maung A, Schuster K, Davis KA. The older they are the harder they fall: Injury patterns and outcomes by age after ground level falls. Injury. 2016; 47(9):1955–1959

[3] Faure A, Graillon T, Pesenti S, Tropiano P, Blondel B, Fuentes S. Trends in the surgical management of odontoid fractures in patients above 75 years of age: Retrospective study of 70 cases. Orthop Traumatol Surg Res. 2017; 103(8): 1221–1228

References

[1] Bhattacharya B, Maung A, Schuster K, Davis KA. The older they are the harder they fall: Injury patterns and outcomes by age after ground level falls. Injury. 2016; 47(9):1955–1959

[2] Ortman JM, Velkoff VA, Hogan H. An Aging Nation: The Older Population in the United States. 2014

[3] Centers for Disease Control and Prevention (CDC). Fatalities and injuries from falls among older adults–United States, 1993–2003 and 2001–2005. MMWR Morb Mortal Wkly Rep. 2006; 55(45):1221–1224

[4] Burge R, Dawson-Hughes B, Solomon DH, Wong JB, King A, Tosteson A. Incidence and economic burden of osteoporosis-related fractures in the United States, 2005–2025. J Bone Miner Res. 2007; 22(3):465–475

[5] Hu R, Mustard CA, Burns C. Epidemiology of incident spinal fracture in a complete population. Spine. 1996; 21(4):492–499

[6] Yoshida G, Yasuda T, Togawa D, et al. Craniopelvic alignment in elderly asymptomatic individuals: analysis of 671 cranial centers of gravity. Spine. 2014; 39(14):1121–1127

[7] Oe S, Togawa D, Nakai K, et al. The Influence of Age and Sex on Cervical Spinal Alignment Among Volunteers Aged Over 50. Spine. 2015; 40(19):1487–1494

[8] Blume SW, Curtis JR. Medical costs of osteoporosis in the elderly Medicare population. Osteoporos Int. 2011; 22(6):1835–1844

[9] Hlubek RJ, Nakaji P. Nonoperative Management of Odontoid Fractures: Is Halo Vest Immobilization Warranted? World Neurosurg. 2017; 98:839–840

[10] Scheer JK, Tang JA, Smith JS, et al. International Spine Study Group. Cervical spine alignment, sagittal deformity, and clinical implications: a review. J Neurosurg Spine. 2013; 19(2):141–159

[11] Reinhold M, Bellabarba C, Bransford R, et al. Radiographic analysis of type II odontoid fractures in a geriatric patient population: description and pathomechanism of the "Geier"-deformity. Eur Spine J. 2011; 20(11):1928–1939

[12] Berger C, Langsetmo L, Joseph L, et al. Canadian Multicentre Osteoporosis Study Research Group. Change in bone mineral density as a function of age in women and men and association with the use of antiresorptive agents. CMAJ. 2008; 178(13):1660–1668

[13] Wang H, Coppola M, Robinson RD, et al. Geriatric Trauma Patients With Cervical Spine Fractures due to Ground Level Fall: Five Years Experience in a Level One Trauma Center. J Clin Med Res. 2013; 5(2):75–83

[14] Faure A, Graillon T, Pesenti S, Tropiano P, Blondel B, Fuentes S. Trends in the surgical management of odontoid fractures in patients above 75 years of age: Retrospective study of 70 cases. Orthop Traumatol Surg Res. 2017; 103(8):1221–1228

[15] Robinson A-L, Möller A, Robinson Y, Olerud C. C2 Fracture Subtypes, Incidence, and Treatment Allocation Change with Age: A Retrospective Cohort Study of 233 Consecutive Cases. BioMed Res Int. 2017; 2017:8321680

[16] Anderson LD, D'Alonzo RT. Fractures of the odontoid process of the axis. J Bone Joint Surg Am. 1974; 56(8):1663–1674

[17] Grauer JN, Shafi B, Hilibrand AS, et al. Proposal of a modified, treatment-oriented classification of odontoid fractures. Spine J. 2005; 5(2):123–129

[18] Rao G, Apfelbaum RI. Odontoid screw fixation for fresh and remote fractures. Neurol India. 2005; 53(4):416–423

[19] Kim DH, Riew KD. Odontoid Fractures: Current Evaluation and Treatment Principles. Semin Spine Surg. 2007; 19:235–243

[20] An HS, Jenis LG. Complications of Spine Surgery: Treatment and Prevention. Lippincott Williams & Wilkins; 2006

[21] Mazur MD, Mumert ML, Bisson EF, Schmidt MH. Avoiding pitfalls in anterior screw fixation for type II odontoid fractures. Neurosurg Focus. 2011; 31(4):E7

[22] Fulkerson DH, Hwang SW, Patel AJ, Jea A. Open reduction and internal fixation for angulated, unstable odontoid synchondrosis fractures in children: a safe alternative to halo fixation? J Neurosurg Pediatr. 2012; 9(1):35–41

[23] Damadi AA, Saxe AW, Fath JJ, Apelgren KN. Cervical spine fractures in patients 65 years or older: a 3-year experience at a level I trauma center. J Trauma. 2008; 64(3):745–748

[24] Daneshvar P, Roffey DM, Brikeet YA, Tsai EC, Bailey CS, Wai EK. Spinal cord injuries related to cervical spine fractures in elderly patients: factors affecting mortality. Spine J. 2013; 13(8):862–866

[25] Schroeder GD, Kepler CK, Kurd MF, et al. A Systematic Review of the Treatment of Geriatric Type II Odontoid Fractures. Neurosurgery. 2015; 77 Suppl 4:S6–S14

[26] Chapman J, Smith JS, Kopjar B, et al. The AOSpine North America Geriatric Odontoid Fracture Mortality Study: a retrospective review of mortality outcomes for operative versus nonoperative treatment of 322 patients with long-term follow-up. Spine. 2013; 38(13):1098–1104

[27] Vaccaro AR, Kepler CK, Kopjar B, et al. Functional and quality-of-life outcomes in geriatric patients with type-II dens fracture. J Bone Joint Surg Am. 2013; 95(8):729–735

[28] Turrentine FE, Wang H, Simpson VB, Jones RS. Surgical risk factors, morbidity, and mortality in elderly patients. J Am Coll Surg. 2006; 203(6):865–877

[29] Smith HE, Kerr SM, Maltenfort M, et al. Early complications of surgical versus conservative treatment of isolated type II odontoid fractures in octogenarians: a retrospective cohort study. J Spinal Disord Tech. 2008; 21(8):535–539

[30] Barlow DR, Higgins BT, Ozanne EM, Tosteson ANA, Pearson AM. Cost Effectiveness of Operative Versus Non-Operative Treatment of Geriatric Type-II Odontoid Fracture. Spine. 2016; 41(7):610–617

[31] Joestl J, Lang N, Bukaty A, Platzer P. A comparison of anterior screw fixation and halo immobilisation of type II odontoid fractures in elderly patients at increased risk from anaesthesia. Bone Joint J. 2016; 98-B(9):1222–1226

[32] Hsu WK, Anderson PA. Odontoid fractures: update on management. J Am Acad Orthop Surg. 2010; 18(7):383–394

[33] Tashjian RZ, Majercik S, Biffl WL, Palumbo MA, Cioffi WG. Halo-vest immobilization increases early morbidity and mortality in elderly odontoid fractures. J Trauma. 2006; 60(1):199–203

[34] Yang Z, Yuan Z-Z, Ma J-X, Ma X-L. Conservative versus surgical treatment for type II odontoid fractures in the elderly: Grading the evidence through a meta-analysis. Orthop Traumatol Surg Res. 2015; 101(7):839–844

[35] Joestl J, Lang NW, Tiefenboeck TM, Hajdu S, Platzer P. Management and Outcome of Dens Fracture Nonunions in Geriatric Patients. J Bone Joint Surg Am. 2016; 98(3):193–198

[36] Pola E, Pambianco V, Colangelo D, Formica VM, Autore G, Nasto LA. Teriparatide anabolic therapy as potential treatment of type II dens non-union fractures. World J Orthop. 2017; 8(1):82–86

8 Thoracic and Thoracolumbar Fractures

Jay Kumar and John H. Shin

Abstract

The thoracic and thoracolumbar regions are common fracture sites in aging adults. Multiple classification systems have been developed to facilitate discussion of different fractures and guide surgical decision-making. The four main types of fracture are compression, burst, flexion-distraction, and fracture-dislocation. Conservative management with analgesics, bracing, medical management, and physical therapy is recommended for most stable fractures without neurologic deficit. Surgical decompression and stabilization is generally appropriate for fractures with neurologic deficit, progressive vertebral column collapse, deformity, and/or persistent pain. In the aging population consideration of medical comorbidities and osteoporosis are paramount in surgical decision-making.

Keywords: Thoracic, thoracolumbar, fracture, trauma, aging, osteoporosis

Key Points

- Vertebrae of the thoracic and thoracolumbar spine are prone to fracture in older adults.
- Current classification systems generally categorize fractures as compression, burst, flexion-distraction, and fracture-dislocation.
- Conservative therapy with analgesics, bracing, medical management and physical therapy is recommended for most stable fractures without neurologic deficit.
- Surgical decompression and stabilization is generally indicated for fractures causing neurologic deficit, progressive deformity, and/or persistent pain.
- Medical co-morbidities should be carefully considered in this patient population.

8.1 Epidemiology

The thoracolumbar region is the longest segment of the human spine and a frequent site of fractures, especially in the aging population. One of the major medical conditions which affects older adults and predisposes this patient population to fractures is osteoporosis. For these patients, any type of fracture may be more severe than expected from the mechanism of injury—for example a fall—given the poor bone density typical of the aging.

Osteoporosis is estimated to affect over 100 million people worldwide and at least 10 million people in the United States.[1] In the United States, about 700,000 osteoporotic vertebral compression fractures occur annually, of which 70,000 result in a hospitalization, with an average duration of eight days.[1] Burst fractures are the second-most common injury to the thoracolumbar spine, after compression fractures, with about 25,000 occurring annually in the United States.[2] In situations of severe trauma, thoracolumbar fractures are often associated with other vertebral and nonvertebral fractures and injuries to internal organs. In these situations, the diagnosis of thoracolumbar spine fracture itself may initially be missed.[3] The sequelae of thoracic and thoracolumbar fracture include pain, deformity, and loss of neurologic function.[4,5,6,7] The goal of therapy is to relieve pain, prevent or reverse neurologic deficit, and prevent bony deformities.

8.2 Biomechanical Considerations

The thoracic and lumbar spine is comprised of the thoracic vertebrae, T1-T12, and the lumbar vertebrae, L1–5. The thoracic vertebrae form a rigid unit with the ribs and sternum compared to the more mobile lumbar vertebral column. The thoracolumbar junction, T10-L2, represents the transition between the kyphosis of the thoracic spine and the lordosis of the lumbar spine. The juxtaposition of the stiff thoracic spine with the relatively more mobile lumbar spine creates a site that is subject to increased forces during traumatic injuries. Thoracolumbar fractures are commonly associated with high-energy situations such as motor vehicle accidents, falls, sports injuries, and violence. Associated injuries are common, and may include pneumothorax, rib and long-bone fractures, and penetrating injuries to the lungs, heart, and visceral organs. Ruling out visceral injuries to other organ systems is critical in the evaluation of these patients, particularly if planning a surgical intervention. Paying attention to the mechanism of injury should provide an index of suspicion for injuries to regional organ systems. For example, a pelvic fracture associated with a traumatic thoracolumbar spine injury could put a patient at risk of injury when positioning the patient prone.

In the aging population, osteoporosis is common, especially in women. The United States Preventative Services Task Force currently recommends screening all women over age 65.[8] Osteoporosis is likely prevalent in many elderly men as well, but the current evidence is insufficient for guidelines. In patients with osteoporosis, the spine is commonly affected, as the amount of bone present in each vertebral body is generally decreased. Typically, the cortical layer of each vertebra is thinned, and the cancellous bone has low trabecular continuity. Osteoporosis can be assessed by bone density tests, but such tests are typically not part of any routine trauma evaluation. Most elderly patients with established primary medical care may have an underlying diagnosis of osteopenia or osteoporosis, for which they are followed longitudinally. In the acute setting of managing and planning the treatment pathway for an acute thoracic or thoracolumbar fracture, the treatment history of the osteoporosis is important to know, as the spine fracture may be the patient's first bone fracture. For long-term management of bone health, this may prompt the patient's primary medical provider to start medical treatment or refer to an endocrinologist for further discussion regarding treatment options. For patients without established medical care at this age, there are usually greater issues of general medical health and chronic medical illnesses which may have not been adequately addressed or managed. In these situations, the spine fracture is a small part of a greater issue. Nonetheless, any new spine fracture in the elderly population should prompt follow-up with a medical provider for evaluation and treatment of osteoporosis.

The aging spine is typically less flexible secondary to spondylosis and resultant osteophyte formation. Other conditions can accelerate this stiffening, including diffuse idiopathic skeletal hyperostosis (DISH) and ankylosing spondylitis. Care should be taken to identify these underlying conditions because the stiffened spine can increase the leverage at the fracture site, leading to more significant risk of instability. Fractures in these patients are more like long-bone fractures and are more likely to benefit from internal fixation.

8.3 Common Injury Types

There have been many attempts to classify traumatic injuries to the spine. One of the first classification systems proposed by Holdsworth et al in 1968 sorted injuries according to mechanism of injury and radiologic findings and was based on a two-column (anterior and posterior) model of the spine.[9,10] Denis et al in 1983 advocated a three-column model consisting of the anterior 2/3 of the vertebral body, the posterior 1/3 of the vertebral body, and the posterior column.[11] In light of the new data provided by CT and MRI scans, further classification systems were proposed.[12,13,14] More recently, in 1994 the AO (*Arbeitsgemeinschaft für Osteosynthesefragen*, German for "Association for the Study of Internal Fixation") Foundation created the "AO Classification," a comprehensive classification based on pathology and morphology.[15] They defined three major types of injuries: A. compression, B. distraction, and C. rotation. Each type has several groups and subgroups based on the pathophysiology and morphology of the injury (▶ Table 8.1). This classification of thoracic and thoracolumbar fractures has facilitated research by providing precise and comprehensive diagnostic criteria but has proved to be cumbersome for routine clinical practice.

More recently, Vaccaro et al in 2005 developed the Thoracolumbar Injury Classification and Severity Score (TLICS) (▶ Table 8.2) by using clinically important criteria of morphology,

Table 8.1 A comprehensive classification of thoracic and lumbar injuries by Magerl et al in 1994

Table 8.1a Type A injuries: groups, subgroups, and specifications

Type A. Vertebral body compression

A1. Impaction fractures

    A1.1. Endplate impaction

    A1.2. Wedge impaction fractures

        1. Superior wedge impaction fracture

        2. Lateral wedge impaction fracture

        3. Inferior wedge impaction fracture

    A1.3. Vertebral body collapse

A2. Split fractures

    A2.1. Sagittal split fracture

    A2.2. Coronal split fracture

    A2.3. Pincer fracture

A3. Burst fractures

    A3.1. Incomplete burst fracture

        1. Superior incomplete burst fracture

        2. Lateral incomplete burst fracture

        3. Inferior incomplete burst fracture

    A3.2. Burst-split fracture

        1. Superior burst-split fracture

        2. Lateral burst-split fracture

        3. Inferior burst-split fracture

    A3.3. Complete burst fracture

        1. Pincer burst fracture

        2. Complete flexion burst fracture

        3. Complete axial burst fracture

Table 8.1b Type B injuries: groups, subgroups, and specifications

Type B. Anterior and posterior element injury with distraction

B1. Posterior disruption, predominantly ligamentous (flexion-distraction injury)

    B1.1. With transverse disruption of the disc

        1. Flexion-subluxation

        2. Anterior dislocation

        3. Flexion-subluxation/anterior dislocation with fracture of the articular processes

B1.2. With type A fracture of the vertebral body

    1. Flexion-subluxation + type A fracture

    2. Anterior dislocation + type A fracture

    3. Flexion-subluxation/anterior dislocation with fracture of the articular processes + type A fracture

B2. Posterior disruption predominantly osseous (flexion-distraction injury)

B2.1. Transverse bicolumn fracture

B2.2. With transverse disruption of the disc

    1. Disruption through the pedicle and disc

    2. Disruption through the pars interarticularis and disc (flexion-spondylolysis)

B2.3. With type A fracture of the vertebral body

    1. Fracture through the pedicle + type A fracture

    2. Fracture though the pars interarticularis (flexion-spondylolysis) + type A fracture

B3. Anterior disruption through the disc (hyperextension-shear injury)

B3.1. Hyperextension-subluxations

    1. Without injury of the posterior column

    2. With injury of the posterior column

B3.2. Hyperextension-spondylolysis

B3.3. Posterior dislocation

Table 8.1c Type C injuries: groups, subgroups, and specifications

Type C. Anterior and posterior element injury with rotation

C1. Type A injuries with rotation (compression injuries with roation)

C1.1. Rotational split fracture

C1.2. Rotational split fractures

    1. Rotational sagittal split fracture

    2. Rotational coronal split fracture

    3. Rotational pincer fracture

    4. Vertebral body separation

C1.3. Rotational burst fractures

    1. Incomplete rotational burst fracture

    2. Rotational burst-split fracture

    3. Complete rotational burst fracture

C2. Type B injuries with rotation

C2.1. B1 injuries with rotation (flexion-distraction injuries with rotation)

    1. Rotational flexion subluxation

    2. Rotational flexion subluxation with unilateral articular process fracture

    3. Unilateral dislocation

    4. Rotational anterior dislocation without/with fracture of articular processes

    5. Rotational flexion subluxation without/with unilateral articular process fracture + type A fracture

    6. Unilateral dislocation + type A fracture

    7. Rotational anterior dislocation without/with fracture of articular processes + type A fracture

C2.2. B2 injuries with rotation (flexion-distraction injuries with rotation)

    1. Rotational transverse bicolumn fracture

    2. Unilateral flexion spondylolysis with disruption of the disc

    3. Unilateral flexion spondylolysis + type A fracture

C2.3. B3 injuries with rotation (hyperextension-shear injuries with rotation)

    1. Rotational hyperextension-subluxation without/with fracture of posterior vertebral elements

    2. Unilateral hyperextension-spondylolysis

    3. Posterior dislocation with rotation

C3. Rotational-shear injuries

C3.1. Slice fracture

C3.2. Oblique fracture

Table 8.2 a. Thoracolumbar Injury Classification and Severity Score (TLICS) by Vaccaro et al in 2005.

Injury morphology

Type	Qualifiers	Points
Compression		1
	Burst	1
Translational/ rotational		3
Distraction		4

Integrity of posterior ligamentous complex

PLC disrupted in tension, rotation, or translation	Points
Intact	0
Suspected/ indeterminate	2
Injured	3

Neurologic status

Involvement	Qualifiers	Points
Intact		0
Nerve root		2
Cord, conus medullaris	Complete	2
	Incomplete	3
Cauda equina		3

Recommendation

Need for surgery	Total Score
Nonsurgical	0–3
Surgeon's choice	4
Surgical	>4

Table 8.3 b Thoracolumbar Injury Classification and Severity Score (TLICS) by Vaccaro et al in 2005

Suggested Surgical Approach

	Posterior Ligamentous Complex	
Neurologic Status	Intact	Disrupted
Intact	Posterior approach	Posterior approach
Root injury	Posterior approach	Posterior approach
Incomplete SCI or cauda equina	Anterior approach	Combined approach
Complete SCI or cauda equina	Posterior (anterior)* approach	Posterior (combined) * approach

*Aggressive decompression in ASIA A patients is practiced in many institutions to optimize any potential for neurologic recovery, reconstruct the vertebral support column, restore CSF flow to prevent syringomyelia, and allow for short-segment fixation

complex. These are by far the most common type of thoracic and thoracolumbar fractures, especially in elderly patients with osteoporosis. With advanced osteoporosis, compression fractures may occur with little or even no axial load. They are more likely to occur in women than men, given the higher rates of osteoporosis among women. A single fracture increases the risk of additional fracture.[19]

These injuries may present with pain around the fracture or in the dermatomal region corresponding to the nerve root at the fracture site. A physical exam may reveal focal tenderness, mild local kyphosis in the case of one fracture or more obvious kyphosis in the case of multiple fractures, and nerve root deficits if the fracture is severe enough to cause foraminal stenosis. In these fractures, there is typically fracture and depression of the superior endplate of the vertebrae, causing a change in the radiographic appearance of the vertebrae (▶ Fig. 8.1). The vertebrae appear wedged in these fractures, with height loss of the anterior column. In the thoracic spine, there may be more than one fracture after a fall or injury. It is common to see consecutive vertebral compression fractures in patients with osteoporosis.

8.3.2 Burst Fractures

A more severe type of compression fracture, known as a burst fracture (AO type A3[15]) describes a compression fracture in which the vertebral body expands in all directions. Both the anterior and middle columns are involved, and the injury may be stable or unstable. Burst fractures are classified differently based on the condition of the superior and inferior endplates of the fractured vertebral body and whether any rotation or lateral flexion accompanies the burst fracture. These fractures often involve the entire vertebrae, and there are several characteristic imaging findings. On an axial CT image, there is often comminution and disruption of the cortical walls of the vertebrae with associated widening or splaying of the pedicles. There may also be retropulsion of the posterior wall of the vertebral body into the spinal canal (▶ Fig. 8.2). The amount of retropulsion into the spinal canal may be severe, and the axial image can be alarming with regards to the degree of retropulsion. The degree of retropulsion is not necessarily associated with the severity of neurologic deficit, if at all present, but careful neurologic examination is critical to assess for any signs of spinal cord or cauda equina compression causing urinary, motor, or sensory deficits.

neurologic status, and the integrity of the posterior ligamentous complex as assessed by CT or MRI imaging.[16,17] A TLICS score of < 4 indicates nonsurgical management, a score of > 4 indicates surgical management, and a score of 4 is equivocal. This score has been verified by other investigators.[18]

The most widely accepted classifications of injuries today all use three-column models. Specifically, the anterior column includes the anterior longitudinal ligament, and the anterior 2/3 of each vertebral body and annulus. The middle column includes the posterior longitudinal ligament and the posterior 2/3 of each vertebral body and annulus. The posterior column consists of the multiple structures forming the posterior housing of the spinal cord, including the pedicles, lamina, facets, spinous processes, and the ligamentum flavum and posterior ligamentous complex (supraspinous ligament, interspinous ligament, ligamentum flavum, and facet capsule).

In what follows, the most common thoracic and thoracolumbar spine injuries in patients are discussed: compression fractures, burst fractures, flexion-distraction fractures, and fracture-dislocation injuries.

8.3.1 Compression Fractures

Compression fractures involve collapse of the vertebral body in the vertical axis and are classified as AO type A.[15] They are generally stable fractures that spare the posterior ligamentous

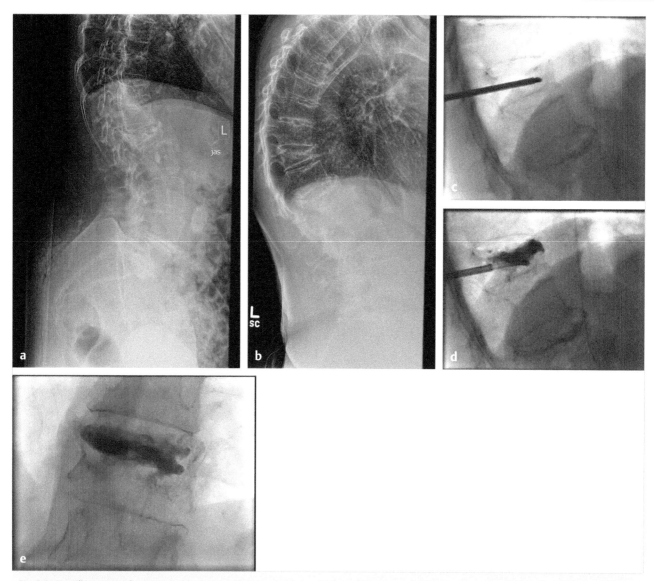

Fig. 8.1 Case illustration of a 79-year-old woman with osteoporosis presenting with acute and chronic compression fractures at T11 and L1 after repeated falls. The patient is neurologically intact. **(a)** Standing lumbar radiograph shows a chronic L1 compression fracture and an acute T11 compression fracture. **(b)** Standing lumbar radiograph 6 weeks later shows interval progression of loss of anterior vertebral body height and further collapse and wedging of the T11 vertebrae. **(c)** Intra-operative lateral radiograph showing needle cannulating the T11 vertebrae during cement augmentation. **(d)** Lateral radiograph showing the cement fill of the T11 vertebrae. **(e)** AP radiograph showing the cement fill.

Patients also may not have any symptoms while on bed rest or in the initial acute assessment while immobile. These patients need to be evaluated once mobilized, as additional weight-bearing and loading of the spine may exacerbate or produce symptoms, which may then prompt more urgent intervention or reconsideration of operative intervention. It is not uncommon for patients to lose bladder function or develop leg weakness once mobilizing from a recumbent to weight-bearing position. This does not necessarily mean that the fracture pattern has changed but demonstrates the general inability of the spine to withstand these loads. Patients may also experience stronger radicular pain when sitting or standing. This is due to further foraminal height loss and compression. This mechanical type of radiculopathy is difficult to treat with bracing alone, because braces do not provide significant resistance to axial load to maintain the height of the foramen and avoid nerve impingement.

Burst fractures are usually associated with high-energy events, including motor vehicle accidents and falls. They are the second most common injury to the thoracolumbar spine after compression fractures, with about 25,000 occurring annually in the United States. The osteoporotic bone of elderly patients can increase the risk of such fractures. Burst fractures may be accompanied by other spine fractures, particularly laminar fractures, which may be associated with dural tear and entrapped nerve roots. Imaging studies, including plain film radiography, CT and MRI scans, may reveal increasing spacing between vertebral bodies, suggesting ligamentous disruption, or direct visualization of ligamentous compromise.

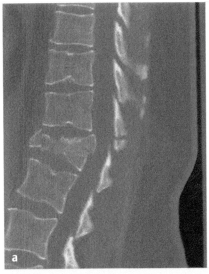 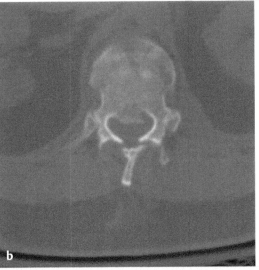 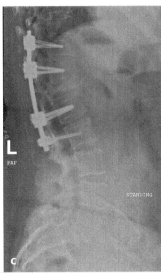

Fig. 8.2 Case Illustration of 67-year-old woman who fell off a horse and presented with an acute T12 burst fracture with pain and urinary retention. (a) Pre-operative sagittal CT shows the loss of height. (b) Pre-operative axial CT shows representative cortical splaying of the vertebral body and retropulsed bone fragment into the spinal canal. (c) Standing lateral radiograph showing the stabilization. Anterior approach was not performed due to medical co-morbidities and previous thoracolumbar approach for abdominal aortic aneurysm.

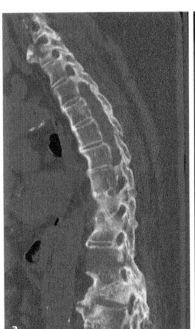 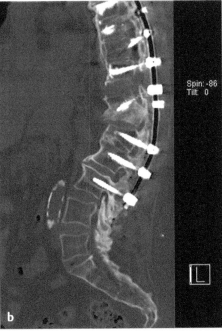

Fig. 8.3 Case illustration of an 84-year-old woman who presented with pain and incomplete spinal cord injury after a fall. (a) Pre-operative CT shows a bony distraction injury at T11 with disruption through the entire vertebral body, pedicle, and posterior elements. (b) Post-operative CT showing reduction of the fracture and multiple points of fixation with pedicle screw fixation. Cement augmentation was also used to supplement bony fixation due to severe ankylosis and osteoporosis.

8.3.3 Flexion-Distraction

Flexion-Distraction injuries (AO type B[15]) occur with sudden flexion of the spine— as in the case of a motor vehicle accident causing acute flexion at the waist—and distraction of the posterior elements of the spine (▶ Fig. 8.3). These fracture types are also called "seatbelt fractures" or, eponymously, Chance fractures. The posterior column is always involved and the middle and anterior column is commonly involved. The instantaneous axis of rotation, or hinge, is created anteriorly to the spine as the abdomen is compressed around an object such as a seatbelt. The fracture may occur through the bone of the vertebral body (AO type B2) or through the ligamentous elements, including the intervertebral disk (AO type B1).[15] Of these two injury patterns, the ligamentous injury is less stable. There is a less common pattern of injury in which the anterior longitudinal ligament is disrupted, in addition to the posterior and middle columns (AO Classification B3[15]). These injuries usually require an impact with significant energy to the abdomen and commonly result from violent trauma, prompting need for thorough assessment by physical examination and imaging of the visceral organs for other injury.

8.3.4 Fracture Dislocations

Fracture dislocations (AO type C[15]) involve disruption of the entire spinal column along the horizontal axis; they are inherently unstable and are generally associated with the highest-energy

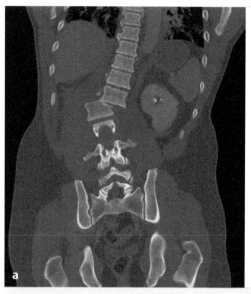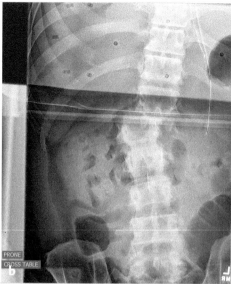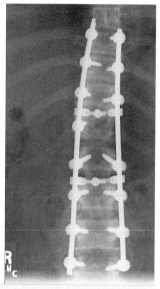

Fig. 8.4 Case illustration of a 75-year-old male who presents with complete acute spinal cord injury after being hit by a motorcycle, resulting in a T12-L1 fracture dislocation injury. **(a)** Pre-operative CT coronal reconstruction showing the dislocation. The T12 vertebral body is dislocated laterally onto L1 with complete disruption of the disco-ligamentous structures. **(b)** Intra-operative AP radiograph showing the dislocation prior to reduction. **(c)** Intra-operative AP radiograph showing the reduction and stabilization with four levels of fixation above and below the injury site.

injuries. These injuries most commonly occur at the thoracolumbar junction, because the juxtaposition of the stiffer thoracic spine and the relatively mobile lumbar spine creates a site that is prone to shear forces. These injuries are associated with a very high risk of injury to the spinal cord, and they most commonly occur at the thoracolumbar junction. In these cases, the dislocation may result in severe deformity of the spinal column in multiple planes. The spine is often rotated and translated as a result of these fractures (▶ Fig. 8.4). Injuries to surrounding visceral organs are also common.

8.4 Treatment Options

For all fractures, treatment options include nonoperative and operative options. A major consideration in the older patient is the morbidity of surgery and the potential complications of surgery. In this patient group, the sequelae of chronic illness such as hypertension, diabetes, obesity, cancer, and osteoporosis all play a role in the decision-making process. Elderly patients may be deconditioned at baseline with poor nutrition, a low level of activity, and poor cardiopulmonary reserve. As such, sometimes surgery is not considered an option, even in the most severe fracture types, due to the patient's underlying medical and functional status. Having an understanding of fracture classification schemes, the mechanism of injury, and the biomechanics of a disrupted spinal column are all essential, but the decision to operate does not necessarily follow a flow-chart diagram in most cases, and reliance on dogmatic algorithms is not recommended.

8.4.1 Nonoperative Treatment

Most thoracic and thoracolumbar spine fractures are stable and do not require surgery. Historically, prolonged bed rest was advised, but bracing is currently a mainstay of conservative management.[20,21,22,23,24] External support may be provided with an over-the-counter brace or a molded orthotic device. These devices permit early ambulation, which is preferred to prolonged bed rest.[21] In some cases, no external support is necessary, and conservative management focuses on pain control and rehabilitation.[24] Even injuries with up to 70% compromise of the spinal canal may not require surgery.[21,24,25,26]

8.4.2 Operative Treatment

While there is consensus regarding the role of conservative management in these simple and stable fractures, some studies suggest that these injuries might benefit from surgery.[27] To help guide surgical decision-making, the angle of kyphosis at the fracture site should be assessed and monitored. Over time, settling may occur and cause the angle of kyphosis at the fracture site to worsen. This has been shown, however, not to correlate consistently with pain.[20,21,23,24,28,29] Surgery should be considered if the angle of kyphosis worsens by more than 10°, or if pain increases significantly.[30] While some flexion-distraction injuries may be eligible in younger patients for conservative management—particularly if the fracture is through the bone—in the aging population, conservative management is less suitable. Fracture-dislocation injuries are by definition unstable and require surgery. In cases in which nonoperative treatment —bracing or casting— is appropriate, operative treatment may still be helpful for those who cannot tolerate months of immobility in an orthosis.[31] In these cases, operative management may allow for earlier mobilization and engagement with rehabilitation while maximizing decompression and alignment.

Here, we discuss nonoperative and operative treatment options for each of the four major categories of thoracic fractures.

8.4.3 Compression Fractures

Most compression fractures can best be managed by nonoperative treatment. The standard treatment is bed rest with encouragement for early mobilization. External support with over-the-counter braces or individually molded orthotics has been and continues to be commonly used. However, there is some evidence that these devices are being used less frequently, and strong evidence that their benefit is lacking.[30]

Operative treatment for compression fractures include minimally invasive augmentation techniques using vertebral cement, namely vertebroplasty and kyphoplasty. In vertebroplasty, a needle is used to inject cement under pressure into the collapsed vertebral body. In kyphoplasty, a balloon is used to expand the collapsed vertebra and create a space for the cement to be injected into.

The most recent guidelines released by the American Academy of Orthopedic Surgeons (AAOS) in 2011 strongly recommend against the use of vertebroplasty.[32] Kyphoplasty is recommended if patients continue to experience severe pain after undergoing 6 weeks of nonoperative management.

8.4.4 Burst Fractures

Burst fractures are considered stable if the posterior ligamentous complex is preserved. If the posterior ligamentous complex is not preserved, or if any neurologic deficit is present, the fracture is likely unstable, and surgery is generally indicated. The ligamentous complex can be imaged with MRI. However, many factors impact the decision to pursue surgery, including the location of the fracture, the degree of vertebral destruction, neurologic involvement, the degree of kyphosis, and the stability of the posterior column. In burst fractures, neurologic involvement is usually caused by retro-pulsed bony fragments impinging upon the spinal canal. However, these fragments can resorb and do not usually cause progressive worsening of neurologic function; moreover, the canal itself can remodel after the fracture, creating a new space for the cord to occupy without impingement.[20,21,22,28,33,34,35]

In patients who are neurologically intact and mechanically stable and/or have a TLICS score of 3 or lower, nonoperative management may be used. External support in the form of a brace or orthosis is commonly used and may provide symptomatic relief, though published evidence of their long-term benefit is scarce.

Operative treatment options include decompression and spinal stabilization.[21,24,26,36,37]

Posterior spinal fusion with pedicle screw fixation and no decompression may be used if there is radiologically confirmed injury to the posterior ligamentous complex or progressive kyphosis without significant compression of the spinal canal.

Anterior decompression of the fracture and spinal stabilization may be used, depending on the degree of vertebral body damage, the extent of spread of fracture fragments, and the angle of kyphosis. If neurologic deficits are present and attributable to vertebral fragments retro-pulsed into the canal, an anterior approach facilitates direct visualization and removal of these fragments. However, in elderly patients, the morbidity of anterior transthoracic or combined retroperitoneal approaches may not be justified. In these patients, especially those with osteoporosis, posterior fixation is preferred, as multiple points of fixation for instrumentation is readily available through a standard posterior approach. As such, several levels above and below the fracture level can be stabilized. Laminectomy can also be performed at the same time through the same incision.

8.4.5 Flexion-Distraction

Flexion-distraction injuries predominantly affect elements of the posterior ligamentous complex furthest away from the anterior-based hinge, and commonly require decompression and stabilization. However, in patients who are neurologically intact and have stable injuries with an intact posterior column, nonoperative management may be attempted. In these cases, external support may be used, such that the spine is supported in extension.

For patients with neurologic deficits, unstable injury patterns, and/or disruption of the posterior ligaments, surgery is indicated with both decompression and stabilization. During the procedure, the canal needs to be visualized directly or with ultrasound to ensure that no fragments are pushed into the canal during surgery. More recently, anterior approaches have been developed.[38,39] To correct the distraction effect of the original injury, a compression strut graft may be used to bring the bony element together and promote union.

8.4.6 Fracture-Dislocation

Fracture-dislocation injuries are unstable, have disrupted ligamentous elements, and require surgery. Operative treatment is superior to nonoperative treatment.[40,41,42] A posterior approach is recommended, followed by reduction, multilevel instrumentation, and fusion. Most fractures of this type can be treated with a posterior approach alone, and anterior approaches are generally not needed. Anterior approaches increases the risk for cerebrospinal fluid fistula into the thoracic or retroperitoneal space.

8.4.7 Minimally Invasive Approaches

There has been increased interest in a growing number of minimally invasive approaches for several currently open procedures. The potential advantages of minimally invasive techniques are reduced postoperative pain, more cosmetically pleasing outcomes, lower periods of immobility, earlier return to activity and ambulation, and potentially decreased duration and dosage of pain medicine.[43]

Importantly, full visualization of the surgical site is increasingly achievable with minimally invasive techniques. Left-sided anterior approaches are generally superior to right-sided approaches, as they do not require elevation of the right hemidiaphragm. Corpectomy, discectomy, decompression, and canal clearance are also all possible.[5,44,45] Bone grafting and cage placement can be achieved with laterally placed supplemental screws. As comfort with minimally invasive techniques has increased, attempts have been made at performing posterior fixation via percutaneous screw placement without fusion, and some studies have found that this approach may be as effective as traditional open approaches with fusion.[46,47,48,49,50]

8.5 Benefits and Risks

The benefits of surgery for thoracic and thoracolumbar fractures include symptomatic relief and the restoration of functional status and natural anatomy. Surgery can often decrease pain and reduce compression of the spinal canal and nerve root foramina. Decompression may relieve neurologic deficit and increase chance of recovery of function. Surgery and instrumentation are also used to provide stability to the fracture site, and prevent worsening of deformity and neurologic deficit.

The risks of any surgery are significant and need to be considered thoughtfully in the decision-making process. In this patient population, the medical co-morbidities may be prohibitive as these patients typically are treated for chronic medical illnesses.

8.6 Pitfalls, Complications And Avoidance

With surgery, postoperative complications can occur despite careful patient selection and detailed operative planning. These include deep vein thrombosis, pulmonary embolism, urinary tract infections, pneumonia, and surgical site infections. Neurologic injury is possible, and may result from trauma to the cord during surgery, excess distraction or compression during fixation, or directly from instrumentation. Similarly, dural tears and cerebrospinal fluid leaks may be created during surgery, particularly during exposure, decompression, and instrumentation.

8.6.1 Compression fractures

The increased angle of kyphosis caused by vertebral compression fractures may affect pulmonary function, with each level of fracture further reducing the functional capacity of the lungs. Compression fractures in elderly patients typically show signs of further collapse within the first several weeks of injury despite bracing. Further loss of height may lead to kyphosis and further pain.

With both vertebroplasty and kyphoplasty, the predominant concern is extravasation of the cement, which can cause a multitude of symptoms depending on the location of the extravasation, and migration of the cement.[51,52] Extravasation of cement into the spinal canal may lead to neurologic injury. Rare cases have been reported of cement entering the cardiopulmonary system.[1,53,54] Kyphoplasty may present less risk of extravasation, because a cavity is created before introduction of cement, allowing the cement to be introduced at lower pressure and higher viscosity.[55,56,57]

8.6.2 Burst Fractures

If the posterior aspect of the vertebral body is retro-pulsed into the spinal canal, the spinal cord may be compressed and injured. Burst fractures may be accompanied by other spine fractures, particularly lamina fractures, which may be associated with dural tear and entrapped nerve roots. In addition to the complications associated with compression fractures, the complications associated with senile burst fractures may include varying degrees of compromise of neurologic function, including paraplegia. Interestingly, the degree to which the spinal canal is involved has not been shown to correlate consistently with the degree of neurologic deficit, however, there is some evidence that narrowing of the canal as determined by axial CT may correlate with an increased risk of presenting with a neurologic deficit.

The risks of pedicle screw fixation include instrumentation failure, pseudo-arthrosis, infection, and need for removal.[21,29,58,59,60] It is also possible that the patient's pain will not be improved, or that the exacerbated natural kyphosis of the thoracic spine may continue to worsen despite operative intervention. Instrumentation failure is an issue and can lead to even more pain for the patient. Osteoporosis does not necessarily affect the ability for the patient to fuse and form new bone around the instrumented levels, but it does affect the purchase and grip of the implants to the bone.

8.6.3 Flexion-Distraction

Decompression and stabilization of flexion-distraction injuries is accompanied by many of the same potential complications as operative treatment for burst fractures. These include pain and worsening spinal deformity including kyphosis, flat back, and scoliosis. Given the pattern of injury, flexion-distraction injuries are particularly prone to nonunion after surgery. Hence it is important to ensure adequate compression by the instrumentation used.

8.6.4 Fracture-Dislocation

Fracture-dislocation injuries have a severe pattern of injury that is particularly prone to causing neurologic injury. In addition to the common complications associated with other thoracic spine fractures— pain, worsening deformity— cauda equina syndrome is a concern.

8.7 Outcomes/Evidence

The outcomes for operative treatment remain controversial, because the majority of available studies are retrospective, and the few prospective studies have small sample sizes. Outcomes seem similar for operative vs. nonoperative management of stable burst fractures. There does seem to be some value in stabilization, but the type of stabilization is unclear. Nonoperative management seems to be effective in most but not all mechanically stable fractures.[22,24,61,62,63] Some factors seem to predict complication rates, including ASIA score, Charlson comorbidity index, and use of steroids.[64] And there is an increasing amount of evidence that minimally invasive procedures may achieve similar results as open procedures.

8.7.1 Compression

The current AAOS guidelines recommend strongly against vertebroplasty for compression fractures.[31] In a study of 78 patients, vertebroplasty did not outperform a sham procedure in pain reduction, physical functioning, quality of life, or perceived improvement at 1 week or at 1, 3, or 6 months.[65] In a multicenter trial of 131 patients who underwent vertebroplasty and a control group that underwent a simulated procedure without cement, both experienced similar improvements in pain and pain-related disability.[66] One prospective 2-year trial found that percutaneous vertebroplasty might provide slightly better pain control at 6 weeks, but not at 12 and 24 months after surgery.[67] Voormolen et al also found some benefit in pain reduction in the immediate short term (2 weeks) after vertebroplasty, but this trial did not assess outcomes after 2 weeks.[68] Rousing et al also found no difference in pain reduction between vertebroplasty and conservative treatment at 3 months.[69]

There is limited evidence in favor of kyphoplasty for compression fractures.[31] In *Lancet*, Wardlaw et al found that balloon kyphoplasty provided moderate benefits relative to conservative management at 12 months in pain reduction, functional status, and quality of life.[70] Grafe et al looked specifically at patients with osteoporosis and also found reduced pain, improved mobility, and lower incidence of additional fracture at 12 months.[71] Other studies have confirmed the benefits in pain reduction compared to nonoperative treatment.[72,73] The symptomatic complication rates and rates of cement leakage for kyphoplasty are superior to those for vertebroplasty.[74,75,76,77,78]

8.7.2 Burst

Since the 1980s, anterior approaches have been developed and evolved to be comparable to more traditional posterior approaches.[79,80,81] Anterior approaches allow for direct visualization of the fracture, which may facilitate more complete removal, followed by restoration of the anterior column by bridging with bone graft or a cage. Several studies have found that these anterior approaches are as effective as posterior approaches, achieve similar or better outcomes in terms of complication rates, reconstruction of the anterior column, shorter operating times, and clinical outcomes.[30,34,37,82,83] For unstable burst fractures, both anterior and posterior approaches have been shown to be effective.[2]

8.7.3 Minimally Invasive Approaches

As minimally invasive approaches have become more widespread, interest in outcomes has increased. One series of 212 patients published by Kim et al found a 90% fusion rate, a mean surgical time of 3.5 hours, and 1.4% conversion rate to open procedures.[43] The overall complication rate was 12%. The rate of complications attributable to the endoscopic technique was 5.7%; these complications included pneumothorax, intercostal neuralgia, and pleural effusions. Another study of 371 patients by Khoo et al found an average surgical time of 3 hours and an overall complication rate of 1.3%.[84] At this point, there does not seem to be a clear long-term difference in outcomes between traditional and minimally invasive techniques.

8.8 Conclusion

Surgery continues to provide significant benefits for certain thoracic and thoracolumbar fractures in the aging population. In particular, unstable fractures that may be associated with neurologic deficit, deformity, and pain are particularly amenable to surgical treatment. Flexion-distraction injuries and fracture-dislocation injuries are very commonly candidates for surgical treatment, while compression fractures and some burst fractures may be stable and not cause neurologic deficit and can be managed conservatively with analgesics, bracing, medication, and physical therapy. Careful consideration of medical co-morbidities is essential in this patient population.

Key References

[1] Magerl F, Aebi M, Gertzbein SD, Harms J, Nazarian S. A comprehensive classification of thoracic and lumbar injuries. Eur Spine J. 1994; 3(4):184–201

[2] Vaccaro AR, Lehman RA, Jr, Hurlbert RJ, et al. A new classification of thoracolumbar injuries: the importance of injury morphology, the integrity of the posterior ligamentous complex, and neurologic status. Spine. 2005; 30(20): 2325–2333

[3] Vaccaro AR, Zeiller SC, Hulbert RJ, et al. The thoracolumbar injury severity score: a proposed treatment algorithm. J Spinal Disord Tech. 2005; 18(3): 209–215

[4] Wood KB, Li W, Lebl DR, Ploumis A. Management of thoracolumbar spine fractures. Spine J. 2014; 14(1):145–164

[5] Rechtine GR, II. Nonoperative management and treatment of spinal injuries. Spine. 2006; 31(11) Suppl:S22–S27, discussion S36

[6] Esses SI, McGuire R, Jenkins J, et al. The treatment of symptomatic osteoporotic spinal compression fractures. J Am Acad Orthop Surg. 2011; 19(3):176–182

References

[1] Kim DH, Vaccaro AR. Osteoporotic compression fractures of the spine; current options and considerations for treatment. Spine J. 2006; 6(5):479–487

[2] Verlaan JJ. Introduction to the surgical treatment of traumatic thoracolumbar fractures. In: Verlaan JJ, ed. Less invasive surgical treatment of traumatic thoracolumbar fractures. Utrecht, The Netherlands: UMC Utrecht: Zuidam & Uithof; 2004:9–24

[3] Dai LY, Yao WF, Cui YM, Zhou Q. Thoracolumbar fractures in patients with multiple injuries: diagnosis and treatment-a review of 147 cases. J Trauma. 2004; 56(2):348–355

[4] Diaz JJ, Jr, Cullinane DC, Altman DT, et al. EAST Practice Management Guideline Committee. Practice management guidelines for the screening of thoracolumbar spine fracture. J Trauma. 2007; 63(3):709–718

[5] Rampersaud YR, Annand N, Dekutoski MB. Use of minimally invasive surgical techniques in the management of thoracolumbar trauma: current concepts. Spine. 2006; 31(11) Suppl:S96–S102, discussion S104

[6] Gertzbein SD. Scoliosis Research Society. Multicenter spine fracture study. Spine. 1992; 17(5):528–540

[7] Levine AM, McAfee PC, Anderson PA. Evaluation and emergent treatment of patients with thoracolumbar trauma. Instr Course Lect. 1995; 44:33–45

[8] Nelson HD, Haney EM, Dana T, Bougatsos C, Chou R. Screening for osteoporosis: an update for the U.S. Preventive Services Task Force. Ann Intern Med. 2010; 153(2):99–111

[9] Holdsworth FW. Diagnosis and treatment of fractures of the spine. Manit Med Rev. 1968; 48:13–15

[10] Holdsworth F. Fractures, dislocations, and fracture-dislocations of the spine. J Bone Joint Surg Am. 1970; 52(8):1534–1551

[11] Denis F. The three column spine and its significance in the classification of acute thoracolumbar spinal injuries. Spine. 1983; 8(8):817–831

[12] Whang PG, Vaccaro AR, Poelstra KA, et al. The influence of fracture mechanism and morphology on the reliability and validity of two novel thoracolumbar injury classification systems. Spine. 2007; 32(7):791–795

[13] Oner FC, Ramos LM, Simmermacher RK, et al. Classification of thoracic and lumbar spine fractures: problems of reproducibility. A study of 53 patients using CT and MRI. Eur Spine J. 2002; 11(3):235–245

[14] Wood KB, Khanna G, Vaccaro AR, Arnold PM, Harris MB, Mehbod AA. Assessment of two thoracolumbar fracture classification systems as used by multiple surgeons. J Bone Joint Surg Am. 2005; 87(7):1423–1429

[15] Magerl F, Aebi M, Gertzbein SD, Harms J, Nazarian S. A comprehensive classification of thoracic and lumbar injuries. Eur Spine J. 1994; 3(4):184–201

[16] Vaccaro AR, Lehman RA, Jr, Hurlbert RJ, et al. A new classification of thoracolumbar injuries: the importance of injury morphology, the integrity of the posterior ligamentous complex, and neurologic status. Spine. 2005; 30(20): 2325–2333

[17] Vaccaro AR, Zeiller SC, Hulbert RJ, et al. The thoracolumbar injury severity score: a proposed treatment algorithm. J Spinal Disord Tech. 2005; 18(3):209–215

[18] Lenarz CJ, Place HM. Evaluation of a new spine classification system, does it accurately predict treatment? J Spinal Disord Tech. 2010; 23(3):192–196

[19] Cohen D, Feinberg P. Secondary osteoporotic compression fractures after kyphoplasty. American Academy of Orthopedic Surgeons Meeting; February 5–9, 2003; New Orleans, LA: Poster no. P312

[20] Weinstein JN, Collalto P, Lehmann TR. Thoracolumbar "burst" fractures treated conservatively: a long-term follow-up. Spine. 1988; 13(1):33–38

[21] Wood K, Buttermann G, Mehbod A, Garvey T, Jhanjee R, Sechriest V. Operative compared with nonoperative treatment of a thoracolumbar burst fracture without neurological deficit. A prospective, randomized study. J Bone Joint Surg Am. 2003; 85-A(5):773–781

[22] Mumford J, Weinstein JN, Spratt KF, Goel VK. Thoracolumbar burst fractures. The clinical efficacy and outcome of nonoperative management. Spine. 1993; 18(8):955–970

[23] Cantor JB, Lebwohl NH, Garvey T, Eismont FJ. Nonoperative management of stable thoracolumbar burst fractures with early ambulation and bracing. Spine. 1993; 18(8):971–976

[24] Shen WJ, Shen YS. Nonsurgical treatment of three-column thoracolumbar junction burst fractures without neurologic deficit. Spine. 1999; 24(4):412–415

[25] Yi L, Jingping B, Gele J, Baoleri X, Taixiang W. Operative versus non-operative treatment for thoracolumbar burst fractures without neurological deficit. Cochrane Database Syst Rev. 2006; 4(4):CD005079

[26] Yazici M, Atilla B, Tepe S, Calisir A. Spinal canal remodeling in burst fractures of the thoracolumbar spine: a computerized tomographic comparison between operative and nonoperative treatment. J Spinal Disord. 1996; 9(5):409–413

[27] Siebenga J, Leferink VJM, Segers MJM, et al. Treatment of traumatic thoracolumbar spine fractures: a multicenter prospective randomized study of operative versus nonsurgical treatment. Spine. 2006; 31(25):2881–2890

[28] Dai LY, Jiang SD, Wang XY, Jiang LS. A review of the management of thoracolumbar burst fractures. Surg Neurol. 2007; 67(3):221–231, discussion 231

[29] Rechtine GR, II. Nonoperative management and treatment of spinal injuries. Spine. 2006; 31(11) Suppl:S22–S27, discussion S36

[30] Wood KB, Li W, Lebl DR, Ploumis A. Management of thoracolumbar spine fractures. Spine J. 2014; 14(1):145–164

[31] Wood KB, Bohn D, Mehbod A. Anterior versus posterior treatment of stable thoracolumbar burst fractures without neurologic deficit: a prospective, randomized study. J Spinal Disord Tech. 2005; 18 Suppl:S15–S23

[32] Esses SI, McGuire R, Jenkins J, et al. The treatment of symptomatic osteoporotic spinal compression fractures. J Am Acad Orthop Surg. 2011; 19(3):176–182

[33] Mehta JS, Reed MR, McVie JL, Sanderson PL. Weight-bearing radiographs in thoracolumbar fractures: do they influence management? Spine. 2004; 29(5):564–567

[34] Dai LY. Remodeling of the spinal canal after thoracolumbar burst fractures. Clin Orthop Relat Res. 2001(382):119–123

[35] Korovessis P, Baikousis A, Zacharatos S, Petsinis G, Koureas G, Iliopoulos P. Combined anterior plus posterior stabilization versus posterior short-segment instrumentation and fusion for mid-lumbar (L2-L4) burst fractures. Spine. 2006; 31(8):859–868

[36] Leferink VJ, Keizer HJ, Oosterhuis JK, van der Sluis CK, ten Duis HJ. Functional outcome in patients with thoracolumbar burst fractures treated with dorsal instrumentation and transpedicular cancellous bone grafting. Eur Spine J. 2003; 12(3):261–267

[37] McLain RF. Functional outcomes after surgery for spinal fractures: return to work and activity. Spine. 2004; 29(4):470–477, discussion Z6

[38] Sasso RC, Renkens K, Hanson D, Reilly T, McGuire RA, Jr, Best NM. Unstable thoracolumbar burst fractures: anterior-only versus short-segment posterior fixation. J Spinal Disord Tech. 2006; 19(4):242–248

[39] Okuyama K, Abe E, Chiba M, Ishikawa N, Sato K. Outcome of anterior decompression and stabilization for thoracolumbar unstable burst fractures in the absence of neurologic deficits. Spine. 1996; 21(5):620–625

[40] Fehlings MG, Perrin RG. The timing of surgical intervention in the treatment of spinal cord injury: a systematic review of recent clinical evidence. Spine. 2006; 31(11) Suppl:S28–S35, discussion S36

[41] Fehlings MG, Perrin RG. The role and timing of early decompression for cervical spinal cord injury: update with a review of recent clinical evidence. Injury. 2005; 36(2) Suppl 2:B13–B26

[42] Fehlings MG, Tator CH. An evidence-based review of decompressive surgery in acute spinal cord injury: rationale, indications, and timing based on experimental and clinical studies. J Neurosurg. 1999; 91(1) Suppl:1–11

[43] Lee MC, Coert BA, Kim SH, Kim DH. Endoscopic techniques for stabilization of the thoracic spine. In: Vaccaro AR, Bono CM, eds. Minimally invasive spine surgery. New York, NY: Informa Healthcare USA; 2007:189–202

[44] Kim DH, Jahng TA, Balabhadra RSV, Potulski M, Beisse R. Thoracoscopic transdiaphragmatic approach to thoracolumbar junction fractures. Spine J. 2004; 4(3):317–328

[45] Beisse R. Video-assisted techniques in the management of thoracolumbar fractures. Orthop Clin North Am. 2007; 38(3):419–429, abstract vii

[46] Palmisani M, Gasbarrini A, Brodano GB, et al. Minimally invasive percutaneous fixation in the treatment of thoracic and lumbar spine fractures. Eur Spine J. 2009; 18(1) Suppl 1:71–74

[47] Lowery GL, Kulkarni SS. Posterior percutaneous spine instrumentation. Eur Spine J. 2000; 9(1) Suppl 1:S126–S130

[48] Wild MH, Glees M, Plieschnegger C, Wenda K. Five-year follow-up examination after purely minimally invasive posterior stabilization of thoracolumbar fractures: a comparison of minimally invasive percutaneously and conventionally open treated patients. Arch Orthop Trauma Surg. 2007; 127(5):335–343

[49] Logroscino CA, Proietti L, Tamburrelli FC. Minimally invasive spine stabilisation with long implants. Eur Spine J. 2009; 18(1) Suppl 1:75–81

[50] Wang ST, Ma HL, Liu CL, Yu WK, Chang MC, Chen TH. Is fusion necessary for surgically treated burst fractures of the thoracolumbar and lumbar spine?: a prospective, randomized study. Spine. 2006; 31(23):2646–2652, discussion 2653

[51] Barr JD, Barr MS, Lemley TC, McCann RM. Percutaneous polymethylmethacrylate vertebroplasty for pain relief and spinal stabilization. Spine. 2000; 25:923–928

[52] Garfin SR, Hardy N. Treatment of vertebral compression fractures. Spine. 2001; 26:1511–1515

[53] Farahvar A, Dubensky D, Bakos R. Perforation of the right cardiac ventricular wall by polymethylmethacrylate after lumbar kyphoplasty. J Neurosurg Spine. 2009; 11(4):487–491

[54] Choe DH, Marom EM, Ahrar K, Truong MT, Madewell JE. Pulmonary embolism of polymethyl methacrylate during percutaneous vertebroplasty and kyphoplasty. AJR Am J Roentgenol. 2004; 183(4):1097–1102

[55] Verlaan JJ, Oner FC, Dhert WJ. Anterior spinal column augmentation with injectable bone cements. Biomaterials. 2006; 27(3):290–301

[56] Bono CM, Sanfilippo J, Garfin SR. Kyphoplasty for the treatment of osteoporotic compression fractures. In: Vaccaro AR, Bono CM, eds. Minimally invasive spine surgery. New York, NY: Informa Healthcare USA; 2007:315–25

[57] Rhyne A, III, Banit D, Laxer E, Odum S, Nussman D. Kyphoplasty: report of eighty-two thoracolumbar osteoporotic vertebral fractures. J Orthop Trauma. 2004; 18(5):294–299

[58] Benson DR, Burkus JK, Montesano PX, Sutherland TB, McLain RF. Unstable thoracolumbar and lumbar burst fractures treated with the AO fixateur interne. J Spinal Disord. 1992; 5(3):335–343

[59] Verlaan JJ, Diekerhof CH, Buskens E, et al. Surgical treatment of traumatic fractures of the thoracic and lumbar spine: a systematic review of the literature on techniques, complications, and outcome. Spine. 2004; 29(7):803–814

[60] Acosta FL, Jr, Aryan HE, Taylor WR, Ames CP. Kyphoplasty-augmented short-segment pedicle screw fixation of traumatic lumbar burst fractures: initial clinical experience and literature review. Neurosurg Focus. 2005; 18(3):e9

[61] Knight RQ, Stornelli DP, Chan DP, Devanny JR, Jackson KV. Comparison of operative versus nonoperative treatment of lumbar burst fractures. Clin Orthop Relat Res. 1993(293):112–121

[62] Kraemer WJ, Schemitsch EH, Lever J, McBroom RJ, McKee MD, Waddell JP. Functional outcome of thoracolumbar burst fractures without neurological deficit. J Orthop Trauma. 1996; 10(8):541–544

[63] Dai LY, Jiang LS, Jiang SD. Conservative treatment of thoracolumbar burst fractures: a long-term follow-up results with special reference to the load sharing classification. Spine. 2008; 33(23):2536–2544

[64] Dimar JR, Fisher C, Vaccaro AR, et al. Predictors of complications after spinal stabilization of thoracolumbar spine injuries. J Trauma. 2010; 69(6):1497–1500

[65] Buchbinder R, Osborne RH, Ebeling PR, et al. A randomized trial of vertebroplasty for painful osteoporotic vertebral fractures. N Engl J Med. 2009; 361(6):557–568

[66] Kallmes DF, Comstock BA, Heagerty PJ, et al. A randomized trial of vertebroplasty for osteoporotic spinal fractures. N Engl J Med. 2009; 361(6):569–579

[67] Diamond TH, Bryant C, Browne L, Clark WA. Clinical outcomes after acute osteoporotic vertebral fractures: a 2-year non-randomised trial comparing percutaneous vertebroplasty with conservative therapy. Med J Aust. 2006; 184(3):113–117

[68] Voormolen MH, Mali WP, Lohle PN, et al. Percutaneous vertebroplasty compared with optimal pain medication treatment: short-term clinical outcome of patients with subacute or chronic painful osteoporotic vertebral compression fractures. The VERTOS study. AJNR Am J Neuroradiol. 2007; 28(3):555–560

[69] Rousing R, Andersen MO, Jespersen SM, Thomsen K, Lauritsen J. Percutaneous vertebroplasty compared to conservative treatment in patients with painful acute or subacute osteoporotic vertebral fractures: three-months follow-up in a clinical randomized study. Spine. 2009; 34(13):1349–1354

[70] Wardlaw D, Cummings SR, Van Meirhaeghe J, et al. Efficacy and safety of balloon kyphoplasty compared with non-surgical care for vertebral compression fracture (FREE): a randomised controlled trial. Lancet. 2009; 373(9668):1016–1024

[71] Grafe IA, Da Fonseca K, Hillmeier J, et al. Reduction of pain and fracture incidence after kyphoplasty: 1-year outcomes of a prospective controlled trial of patients with primary osteoporosis. Osteoporos Int. 2005; 16(12):2005–2012

[72] Kasperk C, Hillmeier J, Nöldge G, et al. Treatment of painful vertebral fractures by kyphoplasty in patients with primary osteoporosis: a prospective nonrandomized controlled study. J Bone Miner Res. 2005; 20(4):604–612

[73] Majd ME, Farley S, Holt RT. Preliminary outcomes and efficacy of the first 360 consecutive kyphoplasties for the treatment of painful osteoporotic vertebral compression fractures. Spine J. 2005; 5(3):244–255

[74] Bouza C, López T, Magro A, Navalpotro L, Amate JM. Efficacy and safety of balloon kyphoplasty in the treatment of vertebral compression fractures: a systematic review. Eur Spine J. 2006; 15(7):1050–1067

[75] Hulme PA, Krebs J, Ferguson SJ, Berlemann U. Vertebroplasty and kyphoplasty: a systematic review of 69 clinical studies. Spine. 2006; 31(17):1983–2001

[76] Eck JC, Nachtigall D, Humphreys SC, Hodges SD. Comparison of vertebroplasty and balloon kyphoplasty for treatment of vertebral compression fractures: a meta-analysis of the literature. Spine J. 2008; 8(3):488–497

[77] Taylor RS, Taylor RJ, Fritzell P. Balloon kyphoplasty and vertebroplasty for vertebral compression fractures: a comparative systematic review of efficacy and safety. Spine. 2006; 31(23):2747–2755

[78] Lee KA, Hong SJ, Lee S, Cha IH, Kim BH, Kang EY. Analysis of adjacent fracture after percutaneous vertebroplasty: does intradiscal cement leakage really increase the risk of adjacent vertebral fracture? Skeletal Radiol. 2011; 40(12):1537–1542

[79] Kaneda K, Abumi K, Fujiya M. Burst fractures with neurologic deficits of the thoracolumbar-lumbar spine. Results of anterior decompression and stabilization with anterior instrumentation. Spine. 1984; 9(8):788–795

[80] Beisse R, Mückley T, Schmidt MH, Hauschild M, Bühren V. Surgical technique and results of endoscopic anterior spinal canal decompression. J Neurosurg Spine. 2005; 2(2):128–136

[81] Been HD. Anterior decompression and stabilization of thoracolumbar burst fractures by the use of the Slot-Zielke device. Spine. 1991; 16(1):70–77

[82] Hitchon PW, Torner J, Eichholz KM, Beeler SN. Comparison of anterolateral and posterior approaches in the management of thoracolumbar burst fractures. J Neurosurg Spine. 2006; 5(2):117–125

[83] Graziano GP. Cotrel-Dubousset hook and screw combination for spine fractures. J Spinal Disord. 1993; 6(5):380–385

[84] Khoo LT, Beisse R, Potulski M. Thoracoscopic-assisted treatment of thoracic and lumbar fractures: a series of 371 consecutive cases. Neurosurgery. 2002; 51(5) Suppl:S104–S117

9 Lumbar Fractures

Carli Bullis, Lauren Simpson, and Khoi D. Than

Abstract

Lumbar spine fractures are among the most common spinal ailments of the aging spine. This is a particularly important problem now, as the elderly population of the United States is rapidly growing. Healthcare costs and hospitalizations for lumbar spine fractures have increased significantly over the past several years. These fractures include compression fractures, burst fractures, chance fractures and, most severely, fracture-dislocation injuries. These fractures are complicated by common comorbidities of the aging spine, such as osteopenia, osteoporosis, diffuse idiopathic skeletal hyperostosis (DISH), and ankylosing spondylitis (AS). Treatment options vary, depending on fracture type and stability, as well as spinal and systemic comorbidities. For stable fractures, conservative management with pain medication, physical therapy, and possibly bracing may be sufficient. More severe fractures may require treatment including kyphoplasty or vertebroplasty, spinal decompression surgeries, percutaneous or open spinal fusions, or even large deformity correction surgeries. Surgery has heightened risks in older adults, but conservative therapy is associated with secondary complications of prolonged immobilization while the injury heals. This chapter will give an overview of common fractures in older adults, as well as treatment modalities and associated risks.

Keywords: Aging spine, lumbar spine fractures, lumbar spine, spine fractures, osteoporosis

---

Key Points

- Increasing aging population is leading to an increase of lumbar spine pathology requiring specialized treatment.
- Osteoporosis is a very common problem that requires nuanced conservative and surgical management.
- With age, bone density decreases, leading to compression of the vertebral body, kyphotic changes in the lumbar spine, and higher rates of fracture.
- Kyphoplasty and vertebroplasty are minimally invasive ways to improve pain and restore bone height in osteoporotic compression fractures.
- When fusion is required, percutaneous pedicle screw placement is often effective and leads to less blood loss, decreased hospital stay, and a trend toward decreased operative time.

9.1 Epidemiology

Lumbar spine fractures are among the most common diagnoses facing spine surgeons as they evaluate and manage today's increasing aging population in the United States. Over the past 5 years, there has been a 17% increase in hospitalizations for lumbar spine fractures. This has been associated with a 24% increase in spinal fusions for lumbar fractures and a 15% increase in hospital charges. For lumbar spine fractures in 2007 alone, there were an estimated 13,000 kyphoplasty/vertebroplasty procedures associated with a total national bill of $450 million. The health care expenditure associated with lumbar spine fractures in totality that year exceeded $1 billion. Given this common and expensive condition, it is prudent to understand lumbar spine fractures in the aging population.[1]

In addition to the economic impact, the recent opioid epidemic has given rise to a new focus on pain management. Most lumbar spine fractures experienced by older adult patients are stable, but they can be quite painful. Finding appropriate pain management options that both respect the medical comorbidities of the patients and decrease the reliance on opioid medications has become increasingly important. There has been a recent increase in minimally invasive management options to treat pain from lumbar spine fractures, which will be highlighted in this chapter.

The goals of treatment for lumbar spine fractures are to reduce pain, prevent further spinal disease and fractures, create stability, and ultimately to increase mobility. This chapter will discuss the biomechanics behind lumbar spine fractures and the treatment options, ranging from medical management to spinal fusions.

9.2 Biomechanical Considerations

The fundamental biomechanics of the spinal column change over the course of a lifetime. Age-related degenerative change, including osteoarthritis, osteoporosis, facet joint arthropathy, and disc dehydration, lead to decreased flexibility, decreased range of motion, and loss of normal physiologic spinal alignment. The accumulation of these changes impacts each region of the spinal column differently. The cervical spine, for example, is most susceptible to uncovertebral joint hypertrophy due to its high degree of mobility. The lumbar spine is more susceptible to compression fractures due to decreased bone mineral density in the setting of increased load bearing from the rostral spine.[2,3]

Many age-related microscopic changes in cartilage and tendinous attachments increase susceptibility to injury, thus predisposing the elderly population for lumbar spine fractures. Cartilage shock-absorbing capacity decreases due to fewer functional proteoglycans that maintain water binding within the tissue. Age-related cartilage stiffness is further promoted by fibrous protein cross-linking. Furthermore, the intervertebral disk avascular matrix relies on transport metabolites, which decrease with age due to millions of load cycles over the course of a lifetime.[4]

The aging population has a high prevalence of low bone mineral density, osteopenia, and osteoporosis. With age comes degeneration of bone density. In the endplates, this causes increased vascularity and subchondral edema, which is seen as Modic type changes on MRI. This causes disruption in the permeability of the intervertebral disks and decreased nutrient transport. The weakening of the endplate leads to concavity, resulting in a more convex shape of the intervertebral disk. The cortex of the bone, however, only carries 10% of the stress of the vertebral body. A larger portion is carried by the inner cancellous bone, which derives its strength from the small bony trabeculae within it. The compressive strength of the vertebral body is exponentially related to the bone mineral density. As a result, small decreases in bone mineral density with age cause a substantial decrease in the vertebral body strength. This is what leads to the degeneration and bony pathology that is so prevalent in the older adults.[3]

9.3 Common Injury Types

9.3.1 Compression

Compression fractures are the most common spinal injury in patients with osteoporosis.[1] The degenerating bone mineral density gives a decreased resistance to compressive forces. Because of the applied forces to the spine in an anterior direction, these compression fractures classically cause anterior wedging. Over time, this causes a loss of lordosis, or even kyphosis, in the lumbar spine.[5] Though these injuries are often stable, they can cause significant pain and spinal deformity. Mild compression fractures can be treated with bracing. This can both help pain and prevent further kyphosis.[6] Vertebroplasty and kyphoplasty are also treatment options, and kyphoplasty can even restore some of the vertebral body height. More extensive fusion surgeries are reserved for very severe and unstable cases. These treatment options will be highlighted later in the chapter.

9.3.2 Burst

Burst fractures are compression fractures that extend through both the anterior and posterior endplates. In other words, on the Denis 3-column classification, they disrupt the anterior and middle columns.[7] Like compression fractures, they are caused by axial loading injury. Those that are stable can be treated conservatively with bracing. Unstable injuries with severe compression, deformity, or ligamentous injury, can be treated surgically in a variety of ways. Fusions, usually extending one level above and one level below the injury, can be performed from the anterior, posterior, or combination approach. Percutaneous instrumentation can be a less invasive surgical option. The hardware acts as an internal brace, allowing the fracture to heal and mobility to be maintained.[7] Severe burst fractures may protrude posteriorly and cause compression of the surrounding neural structures. Rarely, this may lead to neurologic deficits. In such cases, a decompression of the spinal canal is required.

Fracture Dislocation/Chance

Fracture dislocations and chance fractures occur from severe flexion events and represent the most severe types of injury to the lumbar spine. Chance fractures were originally described as osseous injuries that involved a horizontal fracture through the spinal column and neural arch at a single level. We now know that they are often associated with ligamentous injury and can in fact involve more than a single level. They are flexion/distraction injuries, and are most commonly found around the thoracolumbar junction. The classically described mechanism is a car accident, where the seatbelt acts as a fulcrum for flexion. According to a study by Chu et al, 30 to 80% of chance fractures involve intra-abdominal injuries, and 25% have associated spinal cord injury.[8] Purely osseous chance fractures may be treated conservatively with a brace in the absence of neurologic deficits, distraction injury, or comminution. When ligamentous injury is involved, operative intervention is required. This can often be achieved with percutaneous fusion to act as an internal brace while the injury heals.[8]

Spine fractures with distraction or dislocation are very severe injuries that have high rates of neurologic deficits. The risk of these fractures is higher in patients with ankylosing spondylitis (AS), due to increased lever arm from autofusion. With distraction, the facet joints are disrupted, and may become perched or jumped. For both distraction and dislocation injuries, spinal fusions are required to stabilize the spine. The type of fusion can vary and depends on the location in the spine and the fracture type. The important point regarding these fractures is that they are all inherently unstable and require urgent intervention.

9.3.3 Comorbidities – DISH, Ankylosing Spondylitis

AS is the most common spondyloarthropathy seen by spine surgeons. The disease is characterized by an inflammatory process that leads to progressive autofusion of the spine. This causes stiffening and angulation, and manifests in patients with progressive back pain and disability as the disease progresses. The classic "bamboo spine" appearance on imaging refers to the fusion process that takes place in the anterior and posterior endplates. It is also common to have fusion within the posterior column of the spine. The segments of autofusion within the spine lead to a long lever arm that predisposes these patients to fractures from even minor trauma. The disease affects 0.1 to 0.2% of the U.S. population and is more common in men than women, with a ratio of 3:1. Patients with the disease are more than twice as likely to be on disability than the general population. They are also more likely not to have been married or to be divorced, and women with the disease are more likely to not have children.[9]

Diffuse idiopathic skeletal hyperostosis (DISH) is a noninflammatory process of ossification of the spinal ligaments. This affects the anterior longitudinal ligament most profoundly, and while AS begins with the sacroiliac (SI) joint, DISH generally does not involve the SI joint. DISH was considered a relatively benign disease in the past, but with further studies, the disease is associated with many complications, which will be discussed later in the chapter.[10]

9.4 Treatment Options

Generally, conservative therapy should be pursued in those patients who have stable injuries and are neurologically intact. Conservative therapy involves medication for pain relief, physical therapy, bracing, and calcium supplementation. Instability and neurologic deficits from compression of nerve roots, conus medullaris, or cauda equina need to be dealt with surgically.[11] For the aging population, invasive treatment modalities—such as vertebral augmentation, decompressive surgery, or fusions—come with increased operative risks. This population generally has medical comorbidities that can pose potential problems to the patient undergoing general anesthesia. The standard concerns of neurologic deficits, hardware failure, bleeding, and infection also come with these procedures. For the elderly, it can be more difficult to recover from these complications. Osteoporosis also poses an increased concern of hardware failure due to a lack of quality bone to provide hardware purchase. Because of these issues, conservative therapy is preferred in patients who get adequate pain relief with these measures.

9.4.1 Conservative Therapy

Pain Relief

Pain in the setting of an acute compression fracture is typically managed with narcotic medication. In the aging population, it is very important to closely manage the dosing and duration of such medication. Epidural steroid injections can be considered if the pain is still not well controlled with medication.

Another source of pain in patients with compression fractures is radicular pain from pressure on the exiting nerve root. This will follow a typical dermatomal distribution. It is treated initially with antiinflammatory medication and narcotics, if necessary. If the pain is still not well controlled, then a selective transforaminal epidural steroid injection can be considered.[12]

Chronic pain can be treated with anticonvulsant or antidepressant medication. Tricyclic antidepressants are the most studied of these medications. They act by blocking the reuptake of norepinephrine and serotonin. Gabapentin and pregabalin are also very effective medicines for neuropathic pain.

9.4.2 Physical Therapy

Physical therapy has been shown to help people with osteoporotic compression fractures in a number of ways. It can improve posture, help maintain bone mineral density, train the patient to avoid painful triggers, and decrease the risk of further falls. Core exercise is an integral part of physical therapy and helps to strengthen the back extensor muscles. In patients with kyphotic deformity from wedge compression fractures, posture and sagittal alignment is improved and pain is decreased.[12]

Bracing

Braces are a common treatment modality for patients with osteoporotic compression fractures. They function to limit flexion and decrease the load on the anterior column. In creating stability for the spine, they also promote healing and decrease pain. A thoracolumbosacral orthosis, or TLSO brace, is very commonly used for the treatment of stable fractures, particularly osteoporotic compression fractures. There is also literature to support their use in stable burst fractures (those with less than 30° kyphosis, less than 50% loss of vertebral height, and less than 50% canal narrowing from retropulsion).[6] These braces should have at least three points of fixation and put the patient into a small amount of relative extension. Many advocate for obtaining X-rays every 4 to 6 weeks during the healing process to monitor. The braces are generally worn for 8 to 12 weeks, depending on how rapidly the fracture has healed.

Calcium Supplementation

There are multiple modalities of calcium augmentation. Nasal calcitonin is a commonly used supplement. In addition to its antiresorptive effect, it also has an analgesic effect.[1] Medications such as alendronate and risedronate function to prevent calcium resorption. Teriparatide is a newer medication that functions to promote bone formation through direct stimulation of osteoblasts. Park et al studied the use of teriparatide vs. antiresorptive medications in women with single level osteoporotic compression fractures. They found that the compression fractures in both groups of the study progressed with collapse of the injured vertebral body. The degree of collapse, however, was significantly less in the group treated with teriparatide. These patients had less height loss in the anterior and middle columns and also had significantly less kyphosis and lower wedge angle than the group treated with antiresorptive medications.[13]

Vertebroplasty and Kyphoplasty for Osteoporotic Compression Fractures

Vertebroplasty and kyphoplasty are two methods for bone augmentation for patients with vertebral compression fractures (VCF). In the past, treatment for VCFs consisted of open surgery or conservative treatment. The development of both vertebroplasty and kyphoplasty offered an alternative option that was percutaneous and less morbid than surgery. The rates of both procedures increased significantly after their inception in the early 1990s.

Vertebroplasty is the injection of cement into the fracture percutaneously without any attempt to restore height of the vertebral body. Kyphoplasty involves the inflation of a balloon in the fracture to create a cavity. The balloon is then withdrawn and cement is injected into the cavity. Some of the arguments in favor of vertebroplasty are that it is less expensive and may cause less alteration of pressure on adjacent levels, and hence less risk of adjacent level disease. Arguments in favor of kyphoplasty are that it poses less risk of cement embolism (as the cement is contained inside a cavity), and it also gives the ability for some degree of height restoration (▶ Fig. 9.1, ▶ Fig. 9.2).

For both procedures, fluoroscopic guidance is used to pass a large bore needle (typically 11–13-gauge) through the pedicle

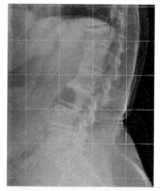
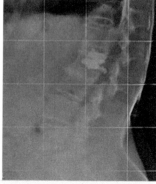

Fig. 9.1 An 85-year-old female presented with 1 year of lower back pain. Radiographs revealed an L2 anterior wedging compression fracture (left). She underwent kyphoplasty at L2 (right). Her pain subsequently resolved.

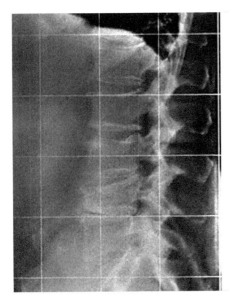

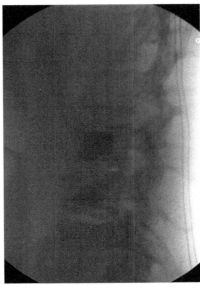

Fig. 9.2 A 65-year-old male presented with pain in his lower back and left lower extremity. He was found to have L3 and L4 compression fractures. He underwent kyphoplasty at both levels. Imaging showed restoration of height, and he had resolution of his lower back and leg pain.

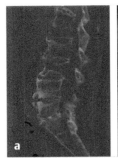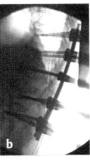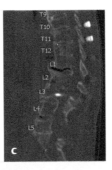

Fig. 9.3 A 76-year-old female with an L1 extension-distraction injury underwent T11-L3 posterior percutaneous instrumentation. Postoperatively, her fracture healed, and she remained neurologically intact. Her hardware was eventually removed. **(a)** Preoperative CT demonstrating the L1 extension-distraction fracture. **(b)** Intraoperative radiograph demonstrating screw placement and reduction of fracture. **(c)** Postoperative CT demonstrating healed L1 fracture.

into the affected vertebral body. In the case of vertebroplasty, barium-opacified polymethylmethacrylate (PMMA) is injected into the fracture until it fills the fracture to oppose the endplates anteriorly and posteriorly.

9.5 Surgical Management

In some cases of lumbar spine fractures, such as those that are unstable or those causing neurologic compromise, surgical spinal fusion is indicated. Patients requiring operative intervention are generally those with fractures resulting in greater than 30° local kyphosis, greater than 50% loss of vertebral body height, or those in which greater than three contiguous levels are involved.[6] Denis's 3-column model is often used to assess for instability. In this model there are three vertical columns within the spine. The anterior column consists of the anterior longitudinal ligament, anterior annulus fibrosis, and the anterior two-thirds of the vertebral body. The middle column consists of the

posterior longitudinal ligament, the posterior annulus fibrosis, and the posterior one-third of the vertebral body. The posterior column consists of the pedicles, facet joints, lamina, spinous processes, and posterior ligaments. If at least two of the three columns of the spine are injured, that segment of the spine is considered unstable.[14] These patients generally require surgical intervention.

As previously mentioned, the medical comorbidities that aging patients have may preclude them from open surgery. Minimally invasive approaches may help decrease blood loss, hospital stay, postoperative pain, and complication rates.[15,16] Minimally invasive techniques involve the percutaneous placement of pedicle screws with the aid of intraoperative imaging and fluoroscopy or stereotactic guidance, as shown in ▶ Fig. 9.3. This allows for smaller incisions and less muscle dissection than open procedures.[17] Studies have shown no statistical difference in neurologic outcomes between the minimally invasive and open approaches. Minimally invasive instrumentation functions as an internal brace to give the fracture time to heal on its own. It is therefore generally reserved for bony fractures that will likely heal with time.[15] Using this form of internal fixation, as opposed to orthotic braces and conservative management, allows the patient to mobilize sooner. This can prevent deconditioning and deep venous thrombosis related to bed rest. It may also decrease the amount of postoperative opioids required.[16]

Kyphotic deformities often result from compression fractures. When this causes intractable pain, severe disability, pulmonary function impairment, or progressive neurologic deficits, open surgical correction with fusion may be required (▶ Fig. 9.4). In elderly patients, this is generally done from a posterior-only approach, if possible, with pedicle screws and rods. This allows for less blood loss and less operative time than a combined anterior-posterior approach. The fusion construct encompasses the area of hyperkyphosis. The upper end of the construct for these deformities will be in the thoracic spine. The region of T5–8, which is the natural kyphotic apex, is avoided because ending a fusion at the apex results in high rates of proximal junctional kyphosis. Because of this, the upper limit of

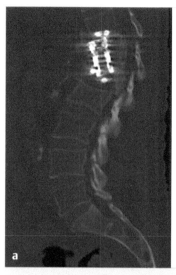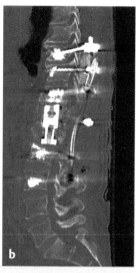

Fig. 9.4 A 60year-old man with a history of a T12 compression fracture, for which he had undergone a prior T12 corpectomy and stand-alone T11-L1 interbody fusion, subsequently developed a fracture and focal kyphotic deformity at L1, resulting in severe back pain and an inability to walk. He underwent an open posterior fusion from T9-L3, including vertebroplasty for pedicle screw augmentation at each level, as well as laminectomies from T11-L3, right T12 costotransversectomy, right T11 and L1 facetectomies, transpedicular corpectomies at T12 and L1, and cage placement spanning from T11-L2. Post operatively, good correction of his deformity was achieved, he had a significant reduction in his back pain, and he became independently mobile.

the construct is usually below T10 or, in higher deformities, between T2 and T5. The lower limit of the fusion has been described by Smith et al as being the sagittal stable vertebra (SSV). This is the vertebral body that first encounters a vertical line drawn from the posterior superior point of the sacrum.[18]

9.6 Benefits and Risks

9.6.1 Conservative

Pain Medication

This population is even more susceptible than younger patients to the cognitive effects of opioid medications, which could lead to further falls and resulting injury, not to mention the usual risks of addiction, nausea, constipation, and respiratory depression.[12] Inflammatory processes causing pain are not typically well controlled by narcotic medication; non-steroidal antiinflammatory medications typically work better for this type of pain. These also come with side effects, most typically being nausea, gastritis, and resulting ulcers.

Gabapentin and amitriptyline come with the side effect of drowsiness and should be titrated up and down when starting and stopping.

Bracing

Keeping patients in braces for too long can also have a negative impact. They can create pressure sores and resultant infection,

and dependence on them can lead to weakening of the axial musculature. The rigidity around the abdomen can lead to decreased lung capacity. There is also an inherent risk of noncompliance and worsening of the fracture, as the braces can be taken off and on.[6]

Older adults are very susceptible to both osteoporotic compression fractures and burst fractures. There is a large amount of literature regarding the treatment of burst fractures, particularly with TLSO. Many advocate for stable burst fractures (AO class A3 and better) to be treated with TLSO braces. As 10 to 20% of all thoracolumbar fractures are burst fractures, the ability to undergo conservative treatment as opposed to surgical treatment can pose a large economic benefit. Wood et al, in a randomized prospective study that controlled for fracture severity and patient disability, found that those patients with burst fractures treated with bracing had a shorter hospital stay and had a cost nearly 4.4 times less than those treated surgically.[11]

Vertebral Augmentation

In the past decade, there has been increasing concern over vertebral augmentation-related complications, including venous embolization, pulmonary cement embolism, cement compression of neurological structures, and adjacent segment fractures. Despite these complications, vertebroplasty, and more often kyphoplasty, are frequent modes of treatment for osteoporotic compression fractures. As previously mentioned, there is less associated blood loss, shorter hospital stay, positive pain reduction, and less anesthetic risk than in open procedures.[1]

Surgical Intervention

Surgical intervention for fractures can prevent worsening or new neurological injuries and also prevent further vertebral body collapse and associated deformity. Patients with unstable fractures have a high risk of neurologic deficit without operative intervention to stabilize their area of injury. In these cases, the benefit of preventing neurologic deterioration generally outweighs the risk of associated medical comorbidities with surgery. Patients with severe compression fractures are slightly more of a grey area in terms of medical decision-making. Without intervention, these patients may develop further collapse of their vertebrae and even kyphotic deformity of the lumbar spine. These patients may benefit from a minimally invasive vertebral augmentation procedure.[1]

Surgical intervention in the aging population comes with risks of complications due to medical comorbidities, and also has a higher cost than nonoperative management. Many of these patients have cardiac and respiratory comorbidities that put them at an increased risk for anesthesia. In terms of the surgical outcomes themselves, there are also risks. Osteoporosis makes fusion more difficult, as there is less bone surface area for screw purchase and thus a higher rate of screw loosening, fractures related to hardware placement, and adjacent segment disease.[19] The cost associated with surgery, as well as vertebroplasty and kyphoplasty, is higher than that of nonoperative management. Goldstein et al found that patients in their study who underwent vertebral augmentation had an overall cost of $26,074, and those who underwent conservative management without augmentation had an average cost of $15,507.[1]

9.7 Pitfalls, Complications and Avoidance

9.7.1 Progressive Kyphosis/Pain

Kyphotic deformity and resulting pain can be an unfortunate progression of degenerative changes and compression fractures, particularly in the setting of osteoporosis. As previously mentioned, kyphoplasty and vertebroplasty have been shown to decrease pain and prevent further vertebral body collapse. Kyphoplasty may even restore vertebral body height.[20] A more conservative approach of bracing and physical therapy may also be chosen in mild cases to prevent further deformity and decrease pain. For severe kyphotic deformities, larger procedures involving posterior osteotomies and fusion may be necessary.[18]

9.7.2 Instrumentation Pullout in the Setting of Osteoporosis

As previously mentioned, osteoporosis leads to poor bone quality and therefore poses a difficulty with spinal instrumentation. The low bone mineral density can lead to pedicle screw pullout or loosening and ultimately hardware failure with posterior instrumentation. With anterior instrumentation, screw pullout and graft subsidence can occur from repetitive cyclic loading. Some of the techniques to mitigate the risk of hardware failure in osteoporotic spines are using larger diameter screws, increasing the points of fixation, adding crosslinks, or bolstering the screws with bone cement. Larger diameter screws provide additional surface area for contact with the bone, which can increase pullout resistance.[21] From a posterior approach, which is most commonly used, additional points of fixation can be achieved through increasing the number of instrumented levels superiorly or inferiorly, or adding double fixation points to levels with the use of hooks and wires.[19,21] Adding crosslinks has been shown to increase the pullout strength of pedicle screws, but that benefit is decreased in the osteoporotic spine. There is also an association with crosslinks and pseudarthrosis, the risks of which may outweigh the benefit of decreased pullout risk. Cement, such as poly(methyl methacrylate), can also be used to increase the hardware strength. This can be done by injecting cement into a pilot hole followed by the screw, injecting the cement through a cannulated screw, or by performing a traditional vertebroplasty or kyphoplasty followed by pedicle screw placement. The cement spreads out the stress of the screw through the bone, decreasing the stress on individual trabeculae.[21,19]

Different screw modalities have also been developed to help increase pullout resistance of pedicle screws. These include screws with a conical shape, expandable screws, and screws that are coated with a thin layer of hydroxyapatite. Conical screws increase the surface area of the screw in contact with the bone.[19] Studies have shown increase in the insertional torque strength, but not an increase in the pullout resistance.[22,23] Screws that have a component that expands in the vertebral body have been shown to increase pullout strength by as much as 50%. That is further increased with the combined use of bone cement. These screws also have a decreased rate of loosening.[24]

Screws that have a thin layer of hydroxyapatite have also been shown to increase pullout strength up to 60%. One downside is that they can be extremely difficult to remove during revision surgery.[19]

Variations in screw insertional technique are also used in osteoporotic bone. Small pilot holes, undertapping the screw tract, bicortical fixation, and hubbing the screws have all been shown to increase screw strength. The use of smaller pilot holes suggests that a small drill bit may be preferable to a rongeur for this step. Bicortical fixation is commonly used. This can be done in pedicle screws by inserting the screw all the way to the anterior endplates. Hubbing the screws, or inserting them until the head abuts the dorsal cortical bone, may prevent "windshield wipering" of the screw through thin osteoporotic bone.[19]

Compression fractures may also be treated with interspinous process spacers. This offers a less invasive alternative to open fusion. The spacer allows for opening of the neural foramen, increased diameter of the spinal canal in extension, and unloading of the facet joints, and it does not increase the rate of adjacent level disease. The device does create a slight flexion at the inserted level. This can cause increased stress anteriorly and could lead to an increase in the compression of the vertebral body. These spacers have been shown, however, to decrease pain resulting from compression fractures.[25]

9.7.3 Unrecognized DISH/AS

AS and DISH are both disorders that affect the aging population, and worsen over time. AS is a rheumatic inflammatory disease closely associated with human leukocyte antigen (HLA)-B27. Most patients (about 80%) will have onset of symptoms before the age of 30. This generally begins in the SI joint.[10] DISH is not an inflammatory disorder, but the definitive cause is not known. Symptom onset is usually after the age of 50.[26] These patients develop ossification of the spinal ligaments, particularly the anterior longitudinal ligament (ALL), and do not usually have SI joint dysfunction.[10]

AS and DISH are closely associated with chance fractures and spinal cord injury. The long lever arm caused by the autofusion that takes place in the diseases causes a greater amount of rotational force in flexion or extension events. This can lead to severe fractures (commonly chance fractures) and spinal cord injury after even relatively minor trauma. The cervical spine is most often affected in these disorders, but fractures of the lumbar spine and corresponding neurologic deficits are also common.[27] Even in the absence of trauma, dysphagia, hoarse voice, and difficult intubations can be complications of the disease process itself.[27]

Aside from the complications from the trauma itself, iatrogenic complications occur in these disorders as well. The ossification of the PLL in DISH can lead to inadvertent dural violation and CSF leak in anterior surgeries.[28] This can make treatment more difficult, and in some cases, it might be necessary to avoid an anterior approach altogether in favor of a posterior fusion. Turning and positioning these patients in the operating room must be done with extreme caution. These patients often have central canal stenosis from hyperostosis, and their fractures are often very unstable. Awkward bending and twisting during turning and positioning processes can cause neurologic injury in and of themselves.[27]

Both AS and DISH patients have higher rates of morbidity and mortality from the disorders themselves compared to the rest of the population. The diseases are even attended by often-overlooked social difficulties. As previously mentioned, these patients are more likely to be unemployed, unmarried or divorced, and have higher rates of depression. All of this has to be taken into consideration when treating these patients. As the aging population increases, these disorders will become even more common.

9.8 Outcomes/Evidence

9.8.1 Conservative

Vertebral Augmentation

There have been a variety of trials comparing outcomes of kyphoplasty, vertebroplasty, and conservative treatment. Some of the outcomes studied include pain reduction, restoration of mobility, reduction of fracture, and adjacent level fractures.[20,29,30,31] The use of vertebroplasty and kyphoplasty varies significantly among surgeons. Many studies, including randomized controlled trials, have been done, but there is still no absolute consensus on their use.

Pain

Older people with acute VCFs can have severe, debilitating pain as a result. Though the pain generally improves with time, it can take months, and being bedridden during that time can lead to deconditioning and further loss of bone mineral density. Doing vertebroplasty or kyphoplasty early may help patients mobilize earlier and avoid some of the complications associated with decreased ambulation. For those patients whose pain is tolerable and whose mobility is at baseline, it may be better to wait 4 to 6 weeks with conservative therapy prior to considering vertebral augmentation.[32]

Many kyphoplasties are performed because of acute, uncontrolled pain. In 2009, a randomized controlled trial in the *New England Journal of Medicine* compared vertebroplasty to conservative treatment. There were 131 patients total, each with 1 to 3 osteoporotic compression fractures. The fractures were determined by history and imaging to be less than 12 months of age. Sixty-eight of the patients were randomized to vertebroplasty, while 63 patients were randomized to conservative therapy. The vertebroplasty group underwent a standard vertebroplasty. The conservative group had local pain medication injected into the soft tissue and periosteum. The PMMA was opened so that the patient was able to smell it, but no cement was injected. The Roland–Morris Disability Questionnaire (RDQ) was used as the primary outcome measure. At one month, there was no significant difference between the groups; both groups were found to have significant improvement in both disability and pain scores. There was, however, a trend toward improvement of pain in the vertebroplasty group. After one month, patients in both groups were allowed to cross over. By 3 months, 51% of the conservative group and 13% of the vertebroplasty group had crossed over. There was no significant difference between the two groups at the end of the study. Some of the criticism of the study involves the lack of a true control group (as both groups underwent the injection of deep local anesthetic), the admission of patients with questionable acute pathology (fractures up to 1 year of age), and the large amount of crossover between groups. This study resulted in a narrowing of the patient group that was indicated for these procedures. The study had similar pain outcomes to many other trials, showing an improvement with both vertebral augmentation and conservative treatment.

Ledlie et al conducted a retrospective review of kyphoplasty in elderly patients with vertebral compression fractures. This study included 96 patients who underwent balloon kyphoplasty for compression fractures associated with osteoporosis. Outcome measures included pain rated on the visual analog scale (VAS), vertebral body height, and mobility status. Preoperative VAS for all 96 patients was 8.6. Postoperative VAS was 2.7 at 1 week (89 patients), 2.3 at 1 month (85 patients), 2.1 at 3 months (73 patients), 1.5 at 6 months (52 patients), and 1.4 at 1 year (29 patients). Truumees et al performed a literature review in 2004 and found that patients had significant pain relief with vertebral augmentation in a select patient population (those with acute and debilitating pain).[32] Tolba et al did a retrospective review to study the outcomes of 67 patients who underwent single or multilevel kyphoplasty. They found a significant decrease in VAS of 3.9.[30]

Restoration of Mobility

Studies have also shown that patients treated with vertebral augmentation may have earlier mobility and increased ambulation. This is particularly notable in patients whose severe acute pain is the cause of limited mobility. Ledlie et al, in addition to pain and restoration of vertebral body height, found that of the 25 who could not ambulate preoperatively, all were ambulatory at 1 year. It is unclear, however, how much of the pain and mobility improvement was from the natural healing process of the acute fractures vs. the kyphoplasty treatment effect, as there was no control group for comparison.[33] The aforementioned 2009 *NEJM* study also found that there was no significant difference in disability between those treated with vertebroplasty and those in the control group. Both groups had improvement, which also supports that the natural healing process itself may play a significant role in the improvement in mobility and disability.[34]

Reduction of Fracture

Reduction of the osteoporotic compression fractures is one of the benefits of kyphoplasty. VCFs lead to kyphosis, which can then lead to decreased mobility, increased pain, and deconditioning with its associated comorbidities. As ▸ Fig. 9.1, ▸ Fig. 9.2 demonstrate, using the balloon to restore height prior to injecting cement can lead to decreased kyphosis.[32] Ledlie et al found that in 20 patients with 36 fractures who underwent kyphoplasty, the mean anterior vertebral body height increased from 66% preoperatively to 89% at 1 month postoperatively. At 1 year, it remained increased at 85% of expected height.[33] There were a number of other studies that showed an increase in vertebral body height after augmentation with kyphoplasty, including Tolba et al, who showed 45% of height regained.[30] A retrospective review by Lee et al in 2014 showed that the vertebral body height was significantly increased in all osteoporotic compression fractures, no matter the degree of preoperative height loss, both immediately after surgery and at 1 year postop. The kyphotic angle, however, was only decreased immediately after the surgery and not at 1 year postop.[29] Kim et al divided their patients into groups according to fracture shape (wedge, v-shaped, and flat), and found that anterior and middle column height loss, as well as kyphotic angle, was restored with kyphoplasty, but not vertebroplasty. They also found that kyphoplasty had a significantly decreased rate of cement extravasation.[20] While a number of studies have shown at least partial reduction of compression fractures and decreased pain medication intake with kyphoplasty, it is difficult to make a concrete connection between the two outcomes. There are likely multiple factors at play with the clinical improvements seen after vertebral augmentation.

9.9 Surgical Intervention

Surgical intervention may be required in cases of unstable fractures and deformity. This may be done through minimally invasive means or through larger, open incisions. There is evidence to support minimally invasive percutaneous pedicle screw placement in the case of unstable thoracolumbar burst fractures. Lee et al showed that radiologic outcomes were favorable with both percutaneous and open pedicle screw placement, but the percutaneous group had earlier pain relief and functional improvement.[35] Percutaneous pedicle screw placement has also been shown to be effective in the case of chance fractures. Both open and percutaneous screw placements improve kyphotic angulation in these cases, and evidence shows no difference between the two types with regard to neurologic outcome. The minimally invasive procedures are associated with a shorter operative time and significantly less blood loss, which are important factors in the aging population with medical comorbidities.[36]

For patients with symptomatic lumbar stenosis from degenerative changes, there is strong evidence to support decompression alone, rather than decompression and fusion. The 2016 randomized controlled trial in the *New England Journal of Medicine* saw no difference in the outcome between the two groups at 2 and 5 years, regardless of the presence of spondylolisthesis. The study did find, however, that the group with decompression alone had shorter hospital stays, less blood loss, and lower hospital costs.[37]

Osteoporosis poses a significant risk of hardware failure and proximal junctional kyphosis. There are multiple surgical techniques, as were detailed earlier in this chapter, which can help increase screw pullout strength. There is evidence to suggest that multiple levels of fixation increase the pullout strength. The use of cement augmentation, both around the screws and even at the adjacent level, may also be beneficial.[19]

9.10 Conclusion

The median age of the U.S. population is increasing, due to aging of the baby boomer generation. There is a greater push for quality measures and lean healthcare spending to temper the large healthcare expenditure of our country. With all this,

the dependence on opioids continues to grow at an alarming rate. These issues all make responsible care of spinal pathology an important focus in medicine today.

Management of lumbar spine fractures in older adults can be a complex problem, with many factors to consider. Options for treatment include conservative management, minimally invasive procedures (vertebroplasty, kyphoplasty, percutaneous instrumentation), or large, open-fusion surgeries. Conservative management removes the risks associated with surgery, which can be particularly important in the case of multiple medical comorbidities, but comes with its own risks which result from prolonged inactivity and immobilization. Minimally invasive options are often a good middle-of-the-road technique. They can allow for healing of the fracture, decrease pain, and allow for earlier mobilization of the patient. Open surgeries may be required in cases of severely unstable fractures or spinal deformity, but these cases should be addressed with caution, and the patient's medical comorbidities should be carefully analyzed. Osteopenia and osteoporosis can further complicate management in this patient population. These should be screened for prior to treatment, and in the case of operative management, measures should be taken to avoid complications from poor bone quality. These may include increased points of fixation, different screw modalities and trajectories, or the addition of bone cement to the screws.

Key References

[1] Goldstein CL, Brodke DS, Choma TJ. Surgical Management of Spinal Conditions in the Elderly Osteoporotic Spine. Neurosurgery. 2015; 77(4) Suppl 4: S98–S107

[2] Chu JK, Rindler RS, Pradilla G, Rodts GE, Jr, Ahmad FU. Percutaneous Instrumentation Without Arthrodesis for Thoracolumbar Flexion-Distraction Injuries: A Review of the Literature. Neurosurgery. 2017; 80(2):171–179

[3] Garfin SR, Yuan HA, Reiley MA. New technologies in spine: kyphoplasty and vertebroplasty for the treatment of painful osteoporotic compression fractures. Spine. 2001; 26(14):1511–1515

[4] Goldstein CL, Chutkan NB, Choma TJ, Orr RD. Management of the Elderly With Vertebral Compression Fractures. Neurosurgery. 2015; 77(4):S33–S45

[5] Ensrud KE, Schousboe JT, Ph D. Clinical practice. Vertebral fractures. N Engl J Med. 2011; 364(17):1634–1642

[6] Fehlings MG, Tetreault L, Nater A, et al. The Aging of the Global Population: The Changing Epidemiology of Disease and Spinal Disorders. Neurosurgery. 2015; 77(4) Suppl 4:S1–S5

References

[1] Goldstein CL, Chutkan NB, Choma TJ, Orr RD. Management of the Elderly With Vertebral Compression Fractures. Neurosurgery. 2015; 77(4):S33–S45

[2] Fehlings MG, Tetreault L, Nater A, et al. The Aging of the Global Population: The Changing Epidemiology of Disease and Spinal Disorders. Neurosurgery. 2015; 77(4) Suppl 4:S1–S5

[3] Papadakis M, Sapkas G, Papadopoulos EC, Katonis P. Pathophysiology and biomechanics of the aging spine. Open Orthop J. 2011; 5:335–342

[4] Smith JS. The Aging of the Global Population: The Changing Epidemiology of Disease and Spinal Disorders. Neurosurgery. 2015; 77(4):1–5

[5] Old JL, Calvert M. Vertebral compression fractures in the elderly. Am Fam Physician. 2004; 69(1):111–116

[6] Rea GL, Zerick WR. The treatment of thoracolumbar fractures: one point of view. J Spinal Disord. 1995; 8(5):368–382

[7] Aono H, Ishii K, Tobimatsu H, et al. Temporary short-segment pedicle screw fixation for thoracolumbar burst fractures: comparative study with or without vertebroplasty. Spine J. 2017; 17(8):1113–1119

[8] Chu JK, Rindler RS, Pradilla G, Rodts GE, Jr, Ahmad FU. Percutaneous Instrumentation Without Arthrodesis for Thoracolumbar Flexion-Distraction Injuries: A Review of the Literature. Neurosurgery. 2017; 80(2):171–179

[9] Ferhan A. Asghar, Gregory P. Graziano and CKI. Youmans Neurological Surgery. 6th ed. Elsevier Inc; 2011

[10] Teunissen FR, Verbeek BM, Cha TD, Schwab JH. Spinal cord injury after traumatic spine fracture in patients with ankylosing spinal disorders. J Neurosurg Spine. 2017; 27(6):709–716

[11] Chang, Victor MD, Holly, Langston T MD. Bracing for thoracolumbar fractures. Neurosurg Focus. 2014; 37(1):1–7

[12] Prather H, Hunt D, Watson JO, Gilula LA. Conservative care for patients with osteoporotic vertebral compression fractures. Phys Med Rehabil Clin N Am. 2007; 18(3):577–591, xi

[13] Park JH, Kang KC, Shin DE, Koh YG, Son JS, Kim BH. Preventive effects of conservative treatment with short-term teriparatide on the progression of vertebral body collapse after osteoporotic vertebral compression fracture. Osteoporos Int. 2014; 25(2):613–618

[14] Denis F. The three column spine and its significance in the classification of acute thoracolumbar spinal injuries. Spine. 1983; 8(8):817–831

[15] Palmisani M, Gasbarrini A, Brodano GB, et al. Minimally invasive percutaneous fixation in the treatment of thoracic and lumbar spine fractures. Eur Spine J. 2009; 18 Suppl 1:71–74

[16] Mobbs RJ, Park A, Maharaj M, Phan K. Outcomes of percutaneous pedicle screw fixation for spinal trauma and tumours. J Clin Neurosci. 2016; 23:88–94

[17] Raley DA, Mobbs RJ. Retrospective computed tomography scan analysis of percutaneously inserted pedicle screws for posterior transpedicular stabilization of the thoracic and lumbar spine: accuracy and complication rates. Spine. 2012; 37(12):1092–1100

[18] Ailon T, Shaffrey CI, Lenke LG, Harrop JS, Smith JS. Progressive Spinal Kyphosis in the Aging Population. Neurosurgery. 2015; 77(4) Suppl 4:S164–S172

[19] Goldstein CL, Brodke DS, Choma TJ. Surgical Management of Spinal Conditions in the Elderly Osteoporotic Spine. Neurosurgery. 2015; 77(4) Suppl 4:S98–S107

[20] Kim KH, Kuh SU, Chin DK, et al. Kyphoplasty versus vertebroplasty: restoration of vertebral body height and correction of kyphotic deformity with special attention to the shape of the fractured vertebrae. J Spinal Disord Tech. 2012; 25(6):338–344

[21] Choma TJ, Rechtine GR, McGuire RA, Jr, Brodke DS. Treating the Aging Spine. J Am Acad Orthop Surg. 2015; 23(12):e91–e100

[22] Kwok AWL, Finkelstein JA, Woodside T, Hearn TC, Hu RW. Insertional torque and pull-out strengths of conical and cylindrical pedicle screws in cadaveric bone. Spine. 1996; 21(21):2429–2434

[23] Bianco RJ, Arnoux PJ, Wagnac E, Mac-Thiong JM, Aubin CÉ. Minimizing Pedicle Screw Pullout Risks: A Detailed Biomechanical Analysis of Screw Design and Placement. Clin Spine Surg. 2017; 30(3):E226–E232

[24] Cook SD, Salkeld SL, Whitecloud TS, III, Barbera J. Biomechanical evaluation and preliminary clinical experience with an expansive pedicle screw design. J Spinal Disord. 2000; 13(3):230–236

[25] Miller JD, Nader R, Frcs C. Treatment of combined osteoporotic compression fractures and spinal stenosis: use of vertebral augumentation and interspinous process spacer. Spine. 2008; 33(19):E717–E720

[26] Whang PG, Goldberg G, Lawrence JP, et al. The management of spinal injuries in patients with ankylosing spondylitis or diffuse idiopathic skeletal hyperostosis: a comparison of treatment methods and clinical outcomes. J Spinal Disord Tech. 2009; 22(2):77–85

[27] Westerveld LA, Verlaan JJ, Oner FC. Spinal fractures in patients with ankylosing spinal disorders: a systematic review of the literature on treatment, neurological status and complications. Eur Spine J. 2009; 18(2):145–156

[28] Lee SH. Spinal subarachnoid hematoma with hyperextension lumbar fracture in diffuse idiopathic skeletal hyperostosis: a case report. Spine. 2009; 34(18):E673–E676

[29] Lee JH, Lee DO, Lee JH, Lee HS. Comparison of radiological and clinical results of balloon kyphoplasty according to anterior height loss in the osteoporotic vertebral fracture. Spine J. 2014; 14(10):2281–2289

[30] Reda Tolba MD. *, Robert B. Bolash, MD*, Joshua Shroll, MD, MPH†, Shrif Costandi M, Jarrod E. Dalton, PhD§, Chirag Sanghvi, MD*, and Nagy Mekhail, MD P. Kyphoplasty Increases Vertebral Height, Decreases Both Pain Score and Opiate Requirements While Improving Functional Status. Pain Pract. 2014; 14(3):91–97

[31] Krüger A, Baroud G, Noriega D, et al. Height restoration and maintenance after treating unstable osteoporotic vertebral compression fractures by cement augmentation is dependent on the cement volume used. Clin Biomech (Bristol, Avon). 2013; 28(7):725–730

[32] Truumees E, Hilibrand A, Vaccaro AR. Percutaneous vertebral augmentation. Spine J. 2004; 4(2):218–229

[33] Ledlie JT, Renfro M. Balloon kyphoplasty: one-year outcomes in vertebral body height restoration, chronic pain, and activity levels. J Neurosurg. 2003; 98(1) Suppl:36–42

[34] Kallmes DF, Comstock BA, Heagerty PJ, et al. A randomized trial of vertebroplasty for osteoporotic spinal fractures. N Engl J Med. 2009; 361(6):569–579

[35] Lee JK, Jang JW, Kim TW, Kim TS, Kim SH, Moon SJ. Percutaneous short-segment pedicle screw placement without fusion in the treatment of thoracolumbar burst fractures: is it effective?: comparative study with open short-segment pedicle screw fixation with posterolateral fusion. Acta Neurochir (Wien). 2013; 155(12):2305–2312, discussion 2312

[36] Grossbach AJ, Dahdaleh NS, Abel TJ, Woods GD, Dlouhy BJ, Hitchon PW. Flexion-distraction injuries of the thoracolumbar spine: open fusion versus percutaneous pedicle screw fixation. Neurosurg Focus. 2013; 35(2):E2

[37] Försth P, Ólafsson G, Carlsson T, et al. A Randomized, Controlled Trial of Fusion Surgery for Lumbar Spinal Stenosis. N Engl J Med. 2016; 374(15):1413–1423

10 External Orthosis Management

Karen A. Petronis

Abstract

The prevalence of spine fracture in the aging patient has increased. Standard fracture management protocols do not always apply to this population due to vast comorbidities including poor bone quality. Spinal segment immobilization through bracing is an option after a comprehensive analysis of the risks and benefits of the device. The decision to use an orthosis requires consideration of the fracture pattern, biomechanical properties of the device, as well as the patient's unique anatomy, medical and cognitive state. Most importantly when the specific brace is selected the goal of the treatment should be defined, as well as a plan to limit complications and associated risks. Bracing in the elderly has limitations due to the coronal and sagittal changes of the aging spine. Each case needs to be treated uniquely as geriatric fracture treatment protocols are almost impossible to generalize to the population.

Keywords: spinal orthosis, aging spine fracture, osteoporotic compression fracture, brace biomechanics, conservative fracture management

Key Points

- The biomechanical principles of bracing guides the orthosis prescription.
- External orthosis management in the aging population adds increased risk to the patient. This is due to the rigid design of the brace, the unique anatomy of the aging spine, and physiologic changes of aging such as skin fragility.
- Determination of a treatment endpoint is necessary.

10.1 Summary

Use of an external orthosis in the aging patient can be an effective method to immobilize one or more spinal motion segments. Reasons to prescribe an orthosis include: fracture management, ligamentous or muscular soft tissue injury, short-term postoperative mobility restriction and to reduce pain by off loading forces from the injured area and support the soft tissue.

Understanding the biomechanical principles of each brace is the first step in the selection process. Currently available braces do not accommodate the coronal and sagittal degenerative changes that occur in the aging spine.

Following trauma, a comprehensive analysis of the risks and benefits of a particular brace, as well as a frank discussion with the patient and caregivers for a mutually agreed upon treatment decision and goals of care is vital. In the aging patient, the decision to brace is complex and not based solely on the fracture type or pattern. A thorough assessment of the potential complications may outweigh the benefits. Thus, not to brace in certain circumstances may be the best option. When an external orthosis is the mutually agreed upon decision, quick brace

application allows for early mobilization and prevention of complications. Long periods of immobility are poorly tolerated by the older adult. Skin fragility should be assessed at baseline to determine whether patient-specific soft tissue features can tolerate the brace application. The risks need to be recognized with a preemptive plan for prevention. When the decision is made to brace, the goal and treatment endpoint should be determined. By keeping the endpoint in mind with critical reevaluation, one can be certain that the orthosis is performing as predicted. Additional aging comorbidities increase the risks, complicating management and medical decision making.

This chapter will provide details regarding the epidemiology, biomechanical principles of bracing, specific features of the spinal orthoses and a plan to evaluate effectiveness based on aging specific criteria.

10.2 Epidemiology

In the aging population, cervical fractures occur at a higher rate than in any other age group. Lomoschitz et al (2002) retrospectively reviewed 225 cervical spine injuries in 149 patients, who were 65 years of age or older. The population was subdivided into two groups, the "young elderly," those 65 to 75 years of age, and the "old elderly," those greater than 75 years of age. In the young elderly, the main cause of fracture was associated with a motor vehicle accident, as opposed to the old elderly, where the injury occurred as a result of a fall from a standing or seated position. Injury to C2 was the most common injury in both groups.[1,2] Guan et al (2017) described the most prevalent fracture pattern to be associated with a forced hyperextension or hyperflexion mechanism of injury.[2] Finally, there is consensus that with cervical fracture in this age group, there is an associated increase in morbidity and mortality.

Limited age-related data is reported on the epidemiology of thoracolumbar fractures. However, in the aged population, osteoporotic compression fractures are common. As noted in previous chapters, the aging population is growing rapidly, leading to increased incidence of fractures in this group. Osteoporotic compression fractures can be a great source of disability, pain, and societal burden.[3] Osteoporosis is described in further detail in chapter 3.

10.3 Biomechanical Considerations

The goal of a spinal orthosis is to immobilize a specific spinal segment or region. The principles of bracing include the ability to offload forces to the affected spinal segment and to stop or attempt to decrease movement at the level of the impairment. Complete immobilization is impossible to achieve because of the dynamics associated with the spine as well as patient specific variables.

Agabegi, et al (2010) have summarized five primary functions of a brace, each of which contributes towards biomechanical optimization, achieving optimal patient outcome.[4] These functions are to serve as a kinesthetic reminder; to distribute total surface contact; to provide three-point fixation; to supply endpoint control; and to increase pressure or fluid compression.

As a kinesthetic reminder, the brace, when applied, restricts movement and alters the position at the area of impairment, acting as a constant tactile stimulus.[5] This constant stimulus creates a learned sensation with a direct link to the spine pathology. A tighter brace provides a greater association. The presence of the brace in theory may also prompt a conscious decision to avoid high-risk behaviors or activities that would impose increased strain. Conversely, a tight brace can cause discomfort or increased pain, which can then lead to noncompliance. If the brace is poorly fit, too heavy, cumbersome or painful to wear, the compliance will be affected, leading to treatment failure.

Total surface contact is measured by the amount of square footage of the brace that is in contact with the body's surface. This contact produces a force that is applied to the soft tissue as well as underlying bone and muscle. When there is a greater surface area contact, the applied force is less at any one point, and there is better control of motion.[4,5] The front and back of the brace should be conformed tightly to the body and secured to prevent movement. The lack of a secure fit leads to biomechanical failure and skin impairment associated with abnormal motion, shear, and friction.

In the aging population, this principle is important, as many patients have preexisting poor tissue perfusion, are malnourished, or are generally deconditioned. In this case, a brace with a larger surface area would be of benefit, as the force would be shared over larger areas of contact. In addition, by decreasing the pressure at any one point, skin impairment will be less likely. On the other hand, when the contact is over excessive soft tissue, as in the obese or edematous individual, the effectiveness of the brace will decrease. As described by Woodard et al, there is an inverse relationship between the thickness of the soft tissue separating the spine from the inner surface of the orthosis and the resulting effectiveness of the immobilization.[5]

Three-point fixation is a principle well known in long bone fracture management and surgical stabilization. To stop motion at the fracture, immobilization needs to occur at the joints both above and below the defect. In the spine, however, this is not as easy to achieve due to the multiple levels of movable spinal segments as well as the regional variability of the cervical, thoracic and lumbar spine. The goal of this principle is to stop motion by providing two points of pressure applied ventrally, one above and one below the pathology, with the third point midway and dorsal to the site of the fracture, or near the axis of rotation for that segment.[6] The axis of rotation is a fulcrum point whereby the vertebral segment rotates. Therefore, when selecting a brace, it is important that the dorsal support is centered at or near the fractured spinal segment's axis of rotation.

Additionally, the length of the brace also has a bearing on stability. A long brace provides a longer lever arm, which internally offers better immobilization with less force required to resist motion, translation, and rotation.[5] In other words, when the two ventral points of fixation are appropriately distanced, with the third dorsal point midway, less force is required to stop motion, as the distance from the fracture is increased. The two

shorter segments provide increased resistance against bending which results in an overall decreased failure rate.

As mentioned, the fourth function of the orthosis is endpoint control. Mechanically, to manage this principle, the brace needs to be anatomically fixed at the proximal and distal end, to stop movement in the middle. Because the spine has so many moving parts, this is difficult to attain, especially in the cervical occipital and lumbar sacral regions. Standard braces have limitations in achieving a firm hold that stops motion at the head and pelvis due to the anatomical contour and surrounding vital structures. Halo immobilization devices have been described as the best method for cervical immobilization because the cephalad endpoint control is achieved by cranial pin fixation. However, even with halo fixation, endpoint control is limited as noted by the resultant abnormal movement within the cervical spine, creating a "snaking effect."[5]

Benzel describes distraction as an important component in the treatment of deformity.[6] A brace that employs distraction lengthens the spine, by pulling caudally and cephalad to the fracture. This allows the fracture ends to realign and hold an anatomical position. Unfortunately, braces are inefficient in this function because of the limitations in endpoint control. The halo vest may provide the best ability to distract.

Pelvic control using a lumbar brace is by definition unattainable unless there is control of the movement at the lumbar sacral junction and both hips. For adequate endpoint fixation in a lumbar fracture, it has been determined that there needs to be at least four to five vertebral levels immobilized distal to the unstable segment.[6] In the lumbar spine, there are not enough levels or distance to provide this degree of immobilization. Spica type designs attempt to incorporate this concept but are inefficient in that there is still unacceptable movement. In addition, with both hips immobilized, patient management is difficult due to discomfort, skin impairment, toileting concerns, and the inability to sit or ambulate.

Lastly, braces also elevate the tissue pressure surrounding the spine. When a brace is securely tightened around the chest and abdomen, it forces the soft tissue and fluids within the body to compress. Woodard et al[5] describes this mechanically as the creation of a fluid-filled cylinder, which can convert the soft tissue into a load-bearing structure. This cylinder can then circumferentially off-load the forces through the axial spine.[5,6,7] Elevating abdominal pressure results in the restriction of motion in the sagittal plane.[5] Interestingly, studies utilizing tight-fitting lumbar braces in cadaveric models do in fact demonstrate a lowering of the intradiscal pressures.[8] The mechanism of increasing tissue pressure to restrict motion is limited in its effectiveness as compared to other methods and can only be used in the thoracolumbar spine where cavity compression can occur.

10.4 Common Injury Types

The upper cervical spine is the most mobile and the most affected by injury in the aging adult. The aging spine typically demonstrates mid to distal cervical segment degeneration, stiffness, and even arthrodesis from normal wear and tear. Therefore, the upper segments are more susceptible to injury. Specific C2 fractures such as odontoid, lateral mass, or hangman can be treated conservatively in a cervical brace. Jefferson burst fractures and other injuries involving the ring of C1 are also typically deemed stable. Subaxial cervical injuries need to be individually evaluated. Many can be treated in a cervical orthosis. The stability of the joints and ligamentous structures must also be considered. Additionally, comorbidities such as diffuse idiopathic skeletal hyperostosis and osteoporosis increase the risk of fracture instability.

In the thoracic and lumbar spine, osteoporotic compression fractures are frequently encountered. Anterior wedge compression fractures are generally classified as stable. They are typically managed with hyperextension orthoses to prevent flexion, thus offloading the anterior column at the site of the fracture.[9] The brace can also provide a splinting effect, decreasing pain and muscle spasm. Based on the neurologic status, bracing is also utilized for fractures types such as a burst, Chance, or extension injury.

10.5 Treatment Options

Spinal braces are organized by the spinal region they immobilize. They can cover one region or incorporate many. The general classification includes cervical occipital, cervical, cervical thoracic, thoracic, thoracolumbar sacral, and lumbar sacral. Combinations of the different braces can be added to treat the entire spine, cervical through the sacrum. The next section will detail the various spinal orthotic devices commonly used. The goal will be to discuss the strengths and weakness associated with the five biomechanical principles as they pertain to each specific orthotic device and to discuss complications and special considerations with respect to the aging spine.

10.5.1 Cervical Orthosis

The cervical orthosis is designed to control motion through four points of fixation, two cephalad and two caudal. The cephalad points are the chin and mandible anteriorly and the occiput posteriorly. Caudally, the points are the sternum and clavicles anteriorly and the spinous process of the upper thoracic spine, usually T3 posteriorly.[4] There is very little total surface contact; thus, the forces are not dispersed over a large area, but restricted to the points of fixation. The applied force at the four points of fixation is great and can lead to skin impairment. A thorough inspection of baseline integument should be performed before brace selection. The cervical brace can successfully achieve the role of a kinesthetic reminder of the pathology due to the pressure at the fixation points and restriction of movement.

End point control in a standard cervical collar is not attainable at the cervical–cranial or cervical–thoracic junction. The mandible plays a role in point fixation; however, with speaking and, particularly, chewing, motion is realized. Distally the sternum and clavicle provide limited fixation to serve as end point control. Any movement of the arms or shoulders causes a reciprocal action of the clavicle which decreases the effectiveness of motion restriction.[4] In the cervical spine, it is impossible to increase the pressure in the soft tissue through brace compressibility. Pressure to the neck and soft tissues can result in complications associated with constriction of the vascular structures, airway and esophagus.

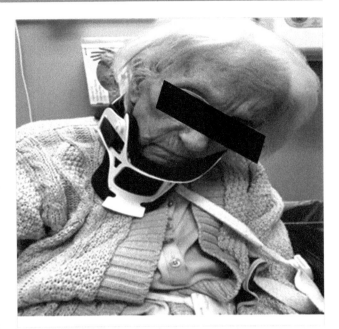

Fig. 10.1 Biomechanical concerns of the cervical collar: lack of endpoint control and excessive lateral bending

The cervical brace is best in restricting motion in the sagittal plane: flexion and extension.[4,5] It performs the worst in rotation and lateral bending due to the minimal control of the mandible. This excessive movement allowed by the collar can be realized by simply observing the aging patient change position, speak and ambulate (▶ Fig. 10.1).

10.5.2 Soft Cervical Collar

The soft foam collars biomechanically provide little resistance to motion; therefore, the role in fracture management is limited.[5] However, some providers feel the soft collar provides enough support when compared to a rigid device for usual activities of daily living.[10] The soft device provides surface contact. However, it provides no point of fixation or endpoint control. The collar can serve as a kinesthetic reminder of the pathology and is lightweight and easy to apply. Comfort is appreciated as the device provides support for the tissues and muscles. The soft designs have various heights; one in particular is 3 inches throughout its entire length (▶ Fig. 10.2). The shorter collar conforms nicely to a kyphotic, cervical spine. The length of the soft collar needs to be addressed, as many standard designs are short, making the fit too tight circumferentially. A collar that can provide up to 20 inches of available length can be fitted to the majority of patients. This is usually tolerated well in patients with a short, thick, kyphotic, or stout neck and one with excessive anterior or posterior soft tissue.

10.5.3 Cervical Thoracic Orthosis

The cervical thoracic orthosis (**CTO**) provides fixation cephalad at the chin/mandible and occiput and caudally at the sternum and thoracic spinous processes/ribs. Some designs offer a head strap that adds better endpoint control. The CTO has adequate

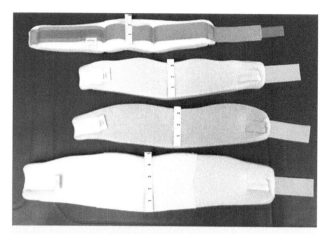

Fig. 10.2 Collar top to bottom: 3 in soft with increased length; small standard soft; medium standard soft; large standard soft.

surface contact; however, compressibility is limited. Motion is best controlled in the sagittal plane with an improved restriction in lateral rotation when compared to the cervical collar.[5] The device is, however, difficult to wear due to the restrictions imposed, causing discomfort and potential for noncompliance.

10.5.4 Halo Vest

The halo vest has been credited with good endpoint control as well as superior immobilization in flexion, extension, lateral bending, and rotation. There is controversy as to which cervical fractures are best managed with halo application. Some feel that this device functions optimally with fractures of the upper cervical spine, or at the cervical–thoracic junction.[5,11] At the mid-cervical region, there is a concern over instability due to the muscle attachments which cause undesired flexion and extension. This instability is described as the "snaking phenomena."[5] Theoretically, the concern for the snaking effect in the elderly may be mitigated because of the advanced degeneration at these middle segments. This age-related factor may provide protection from the abnormal snaking movement.

10.5.5 Thoracic Lumbar Sacral Orthosis

The thoracic spine is stiff, as opposed to the flexible cervical and lumbar regions. Therefore, mobility control needs to be focused on the junctional segments: the cervical thoracic and thoracolumbar regions. Based on the location of the thoracic instability, the closest junction should be immobilized. Literature suggests that injuries above T6 should be managed with a CTO. For injuries below T6, a thoracic lumbar sacral orthosis (TLSO) is recommended. The TLSO is ideal for pathology from T6 to L4. The TLSO provides cephalad points of fixation at the sternum anteriorly and thoraco-lumbar spinous processes posteriorly. Caudally, the pelvis and sacrum provide the points of fixation. Surface contact and compressibility is significant; however, endpoint control is minimal. Three-point bending principles are most times achievable, as the brace has a longer moment arm providing control in lateral bending and to a lesser extent in flexion and extension.[4]

10.5.6 Thoracolumbar Hyperextension Braces

There is a second group of TLSO braces that provide hyperextension. The goal of this category is to offload the anterior vertebral column. This type of brace has been commonly used to treat anterior compression fractures commonly seen in osteoporosis. The goals are similar to those of the standard TLSO braces described above. Extension is realized through the principles of three-point bending. Using the three points of fixation—sternum and pelvis ventrally and thoracic spinous processes dorsal at or near the site of the fracture—creates a force that produces hyperextension. A typical hyperextension orthosis works best in limiting sagittal motion between T10–L2. [2] If the fracture is above T8, the ventral sternal plate should be adjusted cephalad to sit high on the sternum to gain length. Total surface contact and compressibility is limited; however, the length is generally long, providing sufficient lever arm. This brace can create skin impairment at the points of fixation due to the increased pressure and limited total surface contact. Additionally, these devises can be difficult to apply independently, which can lead to poor compliance. Working with an orthotist can help with decision-making and determination of which brace would be most effective. The standard TLSO brace can also be adjusted to provide extension if needed.

Custom Designs

Braces can be custom-molded by the orthotist from molded plastic. The specialty design can better accommodate various body habitus, maximizing total surface contact. Complex or multiple spinal fractures are best served with a unique design to accommodate the instability. A boney Chance or three-column burst fracture may require additional points of fixation. The custom braces are of higher cost and are usually heavy with little flexibility, making application more challenging in the elderly.

10.5.7 Lumbar Sacral Orthosis

The lumbar sacral orthosis (LSO) is designed to control motion from L3 to the sacrum. The LSO seems to provide the best support at L3–4 and is very limited at L4–5 and L5–S1.[5] As discussed, the endpoint control specifically at the lumbar–sacral junction is challenging, if not impossible, to attain. The pelvis contour makes it difficult to achieve point fixation, which is then even further compromised by movement at the hips. The LSO is designed to caudally fix to the anterior pelvis and posterior to the sacrum. Superiorly, there is limited ventral point fixation due to the limitations of the skeletal anatomy. Dorsally, the spinous processes are utilized, as in the TLSO. However, in the lumbar spine, the additional stabilization from the sternum is lost and the 10th, 11th, and 12th ribs provide limited cephalad fixation. The brace imposes a significant restriction in movement and discomfort which can lead to noncompliance.

Compressibility and total contact are the positive aspects of the LSO but again have limitations based on body habitus. The circumferential compression of soft tissue may be the most important part of stabilization in the lumbar spine.[5] Woodard et al (2017) concluded that the TLSO and LSO braces inadequately stabilize individual segments of the lumbar spine, but limit gross motion by altering patient activity.[5] The consequential change in the patient's activity was thought to be the most important mechanism of action. The brace, when properly fit, can also play a role in muscle splinting, with noted modulation of pain.

10.5.8 Lumbar Corset

Given the limitations of the lumbar rigid device, a lumbar corset may be a logical consideration. There are variations in the corset designs, some with features to increase rigidity. However, based on the spinal stability of the patient, the soft elastic binder may be enough. The corset provides some compressibility and muscle support to decrease pain. This device may not provide as rigid a reminder as the LSO, but it does provide a kinetic reminder to decrease trunk motion. The binders are the least expensive, light weight, easily to apply, and can conform to altered alignment. The corset may not be appropriate for all elders but can be considered based on the patient, the pathology and the baseline level of mobility.

Benefits and Risks

The goal of bracing is to stop or minimize motion at the fracture site to allow for optimal healing. Other benefits may include a reduction in pain and possible decrease in high risk behaviors that could lead to secondary injury. The brace as a kinesthetic reminder may alter poor decisions regarding activities that can cause additional harm, such as lifting, bending or climbing.

The risks of bracing are associated with complications and poor endpoint healing results. Long-term effects of prolonged brace wear can lead to deconditioning and increased incidence of skeletal muscle atrophy in the surrounding tissue. The complications associated with bracing are numerous and are discussed in the next section. The most devastating risk of using an orthosis is a decline in neurological status. Frequent evaluation and communication with the patient and or family is needed, so that when changes occur they can be identified quickly. Another risk of bracing is that of treatment failure, as evidenced by nonunion or a poorly healed fracture. This risk is increased in the aged population due to to poor bone quality and preexisting comorbidities that affect bone healing.

10.6 Pitfalls, Complications and Avoidance

10.6.1 Cervical Orthoses

A unique characteristic in the aging cervical and thoracic spine is the alteration of the normal lordotic curve to one of kyphosis.[12] These factors make bracing difficult due to the lack of endpoint control and point fixation associated with the straightening of cervical spine. Standard orthoses are limited in their ability to accommodate the variations from patient to patient. There are a variety of "off the shelf" specialty designs that attempt to account for the stout and/or kyphotic spinal alignment. However, because of the unique patient anatomy, standard braces cannot accommodate the degree of kyphosis and/or potential scoliosis that occurs in the elder spine. Working with

an orthotist can help to provide the best fit for challenging patients.

When the brace is correctly applied, it forces the cervical spine into slight extension. Caution is needed when applying the brace to assess for increased pain or discomfort at the fracture site. As discussed, in the elder there is less motion in the mid and lower cervical spine due to stiffness and potential arthrodesis. Therefore, when the brace is applied, because the distal segments are immobile, the imposed extension may occur at the mobile fracture site. This can then increase the distance between the fracture fragments with potential deleterious effect of worsening the injury. Upright X-rays in the collar can help to confirm fracture reduction and optimal positioning of the fracture fragments.

Another concern regarding the added extension associated with the cervical brace is alteration of the patient's line of vision, limiting the awareness of their immediate environment. Aging patients, who have lost proprioception, rely on visual cues for balance and smooth locomotion. Lack of the ability to look down at their feet can lead to falls and safety concerns. Other deficits in vestibular and somatosensory functions can complicate vertical perception and balance.[4] Many times this instability requires use of a walker or other assistive device. Unfortunately, over time the patient can become dependent on the device making it a permanent adjunct even when brace free. Some acquire increased kyphosis in the thoracic and lumbar spine from leaning forward onto the walker. Consequently, this posture allows for an improved line of vision to counter the effects of the added extension. Evaluation of the patient requiring use of a walker is important to be sure first that it is needed, and then that it is used correctly, to maintain upright posture. The primary goal of the walker should be to reduce falls associated with an alteration in balance and vision.

Skin impairment is a major concern associated with the four points of fixation as well as the tissue at the lateral base of the neck and ears. Pressure from the brace is many times unnoticed due to the patient's lack of sensation or cognition in recognition of the problem. In the acute phase of treatment, it is generally recognized that early removal of the collar decreases the potential for breakdown. Ackland et al (2007) also noted collar removal resulted in fewer ventilator days, decreased ICU stay, decreased length of stay and overall decrease in delirium and pneumonia.[13,14] Data reveals that 6.8% of the ICU patients in a cervical collar for more than 24 hours acquired pressure-related impairment.[15] The probability of a pressure-related skin impairment will increase by 66% for each day in the cervical brace.[14] Infection and risk of sepsis also increase due to skin impairment as well as bodily fluids that collect underneath the device. In this acute phase, based on the fracture pattern and patient condition, continuous use of the collar may not be necessary. Removing the brace when supine can improve tissue perfusion and avoid potential breakdown. If the brace cannot be removed, then use of a pillow back, posterior shell is an option available through some venders. This provides a cushion instead of point fixation at the occiput and spinous processes, which can help with skin impairment at the cost of decreasing the brace's effectiveness. The cushioning is not without risk, as it also provides an environment conducive to moisture formation and shear.

A strategy to reduce pressure-associated complications can be achieved with a liberal brace protocol. This option includes removing the collar when supine or reclined 50°or less. Additionally, allowing the patient to shower without the brace will promote improvement in tissue viability and decrease risk of infection. Aging adults who are alert and can follow directions are able to maintain head alignment with the brace is off. Those with family or social support, who are involved in the patient's care, will add confidence to this decision-making. A liberal protocol can also help reduce muscle deconditioning and stiffness at other cervical motion segments. Prolonged collar utilization can lead to significant loss of motion and even contracture at the fracture site as well as other cervical segments.

Swallowing difficulty while managed in a cervical collar can lead to serious complications. The brace can narrow the pharynx due to the imposed extension. Normal swallowing requires slight flexion. A chin tuck is necessary to facilitate esophageal motility for many aging adults. Choking and aspiration risk, which is a common concern in older individuals, can be made worse with the use of cervical immobilization. Difficulty swallowing leads to dehydration, malnutrition, increase risk of falls, and poor bone healing. If possible, allowing the patient to remove the collar for meals, maintaining a neutral position, may be beneficial. There are adjustments that can be made to the standard cervical brace to decrease the degree of extension by removing padding at the sternal point of fixation. Other options can be explored by collaborating with the orthotist to determine the best brace design and the degree of extension of the anterior shell. This parameter varies among vendors, but a minor alteration in the degree of extension can have significant ramifications related to swallowing function.

10.6.2 Cervical Thoracic Orthosis

Application of the CTO is more challenging, and this should be considered prior to prescribing it for an aging adult. The device can convert a patient who is living independently to one who becomes dependent on others to facilitate brace application. Activities of daily living cannot be overlooked, as an aging adult who lives alone may require family support or a nursing facility to help with daily brace management.

Other specific concerns for CTO use in older individuals include the aforementioned cervical brace risks as well as the thoracic compressibility. The aging patient with thoracic disease poorly tolerates restriction and is at risk for decreased pulmonary capacity. Additionally, those with COPD, have altered body habitus, making the brace application difficult or impossible. The associated barrel chest compromises the ability to achieve adequate points of fixation and makes total contact unattainable.

10.6.3 Halo Vest

While there are proponents for using the halo brace in elderly patients, others feel the complication profile outweighs any benefit.[11,16] Authors have suggested a higher complication rate in patients aged greater than 65 to 70 years.[17] In 2006, Horn et al completed a retrospective review of halo fixation complications specific to those aged 70 years or greater.[16] The authors concluded the device can be used safely. However, they found the rates of serious complications and death to be higher than in younger populations. Although the complication rates may

be correlated to the traumatic or nontraumatic disease process, the authors could not rule out the possibility that the halo vest was the contributing factor. Of the 42 patients followed for three months, 21 had halo alone and 21 had halo plus surgery. There were 31 complications in 23 of the patients, which included, most commonly, respiratory distress, dysphagia, and pin-related complications. However, eight patients died, two from unrelated causes, and the remaining six from respiratory failure or cardiopulmonary collapse. The authors suggest because of the high complication rate, it is difficult to ascertain the contribution of the halo in this age group.[16] Additionally, many authors suggest that there are no significant differences in healing rates between halo immobilization and cervical braces.[2]

Factors to consider when deciding on an immobilization device option should include the impact on the patient's ambulatory ability, any potential alteration in living arrangements, and a thoughtful assessment of associated risks and benefits. Application of the halo on a patient with preexisting sagittal imbalance, i.e., head in front of the pelvis, will place increased stress on the pins and make the posterior shell difficult to fit. Swallowing difficulties are prevalent, leading to suboptimal nutrition and possible aspiration. Pulmonary disease may place the patient at increased risk for respiratory failure. Preexisting conditions such as diabetes and autoimmune disorders can increase the risk for skin impairment and or infection. Finally, bone density data can help to predict potential for cranial pin site complications, such as loosening, migration, or even dural penetration.

10.6.4 Thoracolumbar Orthosis and Lumbar Sacral Orthosis

The TLSO brace is difficult to fit for many reasons associated with body habitus and the common deformities seen in the elderly, again such as kyphosis and scoliosis. Orthoses used in the thoracic and lumbar region are the hardest to manage because of the highly moveable soft tissue. The sternal point of fixation is rarely maintained, especially when the patient changes from supine to sitting or upright posture. Patients may complain of the sternal piece riding more cephalad, which can cause compression of the neck structures. When properly fit, the sternal pad should be stabilized so that with movement, the points of fixation are maintained. To prevent skin impairment, use of a cotton shirt under the brace can absorb perspiration and minimize friction.

The body habitus is an important consideration as to whether the brace will have any effect. If there is excessive tissue or edema, the fixation points will be negated. Conversely, when there is minimal soft tissue or poor integument, there is concern for skin breakdown. Barrel-chested individuals or those with body shapes that are disproportionate, as previously discussed, make finding the proper fit difficult. Ensuring that the brace has total contact is difficult for the same reasons as noted for point fixation. With a deformity (particularly with kyphosis), it may be impossible to provide dorsal support.

Compressibility is possible in the TLSO, which can improve control. However, in the elderly, the degree of compression needs to be cautiously determined, as it may affect breathing and pulmonary capacity. Restricting the abdomen can also comprise GI motility. Additionally, many elders with degenerative scoliotic or kyphotic deformities may not tolerate circumferential compression, thus negating the effectiveness. Finally, the TLSO brace is cumbersome and heavy, which makes it difficult for many elderly patients to handle and properly apply. Reflection of the biomechanical principals and complications should be considered specific to each individual's circumstance. If the goals of the brace are unachievable, other less restrictive options should be considered.

A concern affecting all aged populations with prolonged use of the rigid TLSO or LSO is that of increased lower lumbar sacral pain. This may be a result of lack of endpoint control, whereby the forces in the mid-lumbar spine are offloaded and then increased at the junction. In these circumstances, pain is realized at the L5–S1 region due to increased loading.[18] Clinically, patients will localize pain at the junction as well as over the sacroiliac joints. This pain does not correlate with the fractured spinal level and is most likely the result of the brace. Long-term use can lead to deconditioned paraspinal muscle groups as well as increased stiffness.

In the aging individual, use of a TLSO or LSO can cause progression of an already altered gait. This is particularly true when there is kyphosis and sagittal imbalance. Many older adults because of global instability need to tilt the pelvis forward using the hips and then bend the knees, to achieve the best head position. When the LSO is applied, this adaptive posture is altered, which can affect balance and increase the risk of fall.

Fracture management in the aged population cannot be determined by a standard algorithm. Each patient brings a unique history that impacts this first-line treatment decision-making. The following case studies highlight the difficulties

with management due to the associated bracing risks, pitfalls and complications.

10.6.5 Special Considerations: Knowledge Through Case Examples

The following are four case exemples of the use of spinal orthosis, which demonstrate the complexity of medical decision making, in the aging spine patient.

Case One

One of the most important aspects of providing care to older adults is to determine the plan quickly, to prevent complications of immobility. Following fracture diagnosis, the change in environment and interruption of sleep can lead to confusion and delirium. The following case is an example of a common patient problem, noncompliance.

A 78-year-old female with a history of dementia presented to the emergency department (ED) via ambulance after a fall from a standing height. She arrived alone, unaccompanied by nursing facility staff or family. She complained of neck pain, and a cervical spine CT scan revealed a C7 superior end plate fracture and a left C6 facet fracture. On exam, she was confused, however appropriate with no functional deficit. The patient was immobilized in a rigid cervical collar with the plan to follow up in 2 to 3 weeks. She was discharged back to her long-term nursing facility to familiar environment and care (▶ Fig. 10.3, ▶ Fig. 10.4).

Unfortunately, at the nursing facility, she did not tolerate the collar and became physically violent with staff members who were trying to maintain her immobility. Her cognitive impairment interfered with her understanding and use of the brace, despite the best attempts by staff. After several calls from the facility staff, the decision was made to discontinue the collar. She remained without impairment even after demonstrating excessive cervical range of motion for the first 24 to 48 hours.

The decision for the collar was based on sound principles of fracture management, particularly involving a facet joint.

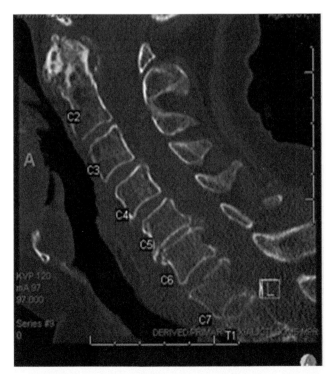

Fig. 10.3 Case One. Sagittal CT: C7 end plate fracture

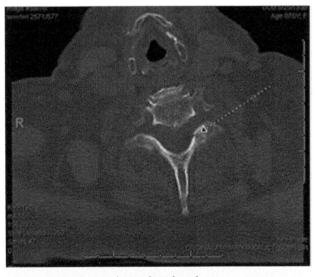

Fig. 10.4 Case One. Axial CT: Left C6 facet fracture

However, if the provider had more information about the patient and the severity of dementia, potentially other options and a frank discussion with the patient's health care power of attorney or guardian as to the risks and benefits of the options may have been considered. A soft device is a reasonable alternative to provide comfort and some degree of protection. Also, a liberal collar protocol may have been decided on, to include removal when supine or reclined as well as at meals with supervision. No collar may also have been reasonable based on the patient's level of activity and supervised environment. In this case, and as noted in many others, the patient demonstrated for us that with this fracture type, no brace is an option, as she did well without untoward sequelae or neurologic loss.

10.6.6 Case Two

There are many options for treatment of osteoporotic compression fractures. The decision regarding bracing is controversial, as it has not shown to decrease the degree of associated kyphosis. To some, the brace may be helpful for pain control. However, based on the fracture location and bone quality, the brace may have no impact biomechanically.

A 72-year-old active female slid off her horse while mounting. CT imaging demonstrated a T4 compression deformity with a Hounsfield unit value of 52, suggesting a low bone density. This patient was well known to the service, having sustained a T3 compression and T6 end plate fracture from a similar event four years prior. She did complain of pain in the upper thoracic region and therefore was provided a CTO. At the thrid week follow-up, she reported that she had not been compliant with the brace. In fact, she disclosed that the only time she had discomfort was when wearing the brace (▶ Fig. 10.5).

The CTO was selected for the upper thoracic fracture, to stabilize the cervical thoracic junction and to offload the anterior column. However, the CT scan demonstrated a baseline cervical thoracic kyphosis, with an acute worsening kyphosis at the new fracture site T4. The sagittal imbalance was not addressed in the decision-making; therefore, the brace could not perform as expected. There was no way to achieve point fixation or surface contact. In this case, based on the literature, no brace with close follow-up would have been optimal. Preventing further kyphosis was not likely, based on the noted poor bone density. The patient was not interested in surgical correction of the kyphosis; in fact, her main concern was the timing of her being able to return to riding her horse.

10.6.7 Case Three

Odontoid fracture management recommendations in the aging spine patient are not clear and vary based on past history and associated comorbidities.[19,20,21] A surgical or conservative treatment plan is formulated after evaluating the mechanism of injury, fracture pattern, and degree of displacement. However, in the aged, medical comorbidities can often eliminate surgery as a possibility. This fact places some of the highest risk fractures in the conservative treatment group.

A 79-year-old female tripped while walking, landing on her face. She complained of neck pain, with no neurologic deficit. A CT scan demonstrated multiple facial fractures as well as a type II dens fracture with posterior displacement of 5 mm, MRI was concerning due to the spinal cord positioning, but there was no frank cord compression (▶ Fig. 10.6, ▶ Fig. 10.7).

Clinical decision-making took into consideration that the fracture had little chance of bony or fibrous union, and therefore surgical stabilization was preferred. Unfortunately, the patient had stage IV peritoneal cancer, which was being treated with chemotherapy. Additionally, she had a recent deep vein

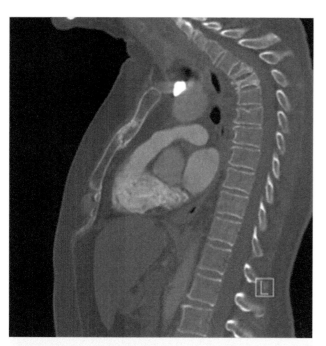

Fig. 10.5 Case Two. Sagittal CT: cervical kyphosis with acute kyphosis at T3 and T4; points of fixation not achievable CTO.

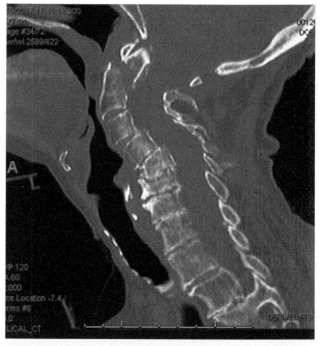

Fig. 10.6 Case Three. Type II dens fracture with 5 mm posterior displacement with severe degeneration distally

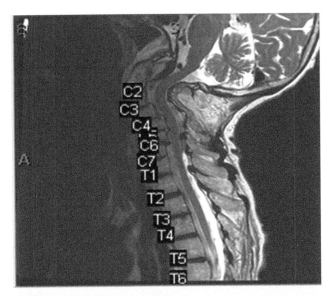

Fig. 10.7 Case Three. Sagittal MRI

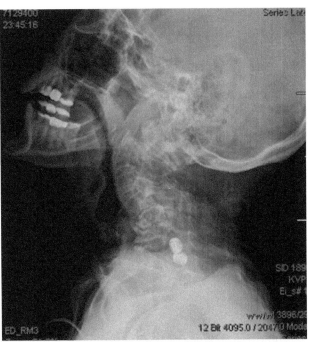

Fig. 10.8 Case Three. X-ray upright in collar demonstrating an increase in posterior displacement (7.5 mm)

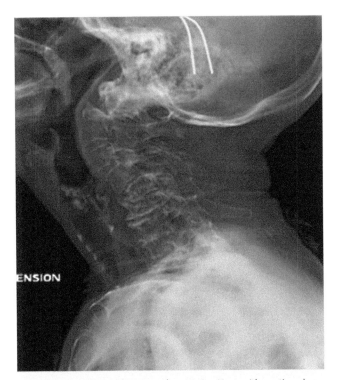

Fig. 10.9 Case Three. Three-month extension X-ray with continued posterior C2 fragment displacement (7.5 mm)

thrombosis with pulmonary embolus, requiring low molecular weight heparin; she was also underweight, with a body mass index of 16.56. Other surgical concerns included pulmonary mycobacterium and multiple lung lesions with innumerable node involvement. Surgical planning was therefore aborted, and she was placed in a rigid cervical collar. Upright X-rays demonstrated a 7.5 mm posterior displacement of the dens fracture, an increase from the supine CT (▶ Fig. 10.8).

At the two week follow-up, the patient's neck pain had subsided, and her main complaint was that of discomfort associated with the brace. At the lateral base of her neck and the occipital area, she was found to have a stage I pressure ulcer. She was advised to remove the collar at night and when reclined in a chair. Hydrocolloid dressings were recommended for the skin impairment. Lateral radiographs continued to display a 7.5 mm displacement of the fracture.

After two months, the patient had more pain associated with the collar, with new skin impairments at the chin and sternum and progression of the breakdown at the occiput and lateral bases of the neck. Protective skin barriers were in place, however, and stage II impairments were noted. At that time, she was provided a soft cervical collar to be used when sedentary. X-rays were unchanged, with no evidence of healing or improvement of fracture displacement.

At month three, she remained neurologically intact, with no neck pain in flexion, extension, or any range of motion. She felt relief when out of the collar. Lateral radiograph continued to reveal the fracture, with no evidence of bone formation. The flexion film showed decreased displacement of the fracture. In both the extension and neutral views, the displacement returned to 7.5 mm. After 3 months of immobilization, the decision to remove the rigid collar and to continue the soft collar as needed (▶ Fig. 10.9, ▶ Fig. 10.10).

Determining the best orthosis for the fracture patterns in the older individual is complex. Retrospectively, for this case, if at the time of the brace prescription other options were explored, potentially there would be a better chance of fracture approximation. The collar, because of the added hyperextension, may have extended the fracture, contributing to the increased fracture displacement. For complex patients, working with an orthotist can help meet patient-specific variables. For some patients, use of the three-inch soft collar may also be reasonable for providing a kinesthetic reminder, minimal to no added extension and a reduction in the risk of skin impairment.

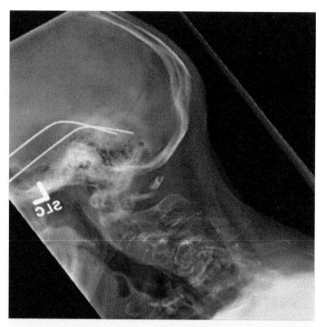

Fig. 10.10 Case Three. Three-month flexion X-ray with reduction of the fracture fragments

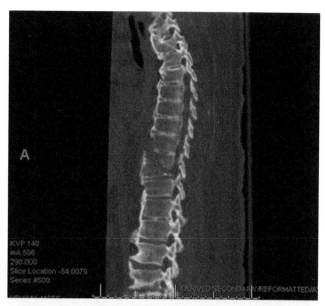

Fig. 10.11 Case Four. Sagittal CT demonstrating extension injury at T 8–9 in the setting of AS

Decisions regarding the endpoint in treatment should be addressed as part of the initial plan. The chance of nonunionization without surgery was realized at the time of diagnosis; however, a fibrous union was anticipated. The consensus definition of a fibrous union is radiographic stability in flexion-extension, with no abnormal motion.[22] Clearly, this fracture has not healed, as it does not meet the fibrous union criteria. However, the patient has remained without deficit and is pain-free with range of motion. Three months of immobilization in the brace has been ineffective radiographically; however, clinically there has been improvement in pain that has been maintained over time. Continued use of the brace would most likely not change the radiographic outcome and would add risk due to the multiple areas of skin impairment. As noted by Molinari el al,[23] when comparing geriatric C2 fracture with surgery vs. collar, healing, and stability did not correlate with improved outcomes in pain, function, or satisfaction.

Treatment endpoint decisions are difficult when anticipated goals are not met. This patient has proven for us that radiographically, a boney or fibrous union is not the only acceptable endpoint, but rather, having neurologic stability without pain can achieve the desired clinical outcome.

10.6.8 Case Four

Establishing a treatment plan for unstable fractures in the acutely ill patient is difficult. Surgery may require postponement due to a patient's medical instability. Continued reassessment is important, as the risks and benefits of surgical decision change over time.

A 72-year-old male with ankylosing spondylitis (AS) fell from standing height following a syncopal event, sustaining a T8–9 three-column injury (▶ Fig. 10.11). Knowledge of the increased mortality associated with spine fracture and AS makes management complex.[24] Other concerns include the risk of bleeding, poor bone density with continued fracture collapse, and concern for sudden neurologic deterioration. Surgical treatment has been favored to prevent pseudoarthrosis and progressive neurological decline.[25]

The patient presented in acute respiratory failure associated with pneumonia and COPD, requiring use of positive pressure to maintain oxygen saturation. Past medical history also included congestive heart failure, coronary artery disease, hypertension, obesity, anxiety, depression, and poorly managed diabetes mellitus. Surgical stabilization of the fracture was not an option due to his medical status. Bracing was also contraindicated due to risk of worsening pulmonary function. Based on the fracture pattern (an extension injury), the patient was managed with the head of bed elevated to at least 60°. This helped to facilitate optimal pulmonary function as well as keep the fracture in the best position (slight flexion) to maximize reduction. Lying flat was restricted to prevent fracture extension, which was poorly tolerated and associated with increased pain. His ICU stay was prolonged due to cardio pulmonary instability. Options for surgical stabilization over the course of treatment were considered; however, they were aborted, as prone positioning was unachievable. The risks and benefits of surgery and bracing in this case were continually reviewed. Eventually, the decision was made to mobilize the patient in a custom-fit TLSO brace designed to fit his body habitus. Obesity interfered with the brace's effectiveness due to excessive tissue and lack of ability to fix to the boney anatomy (▶ Fig. 10.12). The patient fortunately remained neurologically intact, with manageable back pain. At the three-month interval a CT scan was obtained which continued to demonstrate the fracture; however, there was evidence of a fibrous union, and he was weaned from the brace (▶ Fig. 10.13). In this case, decision-making was complicated and repeated at various time intervals during the hospitalization as

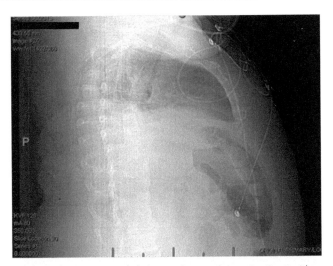

Fig. 10.12 Case Four. Body habitus: edema and excessive tissue with barrel chest; note soft-tissue depth from skin surface to sternum and posterior spine

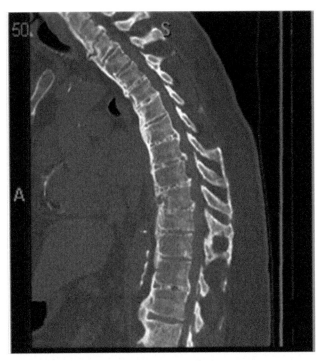

Fig. 10.13 Case Four. CT sagittal at 3 months.

well as through the outpatient clinical course. At each reevaluation, the risks and benefits were weighed, which resulted in a very reasonable patient outcome.

10.7 Outcomes and Evidence

10.7.1 Cervical Bracing

Most of the studies evaluating the outcomes of bracing for cervical spine fractures have been associated with odontoid fracture management. In this population, there is inconsistency in the reports of healing rates and nonunion using the brace, as well as a variation in the criteria used to determine that the fracture has healed. Most authors think surgical fixation, either by an anterior or posterior approach, has the greatest chance for healing.[20,26] Hsu et al (2010) recognized a high nonunion rate with nonsurgical management and postulated that early surgical treatment would improve outcomes. However, after a retrospective review of the surgical clinical outcomes, there was an unexpectedly high morbidity rate following surgery.[27]

Wager et al (2017) summarized many high-powered studies comparing the operative vs. nonoperative treatment groups, concluding that surgery was efficacious, with noted improvements in mortality and functional outcomes, but only in those patients who could undergo general anesthesia.[28] This implies patients in the surgical group were in better health, as they were cleared medically to proceed with surgery. This variation may account for the difference in the mortality outcomes.

Dhall et al (2017) reported that surgical management of C2 fractures in the octogenarian carries an increase in morbidity and postoperative complications during the initial hospitalization. Initially after fracture, the nonsurgical group in this review had a lower rate of complications. Additionally, the surgical group was found to have an increased chance of being discharged to a long-term facility instead of home.[19] Other authors have argued that disposition to long-term facilities are not just specific to the surgery group. These results are similar to those of Molinari et al, who found the conservative group to have a

lower fracture healing rate; however, both the neck disability index scores and visual analogue scores were slightly lower than the surgery group. Complications and mortality rates were lower in fractures with less displacement and in those who were treated in a collar with early mobilization. Interestingly, they found that fracture healing and stability did not correlate with improved outcomes.[23]

Finally, the results from three tertiary referral centers in the Netherlands compared surgical and conservative treatments for odontoid fractures, type II or III. Huybregts et al (2017) reviewed a total of 105 patients and found no radiographic differences in outcomes between the two groups. Most achieved fracture healing. The exact correlation between clinical outcomes and fracture healing (either union or stability) was unclear due to data limitations.[21] Interestingly, the presence of fracture dislocation/angulation or multiple fractures did not negatively influence treatment options; however, healthier patients were more likely to achieve fracture stability.

Until recently, the focus has been on mortality and various definitions of fracture healing. The emphasis has shifted to interpretation of objective patient tools to determine clinical satisfaction. The data continues to be very controversial regarding best practice, and it is recognized that a general algorithm for care will be difficult to achieve.

10.7.2 Thoracolumbar Bracing

There has been a tremendous volume of literature recently indicating that bracing does not add to improved outcomes or fracture healing in osteoporotic compression fractures. Hoshino et al (2013) retrospectively reviewed 362 patients with osteoporotic compression fractures and a mean age of 76.3. All patients were treated conservatively, and through a multivariate logistic regression analysis, they concluded that there was no significant difference between the conservative treatment options, including brace type, hospitalization time, bisphosphonate use after injury, and analgesia requirement.[29] There was prolonged pain, however, in those with middle column compression, for which the study could not prove or disprove that bracing was a benefit. Kim et al (2014) through a prospective randomized trial concluded that Oswestry Disability Index scores for treatment of compression fractures without a brace were not inferior to those with a soft or rigid design.[30] The authors also demonstrated improvement in back pain and progression of the anterior vertebral body compression to be similar among the three groups. An inclusion criterion for this study was age greater than 50 years; the patients were then divided into three groups. The mean age for the no-brace group was 72 +/- 10.4, for the soft-brace group was 66.75 +/- 11, and for the rigid-brace group was 71.75 +/- 7.96, thus demonstrating applicability to the aging population. A host of other studies demonstrate similar findings, indicating that the use of a brace for osteoporotic compression fractures is not always required, as the bracing is not without risk. Others suggest that further validation is needed to determine the role of bracing in all osteoporotic compression fractures.[31]

The value of bracing for thoracic and or lumbar burst fractures has also been addressed in the literature, resulting in conflicting recommendations.[3,31,32,33] A majority of the recommendations have supported that for a stable burst fracture without deficit, outcomes are comparable with or without bracing.[3] However, the study subjects were usually younger in age, where optimal bone density is to be expected. Bailey et al (2014) reviewed 47 patients aged greater than 60 with neurologically stable T11–L3 burst fractures. They found the use of a brace and not using one to be equivalent at the 3-month interval.[32] No statistical differences were revelealed in disease-specific and generic health-related outcomes, patient satisfaction, or length of stay in the hospital. This study is of interest, as it did not include younger age groups, therefore allowing the conclusions to be generalizable to an older population, who inherently have suboptimal bone quality. Additional support is needed, as there are vast differences within the older population. In fact, aging treatment paradigms may require alteration based on each decade of life.

10.8 Conclusion

Bracing in the aging spine is not without risk. Each case needs to be analyzed separately, as each patient brings unique features that cannot be generalized. The selection of the brace should take into consideration the mechanism of injury and fracture pattern, as well as the patient's physical habitus, medical health, and cognitive state. A plan to limit complications should be continually reassessed. The literature suggests that our current bracing designs are not biomechanically able to adequately provide the immobilization that we theorize to be necessary. The limitation of the bracing design and the altered anatomy of aging individuals make generic fracture treatment protocols impossible. Perhaps recommendations for treatment should identify differences based on age. With each decade, there are changes in the aging person's levels of activity, which may allow for less rigid immobilization when compared to the

younger population. Objective validation is needed to identify alternative treatment recommendations that are manageable in older individuals and to provide optimal patient outcomes. In our experience, the aging population have on many occasions provided isolated clinical case studies of noncompliance, which demonstrate that no brace may also be a reasonable option. Continued research is needed to address specific bracing in aging patients and to determine the role of the least restrictive device.

References

[1] Lomoschitz FM, Blackmore CC, Mirza SK, Mann FA. Cervical spine injuries in patients 65 years old and older: epidemiologic analysis regarding the effects of age and injury mechanism on distribution, type, and stability of injuries. AJR Am J Roentgenol. 2002; 178(3):573–577

[2] Guan J, Bisson EF. Treatment of odontoid fractures in the aging population. Neurosurg Clin N Am. 2017; 28(1):115–123

[3] Chang V, Holly LT. Bracing for thoracolumbar fractures. Neurosurg Focus. 2014; 37(1):E3

[4] Agabegi SS, Asghar FA, Herkowitz HN. Spinal orthoses. J Am Acad Orthop Surg. 2010; 18(11):657–667

[5] Woodard EJ, Kowalski RJ, Marcotte N, Benzel EC. Orthosis: Complication Prevention and Management. In: Steinmetz MP, Benzel EC, eds. Spine Surgery Techniques, Complication Avoidance and Management. Phil, PA: Elsevier Science; 2017: 1770–1782

[6] Benzel EC. Spinal Orthotics. In: Benzel EC, ed. Biomechanics of Spine Stabilization Principles and Clinical Practices. New York, NY: McGraw- Hill Inc; 1995:247–258

[7] Morris JM, Lucas DB, Bresler B. Role of the trunk in stability of the spine. Journal of Bone and Joint Surgery. 1961; 43-A(3):327–351

[8] Nachemson A, Morris JM. In vivo measurements of intradiscal pressure: Discometry, a method for the determination of pressure in the lower lumbar discs. J Bone Joint Surg Am. 1964; 46:1077–1092

[9] Newman M, Minns Lowe C, Barker K. Spinal Orthoses for vertebral osteoporosis and osteoporotic vertebral fracture: a systematic review. Arch Phys Med Rehabil. 2016; 97(6):1013–1025

[10] Miller CP, Bible JE, Jegede KA, Whang PG, Grauer JN. Soft and rigid collars provide similar restriction in cervical range of motion during fifteen activities of daily living. Spine. 2010; 35(13):1271–1278

[11] Tashjian RZ, Majercik S, Biffl WL, Palumbo MA, Cioffi WG. Halo-vest immobilization increases early morbidity and mortality in elderly odontoid fractures. J Trauma. 2006; 60(1):199–203

[12] Ailon T, Shaffrey CI, Lenke LG, Harrop JS, Smith JS. Progressive spinal kyphosis in the aging population. Neurosurgery. 2015; 77 Suppl 4:S164–S172

[13] Como JJ, Diaz JJ, Dunham CM, et al. Practice management guidelines for identification of cervical spine injuries following trauma: update from the eastern association for the surgery of trauma practice management guidelines committee. J Trauma. 2009; 67(3):651–659

[14] Ackland HM, Cooper DJ, Malham GM, Kossmann T, Kossmann T. Factors predicting cervical collar-related decubitus ulceration in major trauma patients. Spine. 2007; 32(4):423–428

[15] Powers J, Daniels D, McGuire C, Hilbish C. The incidence of skin breakdown associated with use of cervical collars. J Trauma Nurs. 2006; 13(4):198–200

[16] Horn EM, Theodore N, Feiz-Erfan I, Lekovic GP, Dickman CA, Sonntag VK. Complications of halo fixation in the elderly. J Neurosurg Spine. 2006; 5(1): 46–49

[17] Majercik S, Tashjian RZ, Biffl WL, Harrington DT, Cioffi WG. Halo vest immobilization in the elderly: a death sentence? J Trauma. 2005; 59(2):350–356, discussion 356–358

[18] Díez-Ulloa MA, Gallego-Goyanes A. Prognostic value of an immediate lateral standing X-ray with a TLSO in patients with a thoracolumbar burst fracture. Rev Esp Cir Ortop Traumatol. 2015; 59(3):179–185

[19] Dhall SS, Yue JK, Winkler EA, Mummaneni PV, Manley GT, Tarapore PE. Morbidity and mortality associated with surgery of traumatic C2 fractures in octogenarians. Neurosurgery. 2017; 80(6):854–862

[20] Omeis I, Duggal N, Rubano J, et al. Surgical treatment of C2 fractures in the elderly: a multicenter retrospective analysis. J Spinal Disord Tech. 2009; 22 (2):91–95

[21] Huybregts J, Jacobs W, Arts M, et al. Comparison of surgical and conservative treatments for odontoid fractures in the elderly: results from three tertiary referral centers in the Netherlands. MOJ Orthopaedics and Rheumatology. 2017; 7:00260:1–8

[22] Sime D, Pitt V, Pattuwage L, Tee J, Liew S, Gruen R. Non-surgical interventions for the management of type 2 dens fractures: a systematic review. ANZ J Surg. 2014; 84(5):320–325

[23] Molinari WJ, III, Molinari RW, Khera OA, Gruhn WL. Functional outcomes, morbidity, mortality, and fracture healing in 58 consecutive patients with geriatric odontoid fracture treated with cervical collar or posterior fusion. Global Spine J. 2013; 3(1):21–32

[24] Schoenfeld AJ, Harris MB, McGuire KJ, Warholic N, Wood KB, Bono CM. Mortality in elderly patients with hyperostotic disease of the cervical spine after fracture: an age- and sex-matched study. Spine J. 2011; 11(4):257–264

[25] Lu M-L, Tsai T-T, Lai P-L, et al. A retrospective study of treating thoracolumbar spine fractures in ankylosing spondylitis. Eur J Orthop Surg Traumatol. 2014; 24 Suppl 1:S117–S123

[26] Ishak B, Schneider T, Gimmy V, Unterberg AW, Kiening KL. Early Complications, morbidity, and mortality in Octogenarians and nonagenarians undergoing posterior intra-operative spinal navigation-based C1/ 2 fusion for Type II odontoid process fractures. J Neurotrauma. 2017; 34(24):3326–3335

[27] Hsu WK, Anderson PA. Odontoid Fractures: Update on Management. American Academy of Orthopaedic Surgeon. 2010; 18(7):384–394

[28] Wagner SC, Schroeder GD, Kepler CK, et al. Controversies in the management of geriatric odontoid fractures. J Orthop Trauma. 2017; 31 Suppl 4:S44–S48

[29] Hoshino M, Tsujio T, Terai H, et al. Impact of initial conservative treatment interventions on the outcomes of patients with osteoporotic vertebral fractures. Spine. 2013; 38(11):E641–E648

[30] Kim HJ, Yi JM, Cho HG, et al. Comparative study of the treatment outcomes of osteoporotic compression fractures without neurologic injury using a rigid brace, a soft brace, and no brace: a prospective randomized controlled non-inferiority trial. J Bone Joint Surg Am. 2014; 96(23):1959–1966

[31] Jaffray DC, Eisenstein SM, Balain B, Trivedi JM, Newton Ede M. Early mobilisation of thoracolumbar burst fractures without neurology: a natural history observation. Bone Joint J. 2016; 98-B(1):97–101

[32] Bailey CS, Urquhart JC, Dvorak MF, et al. Orthosis versus no orthosis for the treatment of thoracolumbar burst fractures without neurologic injury: a multicenter prospective randomized equivalence trial. Spine J. 2014; 14(11):2557–2564

[33] Azhari S, Azimi P, Shahzadi S, Mohammadi HR, Khayat Kashani HR. Decision making process in patients with thoracolumbar and lumbar burst fractures with thoracolumbar injury severity and classification score less than four. Asian Spine J. 2016; 10(1):136–142

11 Spinal Cord Injury and Central Cord Syndrome

Suzan Chen, Mohammad Alsharden, Angela A. Auriat, and Eve C. Tsai

Abstract

Corresponding to the marked growth of the aging population is an unfortunate increase in the incidence of older adults who suffer spinal cord injury (SCI). Age-related changes in the vertebral column as well as the spinal cord itself lead to a different presentation of SCI in older adults. Falls, the leading cause of older adult SCI, have a propensity to result in central cord syndrome from hyperextension at the time of the trauma. Management of SCI is challenging because older adults are likely to present with co-morbidities. In addition to co-morbidities present on admission, potential SCI complications from cardiac, pulmonary, skin, renal, and urinary systems can further complicate patient care. All treatment plans and potential complications require management tailored to the individual patient, not to chronological age alone. Conservative and surgical management strategies should always be carefully considered and individualized to patients and their goals of care.

Keywords: Spinal cord injury, central cord syndrome, surgical management, conservative management, epidemiology, pathophysiology

---

Key Points

- There is an increasing incidence of SCI in older adults, with falls being the leading causes of injury
- The pathophysiology of spinal cord injury in the older adult differs from younger patients due to age-related changes of the spinal column
- Central cord syndrome occurs in older adults more frequently and is associated with cervical hyperextension injuries
- Management of older adult SCI patients is complicated by their increased incidence of co-morbidities.
- Cardiac, pulmonary, renal, urinary, integument complications are the most frequent complications seen in older adult SCI patients.
- Conservative and surgical treatments can be considered, and management should be individualized to patients and their goals of care

---

11.1 Epidemiology

There is an estimated global incidence of 67.9 cases of SCI per million population, with a prevalence as high as 116.3/million in the aging population (ago > 65).[1] The economic burden of SCI is an estimated four billion dollars in the United States.[2] Although North American has seen an overall decrease in traumatic SCI due to motor vehicle accidents, the incidence of SCI has not decreased.[3] Globally, in the last decade there is an epidemiological shift in the age of SCI from a younger to an older population, with the average age increasing from 29 years to over 40 years.[4,5,6] It is estimated that patients over 70 years of age will account for the majority of new traumatic spinal cord injuries by 2032.[7]

The most common etiology of SCI is physical trauma, which accounts for an estimated 90% of all SCI.[3] In North America, motor vehicle accidents are the primary cause of SCI among all age groups. While falls are the overall second leading cause of all SCIs it is the leading cause of SCIs in the aging population.[3] Nontraumatic causes of spinal cord injuries account for about 10% of all injuries and can include spinal column degeneration, infection and abscess formation, tumors, and congenital malformation.[3]

Registry data has been helpful in better understanding the differences between the older and the younger population with respect to SCI. In Canada, the Rick Hansen Spinal Cord Injury Registry is a prospective observational registry that collects data from people who have had an SCI.[8] The participating centers in the registry are nationwide and include 18 acute care and 13 rehabilitation hospitals. Recent registry analysis of 1,232 Canadian SCI patients from 2004 to 2013 found an epidemiological divide between the etiology and epidemiology of patients over the age 70 when compared to patients under the age of 70.[9] Older adult patients were more likely to be injured by a fall (83%, compared to 39% of those under the age of 70). Older adults were also found to be less severely injured over all, with 58.2% having Injury Severity Scores (multi-trauma) less than 25 compared to 39.1% for those under age 70. The Injury Severity Score is a standard trauma score that indicates the degree of trauma to major body regions. A score of 25 or more can affect care and is indicative of major trauma to another region in addition to the spine.[10] Older adult patients were also more likely to be American Spinal Injury Association (ASIA) grade C or D (71% vs. 47%) and also more likely to be injured in the cervical level (78% vs. 62%).[9]

Despite being less injured overall, with less severe spinal cord injuries as assessed by ASIA grade, the mortality rate was significantly greater among patients over 70 years of age (4.2% vs. 0.6% in younger patients). In the following sections, we will review how the pathophysiology and management of SCI may be contributing to this increased mortality.

11.2 Pathophysiology and Biomechanical Considerations

Damage from SCI can be classified as primary or secondary injury. Primary injury is characterized as the damage which occurs immediately following the insult to the cord. The physical forces associated with the mechanical trauma include laceration, compression, distraction, and shear. Most spinal cord injuries are caused by a direct insult to the spinal cord as a result of a contusion or traction, and transection of the spinal cord is rare.[3]

Secondary injury is the cascade of events that is initiated by the trauma and results in biochemical and pathological changes that damage axons and neurons secondarily that would have otherwise survived. One of the major treatment aspects to limiting secondary injury is stabilizing the spinal column and removing spinal cord compression such that additional injury does not occur. Other secondary injury mechanisms involve systemic effects, local vascular effects, electrolyte changes, and biochemical changes. Systemic effects of spinal cord injury can result in hypotension and hypoxia due to loss of innervation to supply muscles of vascular tone and muscles for respiration. These systemic effects can lead to loss of autoregulation and loss of microcirculation. The initial trauma can also result in hemorrhage, which can further reduce blood flow and cause ischemic injury.

Electrolyte changes have also been studied with respect to spinal cord injury. Injury can cause an increase in intracellular calcium which can disrupt important cellular processes and can activate destructive processes. Other biochemical changes include the accumulation of neurotransmitters such as the catecholamines, norepinephrine and dopamine. Excitotoxicity is another secondary injury mechanism where neurons are damaged and killed by the overactivation of receptors for the excitatory neurotransmitter glutamate, such as the NMDA receptor and AMPA receptor. Other biochemical secondary injury mechanisms include free radical production, lipid peroxidation, eicosanoid production, pro-inflammatory cytokine release, edema, loss of energy metabolism and apoptosis. Several treatment strategies for spinal cord injury have focused on limiting secondary injury and have undergone or are undergoing clinical trials.[11]

Older adult patients are at increased risk for SCI due to age related degeneration. Degeneration of the spine increases with patient age due to a combination of increased structural load, repetitive microtrauma, and age-related changes to bone, muscle, and intervertebral disc physiology.[12] These degenerative processes typically begin with intervertebral disc wearing, through the loss of proteoglycans and water. Aging and natural wear on intervertebral discs can cause loss of elasticity with progressive loss of disc height and integrity causing disc budging or protrusion. This loss of disc height contributes to the loss of tensile properties of the ligamentum flavum, with buckling of the ligamentum flavum further contributing to narrowing of the spinal canal. Cervical spinal canal space can also be limited by osteophyte development,[12] with hypertrophy of the uncovertebral joints and facet joints and ossification of the posterior ligament. Aging is also associated with loss of vertebral height, further contributing to spinal canal stenosis.[13] Injury can occur with hyperextension, because with extension, there can be further buckling of the ligamentum flavum. This results in an additional 2 to 3 mm loss of the anteroposterior diameter, causing an acute compression of the spinal cord parenchyma and resulting in a central cord injury[3] (▶ Fig. 11.1). Older adult patients with either a narrow spinal canal or large spinal cord (cordcanal mismatch) are at an increased risk for developing spinal cord injury, even in the context of minor spinal cord trauma due to these age-related changes.[14,15]

11.3 Common Injury Types

Complete spinal cord injuries result in a complete loss of motor and sensory function below the level of injury. An incomplete

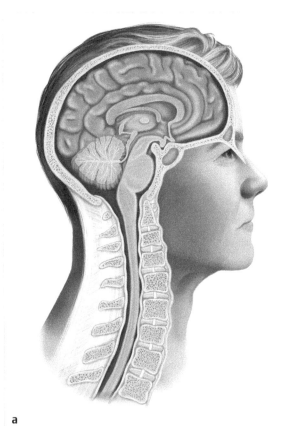
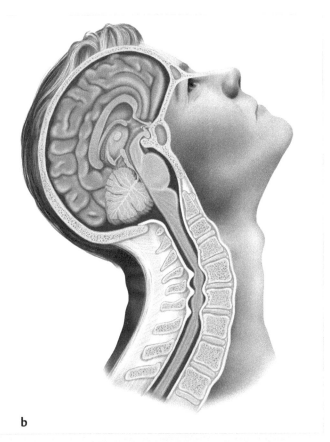

a   b

Fig. 11.1 (a) Neutral neck position compared to (b) loss of the spinal cord parenchyma during extension and resulting in a central cord injury.

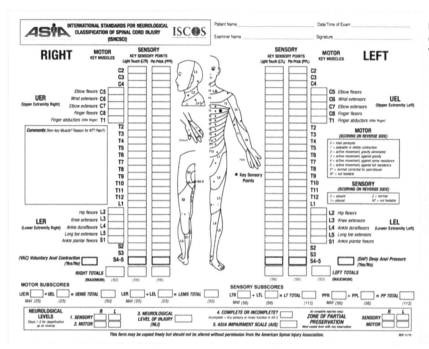

Fig. 11.2 International Standard for Neurological Classification of Spinal Cord Injury (ISNCSCI) Worksheet.

Table 11.1 ASIA Impairment Scale (AIS)

Grade	Classification	Description
A	Complete injury	No motor or sensory function is preserved in the sacral segments S4 or S5
B	Sensory incomplete	Sensory but not motor function is preserved below the level of injury, including the sacral segments
C	Motor incomplete	Motor function is preserved below the level of injury, and more than half of muscles tested below the level of injury have a muscle grade less than 3 (see muscle strength scores, left)
D	Motor incomplete	Motor function is preserved below the level of injury and at least half of the key muscles below the neurological level have a muscle grade of 3 or more
E	Normal	No motor or sensory deficits, but deficits existed in the past

injury preserves some motor or sensory function below the injury level, such as voluntary anal contraction, palpable or visible muscle contraction below the injury level, or sensation below the injury level. An incomplete injury can be mild, such as an altered sensation to a dermatome. The American Spinal Injury Association (ASIA) impairment scale (► Fig. 11.2) is used to classify the severity of the deficit. Incomplete spinal cord injuries can further be classified as incomplete spinal cord injury syndromes, with central cord syndrome being the most common syndrome seen in older adults. One of the key elements to the evaluation of an SCI patient is the assessment of voluntary anal contraction as it can significantly impact prognosis. Other syndromes, such as anterior cord syndrome, Brown-Sequard syndrome, or posterior cord syndrome (Table 11.1, ► Table 11.2) can also occur.

11.3.1 Central Cord Syndrome

Central cord syndrome is the most common incomplete cervical spinal cord injury affecting older adults.[3] Central cord syndrome was first described by Schneider and colleagues in 1954 as a syndrome characterized by a disproportionately greater motor impairment of the upper extremities compared to the lower extremities, bladder dysfunction, and varying levels of sensory loss below the level of the lesion.[16] They also proposed that the pathophysiology of this syndrome was because of mechanical compression injuring the central portion of the spinal cord disrupting the medial lamination of the cortical spinal tracts that control the hand and upper extremity function, but sparing the lateral tracts serving the sacral and lower extremities. However, this pathophysiological mechanism has not been substantiated because the anatomic distribution and function of the corticospinal tract is controversial.[17,18,19]

Central cord type injuries without traumatic fractures tend to be associated with a stenotic central canal of mean diameter less than 14 mm.[20] Patients with greater degrees of canal stenosis have been found to have poorer neurologic recovery.[20] Unlike complete spinal cord injury, which is perceived to be a disorder of the younger population, incomplete spinal cord syndromes like central cord syndrome affect a greater proportion of aging spinal cord injury patients.[9] The pathophysiology of central cord syndrome also shows a bimodal distribution, with the younger population (< 50 years of age) getting injured due to severe spinal column traumatic injuries and the aging population (> 50 years of age) more likely to be injured due to a hyperextension injury in a narrow spondylotic canal.[20]

A recent summary of postmortem evaluations and observations suggests that the greater selective loss of upper extremity than lower extremity motor function is due to selective injury to lateral white matter columns of the spinal cord[3,21,22,23] and not through the direct loss of motor neurons to the hands or

Table 11.2 Incomplete spinal cord injury syndromes

Syndrome	Pathophysiology	Presentation	Prognosis
Central cord syndrome	Spinal cord compression and central cord edema with selective destruction of lateral corticospinal tract white matter.	Upper extremity motor deficit worse than lower extremity with sacral sparing.	Generally good prognosis. Patients usually able to regain some motor function and bowel and bladder control.
Anterior cord syndrome	Injury to the anterior spinal cord caused by direct compression or anterior spinal artery injury. May be due to flexion/compression injury.	Lower extremities affected more than upper extremities. Motor, pain, and temperature deficits. Preservation of proprioception and vibratory sense.	Prognosis poor if there is cord infarction.
Brown-Séquard syndrome	Lateral spinal cord lesion that can be due to penetrating trauma, blunt injury, disc herniation, epidural hematoma, or neoplasm.	Ipsilateral motor, proprioception, and vibratory sense deficits. Contralateral pain, temperature deficits 2 levels below level of injury.	Prognosis dependent on pathology.
Cauda equina syndrome	Commonly due to disc herniation in the lumbar spine.	Low back pain, leg pain, perianal numbness, and bowel and bladder incontinence.	Prognosis has been associated with timing of decompression of neural elements. Delay in decompression can result in worse prognosis.
Posterior cord syndrome	Very rare, can be caused by interruption of the posterior spinal artery.	Loss of proprioception, but preserved motor, pain and light touch.	Prognosis dependent on pathology.

the precise anatomic lamination or location of the corticospinal tracts referred to by Schneider. Histologic evaluation of three patients with central cord injuries found that there was evidence of axonal and myelin loss of the lateral white matter tracts. At 6 weeks post injury, there was considerable loss of the lateral white matter columns, with Wallerian degeneration and marked axonal breakdown.[19] It appears that the greater selective loss of upper than lower extremity function is associated with the selective injury to the lateral white matter columns.

11.4 Treatment Options

Treatment patterns and clinical outcomes can vary with respect to patient age. The initial management of SCI is focused on basic life support and preventing further injury. Protection and maintenance of airway, breathing, and circulation should be performed, as per trauma management guidelines, ideally concurrently with immobilization of the bony spine. Of particular note in elderly patients is that the patient's spine should be immobilized in neutral alignment for the specific patient. In some older adult patients with kyphotic deformities or those with ankylosing spondylitis, extension of the neck to obtain what would be neutral alignment for an individual without kyphosis can result in increased spinal cord injury and neurological deficits.[24] In these patients, the spine should be maintained in its preinjury kyphotic alignment, which can be obtained with the aid of immobilization devices such as blankets under the head, sandbags or halo orthoses.[25] In the context of serious spinal cord injury, the patient may experience hypoventilation and neurogenic, spinal shock (hypotension and bradycardia) for which the patient would need respiratory and hemodynamic stabilization.

11.4.1 Neurological Assessment

After acute respiratory and hemodynamic stabilization of the spinal cord injury patient, neurologic examination is required.

A full neurologic exam, following the International Standards for Neurological Classification of Spinal Cord Injury should be completed, including motor function, light touch sensory function, pin prick sensory function, voluntary anal contraction and bulbocavernosus reflex, in order to properly determine the severity of spinal cord injury and to guide management. While this examination may be challenging in polytrauma patients, it is important for prognostication, as perineal sensation and voluntary anal contraction function can be present even if there is no motor or sensory function of the lower extremities and can significantly impact prognosis for improvement in neurological function. Presence of any sensation or motor function below the level of injury renders the patient an incomplete spinal cord injury, and there is a significantly increased rate of improved neurologic function in incomplete patients versus complete patients.[3]

11.4.2 Imaging

Recommendations for radiographic imaging from the American Association of Neurological Surgeons and Congress of Neurological Surgeons Joint Guidelines Committee for the radiographic assessment of spinal cord injuries have been published.[26] In the patient with a suspected spinal cord injury, high-quality computed tomography (CT) imaging of the cervical spine is recommended. Only if high-quality CT imaging is not available would a 3-view cervical spine series (anteroposterior, lateral, and odontoid views) be recommended. These X-rays should be supplemented with CT (when it becomes available) to further define areas that are suspicious or not well visualized on the plain cervical X-rays.

Magnetic resonance imaging (MRI) can be helpful to identify soft tissue injuries that may not otherwise be seen with CT, such as disc protrusions, hemorrhage, ligamentous hypertrophy and cord contusions. In regards to central cord injury, common radiographs of central cord-injured patients may not show cervical fractures; because the injury mechanism is believed to result from a hyperextension injury with compression of the spinal cord an MRI would be required to assess these patients. Acute MRI imaging performed after a central cord injury can provide detailed images of the spinal cord parenchyma. Specific imaging sequences such as T2-weighted gradient echo studies have shown hyperintense signal at the level of injury as well as the ability to assess the presence of intraparenchymal hemorrhage and spinal canal stenosis.

11.4.3 Acute Stabilization

Conservative options may be considered, more so in the older adult due to the increase in surgical risks that is associated with the increase in aging comorbidities. Conservative, non-operative management options can include bed rest, traction or bracing. Bed rest with immobilization of the fracture can result in numerous complications, including pneumonia, pressure ulcers, gastrointestinal bleeding, urinary tract infections, deep vein thrombosis, pulmonary embolism, spasticity, and deconditioning. Traction can be used to reduce a fracture or dislocation or to decompress the spinal cord and can be performed using serial weights with clinical and radiological (radiographs or fluoroscopic) examination or with manual traction. Lastly, bracing for cervical injuries can allow for immobilization of the fracture and mobilization of the patient, which can decrease the risks associated with bed rest. Bracing options include rigid cervical spine collars and halo-vest immobilization for cervical injuries and thoracolumbosacral orthoses and Jewett bracing for thoracolumbar injuries. Fracture healing can occur with ultimately no further need of the brace. However, with ligamentous injuries, bracing does not repair the ligamentous injury and surgery may be required for definitive repair.

Surgical options of decompression should be considered if there is failure of the conservative options and progressive neurological deterioration. Surgery can also quickly decompress the spinal cord and fuse the unstable spine to allow for early mobilization of the patient to prevent the complications associated with bedrest. While surgical decompression and fusion can stabilize the unstable spine and relieve spinal cord compression, the success rates are mitigated in patients with comorbidities and/or high anesthesia risks.

There are many different surgical approaches used to treat spinal cord injuries, with a unified goal of neural element decompression and stabilization of the vertebral column. Spinal cord decompression and fracture reduction is intended to relieve pressure on the damaged spinal cord and nerve roots, with the goal of reducing secondary spinal cord damage by minimizing edema and ischemia. Decompression is also utilized to remove disc herniation, ligamentum flavum, hematoma, fractured bone, infection, or tumor.

Depending on the stability of the vertebral column, a fusion combined with a decompression may be required. A spinal fusion joins two or more vertebrae and prevents movement between the fused vertebrae. There are many different types and approaches for spinal fusion that can be used to stabilize the injured spine. Most techniques will involve instrumentation to stabilize the spine and the use of a bone graft to fuse the vertebrate and are detailed in other chapters.

In a nation-wide study on the trends of treating central cord syndrome, Brodell and colleagues found that almost 40% of

aging patients presenting with central cord syndrome underwent surgery, in which anterior cervical decompression and fusion was the most common surgical treatment, accounting for almost 50% of patients, while posterior cervical decompression and fusion was used in 18% of the surgical patients. Posterior cervical decompression without fusion was used in 17% of patients.[27]

11.5 Benefits and Risks

Management of SCI has been examined in the older adult. Aging patients have been found to have a greater morbidity, and in-hospital and postdischarge mortality.[9] Older patients have also been found to have poorer functional outcome when compared to younger populations, especially after cervical spinal cord injury.[3] The causes of poor surgical outcome are not clear, as the aging population may not be treated with surgical intervention as often because of the history of poor results, compliance with the patient's goals of care, or because surgical intervention is more likely to lead to poor results.

Ahn et al looked at the effect of older age on treatment decisions and outcomes in patients with traumatic spinal cord injury in a study involving the Rick Hansen Spinal Cord Injury Registry.[9] This study was a prospective, multicenter observational registry which looked at patients from 18 acute care and 13 rehabilitation hospitals across Canada from 2004 to 2013. Of the 1,440 patients included in the analysis, it was found that there were differences in the spinal cord injuries sustained in patients younger than 70 years of age compared to those 70 years of age or older. Older patients were more likely to be injured by a fall, to be less severely injured overall—with Injury Severity Scores less than 25—to have less severe American Spinal Cord Injury Association Impairment (AIS) grades of C or D, and to have an injury at the cervical level. Despite generally having less severe injuries, they tended to have more postoperative complications, such as urinary tract infections, pneumonia, pressure ulcers and deep vein thromboses. They also had a longer acute length of stay and higher in-hospital mortality. Interestingly, the length of stay at rehabilitation hospitals did not differ significantly between the older and younger groups.

While the older-aged patients were less likely to receive acute surgical treatment, age was no longer a factor when neurologic severity and level were adjusted, as surgery was more likely if the injury was from a high-energy trauma or if the patient had an AIS grade of A or B. Patients aged 70 years or more experienced a significantly longer time from injury to arrival at a participating acute care hospital (median 14.5 vs. 8 hours) and there was a significantly longer time from admission to surgery (37 vs. 19 hours). While there was a significant delay from injury to arrival at an acute care hospital and a significant delay from admission to surgery, it is unclear whether or not these delays were associated with the increased mortality that was found to be significantly greater among older than younger patients.

The delays in older patients may be because older patients require a more complex management plan for their comorbid conditions, and clinicians may prefer to manage incomplete cervical spinal cord injuries with a period of initial observation to assess neurologic improvement, especially in patients with central cord injury. However, even with the adjustment for injury severity, neurologic level and trauma severity, there was a delay in time to surgery associated with age. The delay to surgery may also be accounted for insofar as older patients may require more time to optimize their medical status for surgery with measures such as reversing anticoagulation, assessing for cardiovascular risk, and planning for prolonged ventilation. However, in the Ahn et al study, the comorbidity scores for the older and younger patients in the study were similar, suggesting that advanced age alone was associated with delays in both triage and surgical management.

Another significant factor may be because there are more central cord injuries in older adults compared to the younger population. Because the prognosis of patients with central cord injury can be quite good,[26] the delays to surgical intervention may have been because surgeons were waiting to see if there was significant recovery and only operating if there was a plateau in recovery and the patient was optimized. Indeed, Ahn et al[9] found that those with thoracolumbar injuries had the shortest delay to surgery. While age did appear to be associated with delayed triage and treatment, it is unclear as to whether such delays are fundamentally responsible for increases in morbidity and mortality. While decompression may decrease the complications associated with prolonged bedrest, rushing to surgery prior to optimization for surgery in older adults may increase morbidity and mortality from other comorbidities.

Schneider originally observed the natural history of central cord injuries and concluded that good neurologic recovery can be achieved without surgical intervention. Although the initial presentation of central cord syndrome, quadriplegia with perianal and sacral sparing can be quite severe, the prognosis is good when compared to that of complete spinal cord injuries, as 75% of patients can have partial recovery of motor function.[3] Patients with traumatic central cord syndrome usually have some degree of progressive return or recovery of neurologically function, even with conservative treatment alone. Age of the patient at the time of injury seems to have an effect on neurological recovery; unfortunately, patients aged 50 and over tend to recover slower and only achieve limited recovery when compared to patients in the younger population.[21,22] Numerous studies have supported this conclusion.[21,28,29] However, more recent studies have shown that patients who underwent surgical decompression may have a more rapid initial neurologic improvement and shorter hospitalization and rehabilitation periods.[30]

As discussed previously, older adults disproportionately had more cervical spine fractures than any other age group. The management options in aging patients with cervical spine fractures include prolonged bed rest, rigid-collar orthosis or halo vest immobilization and operative fixation, with the later three treatments being the most commonly performed. Prolonged bedrest is often not well tolerated in the aging population because of the risk of increased morbidities, including spasticity, decubitus ulcers, gastrointestinal bleeding, and/or urinary tract infections.[31] Osteoporosis, reduced recovery capacity, and medical comorbidities have also been postulated to contribute to a higher risk for negative outcomes.[31]

11.6 Pitfalls, Complications, and Avoidance

While there is an increase in comorbidities in older adults,[32] it is not clear that this will translate into increased complications in older adults, and so vigilance should be paid to avoid complications. A trend for an increased incidence of secondary complications in older adults has been reported, with the most common secondary complications being infections, psychiatric disorders, pressure sores, and cardiovascular complications.[32] The elderly were also found to have an increase in major postoperative complications (e.g.., urinary tract infection, pneumonia, pressure ulcer, or deep vein thrombosis). Spinal cord injury complications and their possible avoidance are reviewed below.

11.6.1 Cardiovascular

The increase in cardiovascular disease in older adults is of significant concern, as SCI can critically impact even healthy cardiovascular systems. Acute SCI above the level of T6 can involve the descending pathways to sympathetic neurons. This results in impairment in the control of the autonomic nervous system (ANS) and can cause bradycardia, arterial hypotension, and autonomic dysreflexia, which are components of neurogenic shock.[33] An estimated 68% of patients with ASIA A and B develop arterial hypotension, and 35% of all patients need vasopressor support. Additionally, 16% of these patients have been reported to experience cardiac arrest.[34]

The management of these patients must balance adequate perfusion and oxygenation of the spinal cord with the complications associated with maintaining that perfusion. Fluids are often the first line to treat the hypotension associated with trauma and spinal cord injury. However, in patients with limited cardiac function, excessive fluid resuscitation may result in congestive heart failure (CHF). Development of CHF further limits systemic oxygenation, adequate perfusion and thus spinal cord oxygenation. Vasopressors, a mainstay in the treatment of the arterial hypotension and bradycardia associated with high SCI, may also stress an already compromised heart, leading to cardiac ischemia and infarction. Thus, to prevent potential cardiac complications, clinicians may be *less* aggressive with maintaining mean arterial blood pressures at 85 to 90 mm Hg for the first seven days after SCI— which has been described as a level III recommendation in the current guidelines for the clinical management of acute SCI.[35] A low threshold for cardiology consultation is warranted.

11.6.2 Pulmonary

Pulmonary complications pose the greatest patient risk during the first two years post injury[36] and are a primary cause of morbidity and mortality in the SCI population.[37] Complete SCI can be associated with near complete absence of function of the muscles of inspiration, dependent on level of injury. Injury to the cervical and upper thoracic segments of the spinal cord can results in varying degrees of pulmonary complications. High cervical injuries, in the C1-C3 level is associated with paralysis of the diaphragm (C3-C5) and intercostal muscles. Patients with high cervical injures are usually ventilator dependent and may require diaphragmatic pacing.

Patients with mid cervical injuries (C3-C5) will have varying degrees of diaphragmatic and accessory inspiratory muscle function but generally lower lung volumes compared to pre injury. Patients with low cervical injuries (C6-C8) have intact innervation to the diaphragm and accessory neck muscles, but impaired expiratory muscle function due to paralysis of the internal intercostals and abdominal muscles. These patients are still susceptible to ventilatory failure because of increased ventilatory loads due to reduced expiratory capacity. Thoracic level (T1-T12) SCI patients have preserved diaphragmatic function with some loss of intercostal muscle function. Cough function and residual execratory muscle function improve with lower levels of injury.[38]

The older adult with pulmonary comorbidities and limited pulmonary volumes may not have adequate reserves to tolerate the decrease in lung volumes associated with spinal cord injury. A 2012 study regarding 86 patients post SCI found that spinal level, age, and completeness of SCI were all predictors of pulmonary complications. Patients over the age of 65 had a 1.5 times increased risk of pulmonary complications when compared to other age groups.[39] These complications can be reduced with the use of physiotherapy, postural drainage, suction, manual cough support, mechanical insufflation, and mechanical exsufflation.[40] Prevention of pulmonary complications can mitigate the adverse effects of ischemic insults to the injured spinal cord and aid in neurological recovery.[39]

11.6.3 Integumentary Complications

The management of pressure ulcers represents one of the most challenging problems facing all older adult patients with mobility impartments, not just those with spinal cord injury. The U. S. Joint Commission on Patient Safety estimates that over 60,000 American patients die from pressure ulcer complications each year.[41] Immobility caused by SCI renders patients particularly susceptible to decubitus ulcers, which are ulcers over bony prominences in the recumbent and seated positions. These ulcers specifically form in the areas of the sacrum, ischial tuberosities, trochanters, sacrum, heels, malleoli, occiput, scalp, and elbows.[42] Decubitus ulcers occur when external pressure exceeds the capillary pressure of 12 to 32 mm Hg. This commences ulcer development, which starts in the anoxia stage, followed by ischemia and necrosis, but can be reversed if factors causing injury are removed in the ischemic stage.[43]

Tissue injury and ulcer formation can be related to extrinsic environment factors and intrinsic patient factors. Extrinsic factors include pressure, shear, friction, immobility, and moisture.[44] Intrinsic factors relate to the patient's medical condition, such as infectious stage, autonomic control, level of consciousness, nutritional status, sensory and motor deficits, and patient age.[45] Elderly patients are at an increased risk for decubitus ulcers due to the increased incidence of comorbidities, such as diabetes and poor nutritional status.[42] Age-related skin changes, including loss of dermal vessels, loss of epidermis thickness, loss of skin elastic fibers, flattening of the dermalepidermal junction, and increased permeability of the skin may also contribute to skin breakdown and ulcer risk.[46]

Ulcer prevention strategies in the elderly can target both extrinsic and intrinsic factors. Relieving skin pressure over bony prominences for five minutes every two hours can allow adequate perfusion and prevent tissue breakdown caused by immobility.[47]

Advanced Trauma Life Support (ATLS) protocols stress backboard awareness by limiting backboard use for more than two hours and emphasize care to prevent prolonged pressure on bony pressure points, especially in the older adult, may help prevent decubitus ulcers.

11.6.4 Urinary/Renal

Urinary complications continue to be a very frequent type of complication seen in the older adult with SCI. An estimated 81% of SCI patients suffer from urinary dysfunction within one year after injury.[49] This dysfunction substantially lowers a patient's quality of life and can result in severe complications.[50] Improvements in treating urological complications following the SCI has shifted the global clinical picture: Whereas renal failure and urosepsis were previously leading causes of death from SCI,[51] they have been surpassed by pulmonary complications.[37]

The aging kidney is particularly susceptible to nephrotoxic injury and oxidative stress.[52] Although kidney disease has been shown to be a predictor of mortality in chronic SCI patients regardless of age,[53] chronic kidney disease in patients with SCI has an adjusted hazard ratio of mortality of 3.16 in patients aged 50 to 64, 2.38 in patients aged 65 to 80, and 1.61 in patients over 80 years of age.[54] Treatment guidelines suggest that SCI patients be followed up regularly for kidney dysfunction with an individually tailored approach. A one year follow-up schedule is reasonable for SCI patients with no additional risk factors or symptoms of renal deterioration.[55] For patients who report changes in bladder behavior or complications of neurogenic bladder dysfunction, more frequent monitoring may be required.

11.6.5 Deep Vein Thrombosis/ Pulmonary Embolism

Deep vein thrombosis (DVT) and subsequent pulmonary embolism (PE) is the third leading cause of death after SCI.[37] The incidence of PE has been estimated to be 4.6%. A study of the incidence of DVT after SCI found a greater incidence of DVT in patients 65 and over (30.6%) compared to patients under 65 (26.8%), but this difference was not found to be statistically significant.[56] For the prevention of DVT, patients with SCI given mechanical prophylaxis without anticoagulation had a higher incidence of DVT compared with those given routine pharmacologic prophylaxis. Therefore, it is recommended that pharmacologic anticoagulation should be used as the initial DVT prophylaxis measures unless there are contraindications such as active bleeding[57] or imminent surgery.

11.6.6 Psychologic and Social

Although depression is one of the most common psychological conditions in older adults and in the SCI population, recent studies have not found that older-adult SCI patients are at an increased risk for depression compared to patients of all age groups.[58] However, there was a higher reported probabiliy of depression in patients who are female, tetraplegic, had suicidal ideation, had history of suicide attempt, whose education level was low, or whose primary care taker was a family member other than the patient's spouse or parents.[58] The routine evaluation of mental health is highly recommended in the older-adult spinal cord injury population. Mental health among the aging patient with long-term SCI may be supported through rehabilitation programs. Comprehensive rehabilitation programs educate patient and caregivers, strengthening the ability to understand and confront life stressors; they also promote injury acceptance, provide adequate pain management, and encourage leisure-time physical activity.[59]

11.6.7 Discussion of Goals of Care

Addressing goals of care is essential with any patient. It is essential in the SCI population to determine the patient's values and his/her wishes or preferences for care. Skilled case managers, who are usually nurses or social workers, can help balance the needs of the patient and family, ensure quality of care, and assist with the optimal use of health care services and resources.[60]

End of life decisions are frequently addressed in older adults.[61] Death after SCI has been seen more in older adults with high cervical and motor complete injuries when compared to survivors. When the circumstances of the death were investigated, 63% of these deaths were due to end-of-life decisions, with almost 90% of those decisions being the withdrawal of treatment, and the remainder being no treatment.[62]

11.7 Outcomes/Evidence

As the reported mortality rates range in older adults from 26% to 100%, the optimal course of treatment, conservative or surgical, is controversial.[63] Daneshvar et al performed a retrospective cohort study at two Level I trauma centers to look at factors affecting mortality in elderly patients, defined as 60 years of age or greater, with SCI related to cervical spine fractures. It was found that the mortality rate was 38%, with respiratory failure as the leading cause of death. Interestingly, preinjury medical comorbidities, age, and operative versus nonoperative treatment did not affect mortality. However, injury level and severity of risk were associated. Injury at C4 or above was associated with a 7.1 times higher risk of mortality compared with injuries below C4. Complete injury was associated with a 5.1 times higher risk. This increase in mortality with high-level complete injuries may reflect an increased rate of withdrawal of care. Neurologic recovery was not common in the cohorts assessed in this study. No other factors examined were found to be related to ambulatory disposition at discharge, including sex, age, medical comorbidities, associated injuries vs. no other injuries, fracture type (dislocation vs. no dislocation), operative vs. nonoperative treatment, anterior vs. posterior surgery, single-side vs. 360° surgery, and delay of greater than or less than two days for treatment.

Other factors that may contribute to the poorer outcome in older adults may be comorbidities rather than age itself. Older patients are more likely to have various comorbid conditions, such as cardiovascular disease, respiratory disorders, cerebrovascular disease, and dementia.[9] These conditions can increase the risk of perioperative adverse events. Anticoagulant therapy

for various cardiac and cerebrovascular indications may delay timely surgical intervention,[9] especially with the use of anticoagulants that do not have a reversal agent. Elderly patients also have an increased risk of postoperative and medication-related adverse events, such as delirium, which impede recovery from surgery.

While there are proponents for early spinal decompression for patients with spinal cord injury,[64,65] an optimal window for the timing of surgical management has not been established, especially in older adults. A systematic review and quality-adjusted meta-analysis of studies evaluating the effects of the timing of spinal surgery after traumatic spinal cord injury was performed by van Middendorp et al. They found that although "early" spinal surgery has been reported to improve both neurologic and length-of-stay outcomes, the evidence to support this claim lacked robustness due to heterogeneity within and between original studies.[66] Indeed, funnel plots showed significant proof of publication bias. The perceived risks and overall ambiguity about the optimal timing of treatment for spinal cord injury in the aging population may further delay surgical intervention. While delays may be associated with the time it takes to deliberate before making a therapeutic decision, they may also occur due to the time it takes to optimize the patient medically to undergo surgery (e.g., delay associated with reversal of anticoagulation).

Older adult patients, whether treated medically or surgically, tend to have more complications than younger patients due to multiple factors, including medical comorbidities. These complications include pneumonia, bed sores, a longer hospital stay, urinary tract infections, and gastrointestinal bleeding. While patients with high-energy trauma and severe spinal cord injuries have been found to have surgical treatment regardless of age,[27] it is unclear that delay in surgical treatment in patients with central cord syndrome increases management complications.

Additionally, older patients are more likely to be affected by osteoporosis that could affect the bone's healing and subject them to failure of the instrumented fusion postsurgery.[67] Osteoporosis was found to affect 14.5% of males and 51.3% of females who underwent spine surgery in patients above 50 years or age. While it has been recommended that all patients over 50 years of age undergo an evaluation for treatment for osteoporosis,[68] this is not practical in a trauma population.

The mortality of older patients with SCI is 38%. Mortality was associated with the level of injury and whether the patient sustained a complete or incomplete injury. There was no association between mortality and operative vs. nonoperative options, nor between mortality and early vs. delayed surgery.[9] The increased mortality risk among older patients is likely related to this group's elevated rate of comorbidities. Several comorbidities were associated with a significant increase in mortality, including congestive heart failure, weight loss, coagulation deficiency, and uncomplicated diabetes mellitus. These risk factors should be included in the surgical decision-making process.

11.8 Conclusion

With the growing aging population sustaining spinal cord injuries, the optimal management of this population continues to be a challenge. The pathophysiology in the older adult differs from that of the younger population in that older adults tend to have more severe injuries from less severe trauma. However, the morbidity and mortality in the older adult with SCI has been found to be increased, and this may be associated with the increase in co-morbidities and degenerative changes seen in the aging spine. The optimal management of the aging patient is unclear, and current management should include consideration of both conservative and surgical measures tailored to the individual patient's health state rather than chronological age.

References

[1] Smith S, Purzner T, Fehlings M. The Epidemiology of Geriatric Spinal Cord Injury. Top Spinal Cord Inj Rehabil. 2010; 15:54–64

[2] Ma VY, Chan L, Carruthers KJ. Incidence, prevalence, costs, and impact on disability of common conditions requiring rehabilitation in the United States: stroke, spinal cord injury, traumatic brain injury, multiple sclerosis, osteoarthritis, rheumatoid arthritis, limb loss, and back pain. Arch Phys Med Rehabil. 2014; 95(5):986–995.e1

[3] Harrop JS, Sharan A, Ratliff J. Central cord injury: pathophysiology, management, and outcomes. Spine J. 2006; 6(6) Suppl:198S–206S

[4] Knútsdóttir S, Thórisdóttir H, Sigvaldason K, Jónsson H, Jr, Björnsson A, Ingvarsson P. Epidemiology of traumatic spinal cord injuries in Iceland from 1975 to 2009. Spinal Cord. 2012; 50(2):123–126

[5] Oliver M, Inaba K, Tang A, et al. The changing epidemiology of spinal trauma: a 13-year review from a Level I trauma centre. Injury. 2012; 43(8):1296–1300

[6] Pirouzmand F. Epidemiological trends of spine and spinal cord injuries in the largest Canadian adult trauma center from 1986 to 2006. J Neurosurg Spine. 2010; 12(2):131–140

[7] Lewis RNV, Zhong G. What will traumatic spinal cord injury care look like in 20 years in Canada? Resource planning by forecasting. Can J Surg. 2013; 56: S65–S66

[8] Institute RH. Rick Hansen SCI Registry., < http://www.rickhanseninstitute. org/work/our-projects-initiatives/rhscir. > (2018)

[9] Ahn H, Bailey CS, Rivers CS, et al. Rick Hansen Spinal Cord Injury Registry Network. Effect of older age on treatment decisions and outcomes among patients with traumatic spinal cord injury. CMAJ. 2015; 187(12):873–880

[10] Baker SP, O'Neill B, Haddon W, Jr, Long WB. The injury severity score: a method for describing patients with multiple injuries and evaluating emergency care. J Trauma. 1974; 14(3):187–196

[11] Meurer WJ, Barsan WG. Spinal cord injury neuroprotection and the promise of flexible adaptive clinical trials. World Neurosurg. 2014; 82(3–4):e541–e546

[12] Gibson J, Nouri A, Krueger B, et al. Degenerative Cervical Myelopathy: A Clinical Review. Yale J Biol Med. 2018; 91(1):43–48

[13] Nouri A, Tetreault L, Singh A, Karadimas SK, Fehlings MG. Degenerative Cervical Myelopathy: Epidemiology, Genetics, and Pathogenesis. Spine. 2015; 40 (12):E675–E693

[14] Karadimas SK, Gatzounis G, Fehlings MG. Pathobiology of cervical spondylotic myelopathy. Eur Spine J. 2015; 24 Suppl 2:132–138

[15] Beattie MS, Manley GT. Tight squeeze, slow burn: inflammation and the aetiology of cervical myelopathy. Brain. 2011; 134(Pt 5):1259–1261

[16] Schneider RC, Cherry G, Pantek H. The syndrome of acute central cervical spinal cord injury; with special reference to the mechanisms involved in hyperextension injuries of cervical spine. J Neurosurg. 1954; 11(6):546–577

[17] Jimenez O, Marcillo A, Levi AD. A histopathological analysis of the human cervical spinal cord in patients with acute traumatic central cord syndrome. Spinal Cord. 2000; 38(9):532–537

[18] Levi AD, Tator CH, Bunge RP. Clinical syndromes associated with disproportionate weakness of the upper versus the lower extremities after cervical spinal cord injury. Neurosurgery. 1996; 38(1):179–183, discussion 183–185

[19] Quencer RM, Bunge RP, Egnor M, et al. Acute traumatic central cord syndrome: MRI-pathological correlations. Neuroradiology. 1992; 34(2):85–94

[20] Ishida Y, Tominaga T. Predictors of neurologic recovery in acute central cervical cord injury with only upper extremity impairment. Spine. 2002; 27(15): 1652–1658, discussion 1658

[21] Penrod LE, Hegde SK, Ditunno JF, Jr. Age effect on prognosis for functional recovery in acute, traumatic central cord syndrome. Arch Phys Med Rehabil. 1990; 71(12):963–968

[22] Dai L, Jia L. Central cord injury complicating acute cervical disc herniation in trauma. Spine. 2000; 25(3):331–335, discussion 336

[23] Roth EJ, Lawler MH, Yarkony GM. Traumatic central cord syndrome: clinical features and functional outcomes. Arch Phys Med Rehabil. 1990; 71(1):18–23

[24] Thumbikat P, Hariharan RP, Ravichandran G, McClelland MR, Mathew KM. Spinal cord injury in patients with ankylosing spondylitis: a 10-year review. Spine. 2007; 32(26):2989–2995

[25] Papadopoulos MC, Chakraborty A, Waldron G, Bell BA. Lesson of the week: exacerbating cervical spine injury by applying a hard collar. BMJ. 1999; 319 (7203):171–172

[26] Ryken TC, Hadley MN, Walters BC, et al. Radiographic assessment. Neurosurgery. 2013; 72 Suppl 2:54–72

[27] Brodell DW, Jain A, Elfar JC, Mesfin A. National trends in the management of central cord syndrome: an analysis of 16,134 patients. Spine J. 2015; 15(3): 435–442

[28] Merriam WF, Taylor TK, Ruff SJ, McPhail MJ. A reappraisal of acute traumatic central cord syndrome. J Bone Joint Surg Br. 1986; 68(5):708–713

[29] Schaefer DM, Flanders A, Northrup BE, Doan HT, Osterholm JL. Magnetic resonance imaging of acute cervical spine trauma. Correlation with severity of neurologic injury. Spine. 1989; 14(10):1090–1095

[30] Chen TY, Dickman CA, Eleraky M, Sonntag VK. The role of decompression for acute incomplete cervical spinal cord injury in cervical spondylosis. Spine. 1998; 23(22):2398–2403

[31] Alander DH, Parker J, Stauffer ES. Intermediate-term outcome of cervical spinal cord-injured patients older than 50 years of age. Spine. 1997; 22(11): 1189–1192

[32] Krassioukov AV, Furlan JC, Fehlings MG. Medical co-morbidities, secondary complications, and mortality in elderly with acute spinal cord injury. J Neurotrauma. 2003; 20(4):391–399

[33] Oh YM, Eun JP. Cardiovascular dysfunction due to sympathetic hypoactivity after complete cervical spinal cord injury: a case report and literature review. Medicine (Baltimore). 2015; 94(12):e686

[34] Popa C, Popa F, Grigorean VT, et al. Vascular dysfunctions following spinal cord injury. J Med Life. 2010; 3(3):275–285

[35] Ryken TC, Hurlbert RJ, Hadley MN, et al. The acute cardiopulmonary management of patients with cervical spinal cord injuries. Neurosurgery. 2013; 72 Suppl 2:84–92

[36] DeVivo MJ, Kartus PL, Stover SL, Rutt RD, Fine PR. Cause of death for patients with spinal cord injuries. Arch Intern Med. 1989; 149(8):1761–1766

[37] Krause JS, Cao Y, DeVivo MJ, DiPiro ND. Risk and Protective Factors for Cause-Specific Mortality After Spinal Cord Injury. Arch Phys Med Rehabil. 2016; 97 (10):1669–1678

[38] Schilero GJ, Bauman WA, Radulovic M. Traumatic Spinal Cord Injury: Pulmonary Physiologic Principles and Management. Clin Chest Med. 2018; 39(2): 411–425

[39] Aarabi B, Harrop JS, Tator CH, et al. Predictors of pulmonary complications in blunt traumatic spinal cord injury. J Neurosurg Spine. 2012; 17(1) Suppl:38–45

[40] Tollefsen E, Fondenes O. Respiratory complications associated with spinal cord injury. Tidsskr Nor Laegeforen. 2012; 132(9):1111–1114

[41] Dorner B, Posthauer ME, Thomas D, National Pressure Ulcer Advisory Panel. The role of nutrition in pressure ulcer prevention and treatment: National Pressure Ulcer Advisory Panel white paper. Adv Skin Wound Care. 2009; 22 (5):212–221

[42] Allman RM. Pressure ulcers among the elderly. N Engl J Med. 1989; 320(13): 850–853

[43] Kosiak M. Etiology of decubitus ulcers. Arch Phys Med Rehabil. 1961; 42:19–29

[44] Bauer J, Phillips LG. MOC-PSSM CME article: Pressure sores. Plast Reconstr Surg. 2008; 121(1) Suppl:1–10

[45] Fuhrer MJ, Garber SL, Rintala DH, Clearman R, Hart KA. Pressure ulcers in community-resident persons with spinal cord injury: prevalence and risk factors. Arch Phys Med Rehabil. 1993; 74(11):1172–1177

[46] Carter DM, Balin AK. Dermatological aspects of aging. Med Clin North Am. 1983; 67(2):531–543

[47] Dinsdale SM. Decubitus ulcers: role of pressure and friction in causation. Arch Phys Med Rehabil. 1974; 55(4):147–152

[48] Kool DR, Blickman JG. Advanced Trauma Life Support. ABCDE from a radiological point of view. Emerg Radiol. 2007; 14(3):135–141

[49] Stover SL, DeVivo MJ, Go BK. History, implementation, and current status of the National Spinal Cord Injury Database. Arch Phys Med Rehabil. 1999; 80 (11):1365–1371

[50] Sahai A, Cortes E, Seth J, et al. Neurogenic detrusor overactivity in patients with spinal cord injury: evaluation and management. Curr Urol Rep. 2011; 12 (6):404–412

[51] Hartkopp A, Brønnum-Hansen H, Seidenschnur AM, Biering-Sørensen F. Survival and cause of death after traumatic spinal cord injury. A long-term epidemiological survey from Denmark. Spinal Cord. 1997; 35(2): 76–85

[52] Wang X, Bonventre JV, Parrish AR. The aging kidney: increased susceptibility to nephrotoxicity. Int J Mol Sci. 2014; 15(9):15358–15376

[53] Greenwell MW, Mangold TM, Tolley EA, Wall BM. Kidney disease as a predictor of mortality in chronic spinal cord injury. Am J Kidney Dis. 2007; 49(3): 383–393

[54] Yu SC, Kuo JR, Shiue YL, et al. One-Year Mortality of Patients with Chronic Kidney Disease After Spinal Cord Injury: A 14-Year Population-Based Study. World Neurosurg. 2017; 105:462–469

[55] Przydacz M, Chlosta P, Corcos J. Recommendations for urological follow-up of patients with neurogenic bladder secondary to spinal cord injury. Int Urol Nephrol. 2018; 50(6):1005–1016

[56] Do JG, Kim H, Sung DH. Incidence of deep vein thrombosis after spinal cord injury in Korean patients at acute rehabilitation unit. J Korean Med Sci. 2013; 28(9):1382–1387

[57] Chung SB, Lee SH, Kim ES, Eoh W. Incidence of deep vein thrombosis after spinal cord injury: a prospective study in 37 consecutive patients with traumatic or nontraumatic spinal cord injury treated by mechanical prophylaxis. J Trauma. 2011; 71(4):867–870, discussion 870–871

[58] Khazaeipour Z, Taheri-Otaghsara SM, Naghdi M. Depression Following Spinal Cord Injury: Its Relationship to Demographic and Socioeconomic Indicators. Top Spinal Cord Inj Rehabil. 2015; 21(2):149–155

[59] Jörgensen S, Ginis KA, Iwarsson S, Lexell J. Depressive symptoms among older adults with long-term spinal cord injury: Associations with secondary health conditions, sense of coherence, coping strategies and physical activity. J Rehabil Med. 2017; 49(8):644–651

[60] Emerich L, Parsons KC, Stein A. Competent care for persons with spinal cord injury and dysfunction in acute inpatient rehabilitation. Top Spinal Cord Inj Rehabil. 2012; 18(2):149–166

[61] Deyaert J, Chambaere K, Cohen J, Roelands M, Deliens L. Labelling of end-of-life decisions by physicians. J Med Ethics. 2014; 40(7):505–507

[62] Osterthun R, van Asbeck FW, Nijendijk JH, Post MW. In-hospital end-of-life decisions after new traumatic spinal cord injury in the Netherlands. Spinal Cord. 2016; 54(11):1025–1030

[63] Daneshvar P, Roffey DM, Brikeet YA, Tsai EC, Bailey CS, Wai EK. Spinal cord injuries related to cervical spine fractures in elderly patients: factors affecting mortality. Spine J. 2013; 13(8):862–866

[64] Fehlings MG, Vaccaro A, Wilson JR, et al. Early versus delayed decompression for traumatic cervical spinal cord injury: results of the Surgical Timing in Acute Spinal Cord Injury Study (STASCIS). PLoS One. 2012; 7(2):e32037

[65] Dvorak MF, Noonan VK, Fallah N, et al. RHSCIR Network. The influence of time from injury to surgery on motor recovery and length of hospital stay in acute traumatic spinal cord injury: an observational Canadian cohort study. J Neurotrauma. 2015; 32(9):645–654

[66] van Middendorp JJ, Hosman AJ, Doi SA. The effects of the timing of spinal surgery after traumatic spinal cord injury: a systematic review and meta-analysis. J Neurotrauma. 2013; 30(21):1781–1794

[67] Donovan WH, Cifu DX, Schotte DE. Neurological and skeletal outcomes in 113 patients with closed injuries to the cervical spinal cord. Paraplegia. 1992; 30 (8):533–542

[68] Chin DK, Park JY, Yoon YS, et al. Prevalence of osteoporosis in patients requiring spine surgery: incidence and significance of osteoporosis in spine disease. Osteoporos Int. 2007; 18(9):1219–1224

12 Cervical Spondylosis with Myelopathy

Daniel Eddelman and John E. O'Toole

Abstract

Cervical spondylosis with resultant myelopathy and/or radiculopathy is an increasingly prevalent disease in our growing aging population. As such, clinicians and surgeons alike must be well-equipped for the medical and surgical management of this clinical entity. This chapter examines the epidemiology of cervical spondylotic myelopathy and details the biomechanics, pathophysiology, and natural history of the disease process. The chapter explores the multitude of non-surgical and surgical treatment options and their respective risks and benefits, highlighting both the challenges inherent in decision-making and the evidence in the existing literature. After reading this chapter, the reader should have an understanding of cervical spondylotic myelopathy, should know how this disease behaves and progresses, and should have a foundation on which to make evidence-based management decisions.

Keywords: Cervical spondylosis, myelopathy, spinal cord, degenerative disease, anterior cervical discectomy, posterior cervical fusion, corpectomy, non-operative treatment

---

Key Points

- Cervical spondylosis is the leading cause of spinal cord dysfunction in aging patients
- Cervical spondylosis is a degenerative process resulting from static, dynamic, and histopathologic factors
- Anywhere from 20 to 63% of patients with cervical spondylotic myelopathy will suffer worsening neurological function 3 to 6 years from diagnosis; however, it is still unclear which patients will deteriorate
- With appropriate counseling, patients with mild CSM may be considered for nonoperative management
- Patients with moderate-to-severe CSM generally should be offered surgical management
- Surgical treatment for CSM involves decompression of the spinal cord with or without fixation (fusion) of the affected vertebral levels
- Surgery may be performed from an anterior, posterior, or combined approach; surgical decision-making should be tailored to each individual case

---

12.1 Epidemiology

Cervical spondylosis is a chronic, progressive degenerative disease of the spine and is the leading cause of spinal cord dysfunction in the aging population worldwide.[1,2] Spondylosis refers to the cascade of degenerative changes which happens throughout the aging spine. In contrast to inflammatory conditions, spondylosis is a naturally-occurring process as a result of chronic, normal compressive forces on the spine. The end result of these degenerative changes is narrowing of the spinal canal that can lead to compression and subsequent dysfunction of the cervical spinal cord (▶ Fig. 12.1a and b). The term cervical spondylotic myelopathy (CSM) is used specifically to describe the phenomenon of cervical spinal cord dysfunction due to the process of cervical spondylosis. CSM presents insidiously with symptoms, including gait instability, bladder dysfunction, and difficulty with finger fine motor tasks; classic signs are upper motor neuron dysfunction referable to the highest level of compression, which include motor weakness, hyperreflexia, and diminished proprioception sense. In order to objectively quantify the functional status of patients with CSM, a number of numeric scales have been created. Perhaps the most commonly used of these scales is the modified Japanese Orthopedic Association (mJOA) scale (▶ Fig. 12.2). The mJOA scale is an investigator-administered, 18 point scale which assesses motor dysfunction of the upper and lower extremities, sensory dysfunction of the upper extremities, and urinary sphincter dysfunction. A full 18 points indicates no neurologic dysfunction, and the score decreases with increasing severity of neurologic injury. In order to standardize the clinical assessment of CSM, the scale has been further divided into ranges for mild (15–17), moderate (12–14), and severe (0–11) myelopathy[3]

The prevalence of spondylotic changes throughout the cervical spine has been reported in a number of studies. Gore et al[4] examined lateral cervical radiographs of 200 asymptomatic patients aged 60 to 65 and found evidence of degenerative changes in 95% of men and 70% of women. Boden et al[5] examined magnetic resonance imaging (MRI) studies in 63 asymptomatic patients and found evidence of disc degeneration in 25% of patients younger than 40 but in 60% of those aged older than 40. Ernst et al[6] reported a 73% prevalence of bulging discs and 37% prevalence of annular tears on MRI of 30 asymptomatic patients. In a larger study, Nakashima et al[7] prospectively examined MRI studies of 1,211 healthy volunteers aged 20 to 70 years. They reported evidence of disc bulge in 87.6% of patients, which significantly increased with age in terms of severity, frequency, and number of levels. In contrast, only 5.3% of asymptomatic subjects had evidence of spinal cord compression; however, this number also increased with age, particularly after age 50. A follow-up study by Kato et al[8] demonstrated a significant decrease in the diameter of the spinal canal, dural tube, and spinal cord in correlation with increasing age. These studies collectively support that cervical spondylosis is primarily a disease of the aging population.

The prevalence of CSM remains significantly more challenging to elucidate. While the vast majority of aged patients have been shown to have evidence of spondylotic changes on imaging studies, it is not entirely clear what fraction of these patients will progress to symptomatic myelopathy. The picture is further complicated by the lack of a universal classification of cervical degenerative disease throughout the literature. Specifically, there is considerable controversy as to whether ligamentous conditions such as ossification of the posterior longitudinal ligament (OPLL) should be included within the category of true CSM. Indeed, OPLL is a known etiology of cervical spinal cord compression and myelopathy, and for that reason it

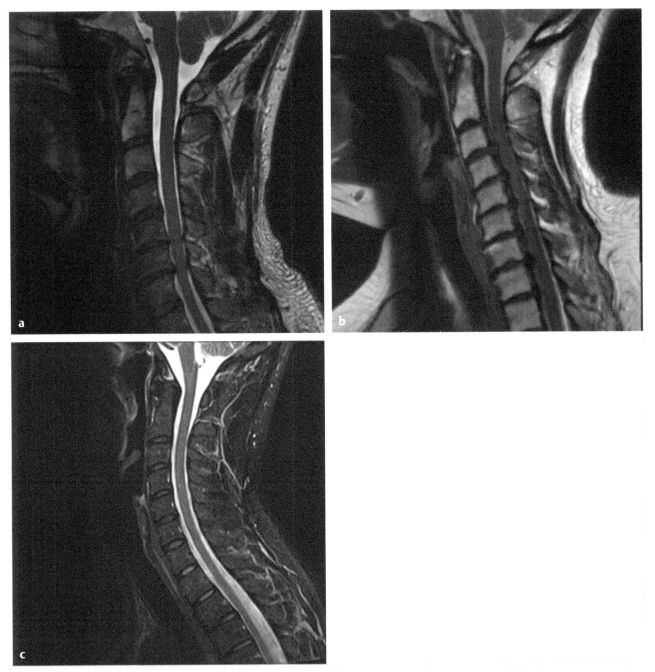

Fig. 12.1 sagittal T2 MRI showing multilevel degenerative changes characteristic of cervical spondylosis **(a)** without and **(b)** with cord compression. **(c)** Sagittal T2 MRI of normal cervical spine.

is sometimes included in epidemiologic studies of CSM. Recent studies[9,10] have even suggested a more overarching term–Degenerative Cervical Myelopathy (DCM) - to encompass the wide range of degenerative spinal disorders which result in cervical cord compression. Those authors define spondylotic changes (e.g. disc degeneration and facet arthropathy) and ligamentous aberrations (OPLL) as two separate categories, both of which fall within the overarching term "DCM". The lack of consistency throughout previous literature partially explains the difficulty in knowing the true prevalence of CSM. For the purposes of this chapter, we define CSM as cervical myelopathy as a result of degenerative spondylosis, not including OPLL.

Despite these challenges, it is well known that CSM is the most common cause of spinal cord dysfunction in the aging population. In a study by Moore and Blumhardt,[11] CSM was the most common (23.6%) cause of nontraumatic paraparesis or tetraparesis in adults. It more commonly affects men than women, with a reported ratio of 2.7:1, and the average age of diagnosis has been reported as 64 years of age.[12] Some studies have attempted to estimate the prevalence and incidence of CSM from nontraumatic spinal cord injury (SCI). In a literature review, New et al[13] reported that degenerative diseases constituted 59% of nontraumatic SCI in Japan, 54% in the United States, and 31% in Europe. However, the authors noted a relative

Motor dysfunction score of the upper extremity
    0 – Inability to move hands
    1 – Inability to eat with a spoon, but able to move hands
    2 – Inability to button shirt, but able to eat with a spoon
    3 – Able to button shirt with great difficulty
    4 – Able to button shirt with slight difficulty
    5 – No dysfunction

Motor dysfunction score of the lower extremity
    0 – Complete loss of motor and sensory function
    1 – Sensory preservation without ability to move legs
    2 – Able to move legs, but unable to walk
    3 – Able to walk on flat floor with a walking aid (cane or crutch)
    4 – Able to walk up and/or down stairs with hand rail
    5 – Moderate to significant lack of stability, but able to walk up/down stairs without hand rail
    6 – Mild lack of stability but walks with smooth reciprocation unaided
    7 – No dysfunction

Sensory dysfunction score of the upper extremities
    0 – Complete loss of hand sensation
    1 – Severe sensory loss or pain
    2 – Mild sensory loss
    3 – No sensory loss

Sphincter dysfunction score
    0 – Inability to micturate voluntarily
    1 – Marked difficulty with micturition
    2 – Mild to moderate difficulty with micturition
    3 – Normal micturition

Fig. 12.2 The modified Japanese Orthopedic Association (mJOA) score

paucity of quality studies in this field, as well as a lack of consistency in classification of nontraumatic SCI. For instance, many studies included only paraplegia/tetraplegia as SCI, likely missing a great deal of patients with milder myelopathy from degenerative disease. Furthermore, these studies included all cases of nontraumatic SCI, not just cervical disease. Other studies have attempted to estimate epidemiological trends for CSM based on hospital admission rates. A study by Boogaarts and Bartels[14] estimated the prevalence of CSM as 1.6 per 100,000 based on the surgically-treated cases at their institution from 2009 to 2012. A retrospective, 12-year, nationwide database analysis by Wu et al[1] estimated an overall prevalence of CSM-related hospitalizations of 4.04 per 100,000; of note, this study included cases of OPLL, which is well-known to be more common in Asian populations.[2] While these are some of the only estimates reported, significant limitations must be considered. First, geographical restrictions limit the extrapolation of these estimates to a more global scale. Furthermore, estimating prevalence of CSM based on surgical treatment or hospitalization likely excludes a large portion of patients with milder, less-symptomatic CSM (i.e. those not requiring hospitalization or surgery); this almost certainly underestimates the true prevalence.

12.1.1 Natural History

When considering treatment options for CSM, it is essential that clinicians be familiar with the natural history of the disease. This knowledge allows for management of patient's expectations, as well as an accurate assessment of the relative risks and benefits of existing treatment options. In regards to

the management of CSM, in particular, knowledge of the natural history of progression is of critical importance in deciding between nonsurgical vs. surgical treatments. The natural history of CSM remains rather challenging to investigate for a number of reasons, including heterogeneity of populations and the subjectivity of questionnaires used to grade myelopathy and quality of life (QOL) outcomes. Furthermore, the natural history of CSM is only approximated by studies using various combinations of nonoperative interventions. Still, recent literature does provide us with some insight into the natural progression of CSM. In a prospective cohort study by Bednarik et al,[15] 199 patients with clinically "silent" asymptomatic spondylotic cervical cord compression on MRI were followed for at least 2 years. In this study, 22.6% of patients progressed to symptomatic CSM within the follow-up period; 35.5% of these patients progressed within the first 12 months. In a more recent study by Sumi et al,[16] 60 patients with mild CSM (JOA score 13) were followed prospectively for a mean of 78.9 months (records were available at follow up for 55 patients). Clinical deterioration (defined by a decline in JOA score below 13 with a decrease of at least 2 points) occurred in 25.5% of cases, while 74.5% remained stable without any deterioration over more than 5 years. A retrospective review by Oshima et al[17] investigated patients with mild myelopathy (defined by motor JOA score of ≥ 3 in both upper and lower extremities) in addition to cervical cord compression with increased T2 signal intensity on MRI. Of the 45 patients in this study, 16 (35.6%) deteriorated and underwent surgery, 2 (4.4%) worsened after minor trauma, while 27 (60%) remained neurologically stable. Shimomura et al[18] prospectively followed 70 patients with mild CSM for an average of 35.6 months; 56 patients were observed for the duration of the study. Eleven of these 56 patients (19.6%) deteriorated to moderate or severe myelopathy. A retrospective cohort study by Yoshimatsu et al[19] found a 62% rate of deterioration in patients with mild CSM who were managed conservatively. In a prospective series by Kadanka et al,[20] the authors reported a progressive worsening of activities of daily living (ADL) scores over time, with 56% of patients deteriorating after 10 years of follow-up.

Numerous studies have attempted to identify clinical or imaging predictors of progression in patients with CSM. A study by Shimomura et al[18] evaluated prognostic indicators of neurological deterioration and found only circumferential cord compression (as opposed to partial compression) as the only statistically significant predictor. They found no association with age, sex, developmental factor, dynamic factor, or high intensity signal on T2 MRI. Oshima et al[17] evaluated risk factors for patients with CSM treated nonoperatively to convert to surgical treatment. They reported that (a) total cervical range of motion (ROM) greater than 50°, (b) segmental kyphosis in the maximum compression segment, or (c), the presence of a local slip were associated with increased risk of requiring surgery. Age greater than 60, sex, C2-C7 alignment, spinal cord diameter less than 50%, developmental canal stenosis, and segmental ROM were not associated with increased risk of surgery.

In summary, the proportion of patients with CSM who deteriorate by at least one point on the JOA scale 3 to 6 years after initial diagnosis ranges from 20–62%, while the proportion of patients with worsening ADL scores may be as high as 56% at 10 years.[21] However, while there is some weak evidence supporting patient risk factors for deterioration, it is still mostly unclear which patients are more likely to progress.

12.2 Biomechanics and Pathophysiology

Cervical spondylotic myelopathy results from a combination of three factors—static, dynamic, and histopathologic—that contribute to compression and dysfunction of the cervical spinal cord.[2,21,22,23]

12.2.1 Static Factors

The degenerative process of cervical spondylosis is thought to begin with desiccation, or loss of normal water content, of the nucleus pulposus of the intervertebral discs. Normally, the nucleus pulposus, comprised largely of proteoglycans, has a relatively high water content. This gives the nucleus pulposus a viscoelasticity which allows it to convert great axial load into hoop stress contained within the surrounding annulus fibrosus.[9] With aging, the water content of the nucleus pulposus decreases. This, in combination with the repetitive, chronic biomechanical forces of daily use, results in disc degeneration and flattening. Subsequently, the uncovertebral processes become flattened, and the load-bearing capacity of the vertebrae is altered.[2,23] As a result, there is increased stress on the articular cartilage endplates of the vertebral bodies, and hypermobility of the facet joints. It is thought that these structural changes result in uneven forces exerted on the vertebrae, leading to

compensatory osteophyte formation in an attempt to stabilize the uneven segment. The loss of disc height is also thought to result in the buckling and hypertrophy of the ligamentum flavum, as well as in the straightening of cervical lordosis or even progression to kyphosis. The combination of these factors ultimately results in stenosis of the spinal canal and compression of the spinal cord.

12.2.2 Dynamic Factors

While static factors involved in the cervical degenerative process are the primary event in CSM, dynamic factors are also important to understand in the development of this disease. Because cervical spine flexion and extension affect the sagittal diameter of the spinal canal, they both can contribute significantly to CSM. Flexion can induce compression of the cervical cord against ventral bone spurs or bulging discs, a phenomenon that is compounded in the case of cervical kyphosis.[24] Extension can result in buckling of the ligamentum flavum, which leads to dorsal compression of the spinal cord.[22,24,25] Furthermore, instability of cervical segments from ligamentous laxity can result in subluxation during flexion or extension, leading to a pincer phenomenon causing more damage to the spinal cord.[22]

12.2.3 Histopathologic Factors

As discussed above, the combination of static and dynamic mechanical factors results in narrowing of the spinal canal, followed by chronic compression and repetitive trauma to the cervical spinal cord. Secondary to this structural damage, the spinal cord has been shown to undergo multiple histopathological and vascular changes, resulting in ischemia/infarction and other cytotoxic processes. Much of our preliminary understanding of this process comes from extrapolation from models of acute SCI. However, the pathophysiologic process of CSM differs from traumatic SCI in that there is no acute mechanical insult; there is an absence of hemorrhagic necrosis of the cord; and the progressive nature of the disease results in compensatory changes within the cord.[26] Current knowledge suggests that progressive compression of the cervical spinal cord leads to a chronic hypoxic/ischemic insult due to compression of spinal arteries and resultant decrease in blood flow.[2] This ischemic state results in damage to oligodendrocytes and neurons, which elicits a unique immune response. Inflammation combined with the chronic hypoxemic state is thought to cause endothelial cell loss and compromise of the blood-spinal cord barrier, which results in edema and entry of neurotoxic substances.[2,23,26] In particular, glutamate neurotoxicity is thought to play a significant role in the pathophysiology of CSM by causing neuronal degeneration, as demonstrated by Karadimas et al in a study utilizing a novel animal model.[27] Other studies have added evidence that apoptosis of neurons and oligodendrocytes further contributes to the pathobiology of CSM.[28] Further research is necessary to more fully understand the molecular pathways and cytotoxic changes involved in CSM. A better understanding of the pathophysiologic processes could implicate potential pharmaceutical therapies to augment or delay the need for surgical treatment.

12.3 Treatment Options

12.3.1 Nonsurgical Treatment

Nonsurgical treatment options reported in the literature vary widely. These range from bedrest and discouragement of high-risk activities to cervical traction and spinal injections. Most of the nonsurgical treatment methods described in the literature involve a combination of techniques. Kadanka et al[20,29] utilized intermittent soft collar, anti-inflammatory medications, intermittent bedrest, and avoidance of high-risk activities and environments. Sampath et al[30] used pain medications (either narcotic or nonsteroidal), steroids, bed rest, home exercise, cervical traction, neck bracing, and various spinal injections (epidural, facet, nerve blocks). Yoshimatsu et al[19] utilized cervical traction (3–4hrs per day), immobilization with cervical orthosis, medications, exercise therapy, and thermal therapy.

12.3.2 Surgical Treatment

Surgical treatment strategies include anterior (ventral), posterior (dorsal), or combined approaches. The goal of surgical treatment is to decompress the spinal cord and stabilize the cervical spine if dynamic injury to the spinal cord is suspected. In deciding on a surgical approach, several variables must be considered by the surgeon, including the area of compression (ventral vs. dorsal), sagittal alignment, focal vs. diffuse disease, the presence of radiculopathy or axial pain, age, comorbidities, and surgeon familiarity with each specific procedure.

A multitude of techniques may be used via the anterior cervical approach. These include single or multiple discectomy or corpectomy (or a hybrid combination of the two), most often in conjunction with anterior plate fixation and fusion. Alternative anterior nonfusion options include cervical disk arthroplasty and oblique minimally destructive corpectomies. These techniques aim to avoid the complications associated with fusion, including adjacent segment disease and altered cervical alignment. Anterior techniques tend to be used when fewer levels are involved (focal disease), when compression is more ventral in nature, and in cases of significant kyphosis.

The two most common posterior cervical procedures are laminoplasty or laminectomy with fusion. While laminectomy alone was used more commonly in the past, accumulating evidence of postlaminectomy kyphosis (in the absence of fusion) has led to a general trend away from this procedure. In general, posterior decompression procedures are more commonly reserved for multi-level, diffuse disease or cord compression that is primarily dorsal.

12.4 Benefits and Risks

As explored in more detail below, the relative benefits and risks of treatment options for CSM depend heavily upon the patient's presenting mJOA status, the treatment option selected, and patient-specific factors (e.g., age or co-morbidities). Just as it has been difficult to ascertain the true natural history of CSM due the heterogeneity inherent in both the disease and the patients affected, it is also challenging to clearly elucidate the real benefits attained or risks assumed for any given CSM treatment. Clinical decision-making for these patients must, therefore, involve a synthesis of 1) the data available from longitudinal (though retrospectively analyzed) clinical studies, 2) surgeons' expertise and appraisal of the individual patient, and 3) patient preferences.

12.5 Pitfalls, Complications, and Avoidance

Though this chapter does not focus on specific surgical techniques, several general "pearls" can be offered. When deciding between nonoperative and operative treatment, patients with moderate or severe mJOA scores should, if possible, be offered surgery. Patients with asymptomatic or mild disease should be counseled on what is known of the natural history of CSM and offered the options of nonoperative vs. operative intervention. In managing patients' expectations for surgery, it should be made clear that the primary goal of surgical intervention is prevention of worsening of neurological status, and that improvements in mJOA scores, though likely, are not guaranteed. When selecting the procedure for patients undergoing surgery, those with significant kyphosis and/or greater than 50% canal compromise from ventral disease are likely to benefit from an anterior approach, either alone or combination anterior-posterior. Finally, when CSM patients have an accompanying deformity, surgeons should consider obtaining standing full spine X-rays to assess and document sagittal plane derangements both for the cervical region and globally.

12.6 Outcomes/Evidence

Evidence for outcomes of treatment for CSM centers mostly around comparative studies (▶ Table 12.1). Outcomes are challenging to assess, given the heterogeneity of populations and treatment modalities, but the literature does provide some insight.

12.6.1 Nonoperative Treatment vs. Surgery

Kadanka et al[20] followed patients with mild CSM (mJOA score > 12) in a randomized controlled trial comparing nonoperative treatment (mentioned above) with surgery (anterior discectomy, corpectomy, or laminoplasty) over a 10-year period. The authors evaluated four primary outcomes: mJOA score, timed 10-minute walk, and ADL as scored by the clinician and the patient. There was no statistically significant difference in any of these outcome measures over the 10-year follow-up period, suggesting surgical treatment is no more effective than conservative therapies in patients with mild CSM. However, it should be noted that within both groups there were patients who declined, and others who improved. In another study by Kadanka et al examining the same study population,[31] the authors attempted to identify predictive factors for outcomes after both conservative and surgical treatments. They found that positive response to conservative treatment after 3 years was more likely in patients with older age, lower body height, higher anterior-posterior spinal cord diameter, lower entry mJOA score, and normal central motor conduction time.

Table 12.1 Summary of surgical outcomes evidence (please see body of chapter for references)

Comparison	Conclusions
Conservative (nonoperative) vs. Surgical Treatment	For moderate-to-severe CSM, surgical treatment may be superior to conservative management
	Surgery may be superior to conservative therapy, though unclear for which entry mJOA scores
	No significant difference in outcomes for patients with mild CSM (mJOA > 12)
Rigorous vs. Nonrigourous Conservative Treatment	Rigorous nonoperative treatment is more effective than non-rigorous or no treatment
Anterior vs. Posterior Surgery	Anterior decompression provides greater improvement in postoperative neural function for patients with < 3 levels
	Anterior decompression and laminoplasty provide similar long-term effectiveness
	Laminoplasty a has higher rate of postoperative neck pain and kyphosis compared to anterior decompression
	Both procedures are effective in improving outcomes for patients with CSM
Laminoplasty vs. Laminectomy + Fusion	Insufficient evidence to suggest superior outcomes or safety of either procedure
	Laminoplasty is contraindicated in cases of instability or kyphosis
	All three procedures provide significant improvement in clinical outcomes, as well as radiographic improvement in sagittal alignment
ACDF vs. Corpectomy vs. Hybrid	All three procedures have acceptable risk of complications and may be used in the appropriate patient
	Multi-level discectomy is recommended in cases of minimal retro-vertebral disease
	Discectomy-corpectomy hybrid is recommended (if possible) over corpectomy alone in cases of multi-level retro-vertebral disease

Positive response to surgical treatment was associated with slower 10-minute walk time, and lower entry mJOA score. It is important to mention here that both studies are somewhat underpowered to draw any significant conclusions.

Two cohort studies compared nonoperative treatment with surgical treatment in patients with moderate to severe CSM. A prospective study by Sampath et al[30] compared outcomes in non-operative and surgical treatment groups with a 1-year follow-up. They found statistically significant improvement in pain and functional status, and no improvement in neurological symptoms in the surgical cohort. On the other hand, they found significant worsening in ability to perform ADL and nonsignificant worsening of neurological symptoms in the conservative cohort in comparison to baseline. Although no direct comparisons were made between cohorts, the results suggest that surgery may be more effective in treating CSM. It should be noted that the surgical cohort had more severe myelopathy at baseline

compared to the conservative cohort, which may have made this group more likely to improve. A retrospective study by Yoshimatsu et al[19] compared outcomes in 32 patients who elected to undergo surgical treatment for CSM with 69 patients who elected for nonoperative care. Patients who chose surgery had more severe CSM (mJOA 9.1) compared with those who chose conservative management (mJOA > 12). The authors found that 78% of patients who underwent surgery had improved mJOA scores at a mean follow-up of 29 months, compared to only 23% in the nonoperative group. These results again suggest that surgical treatment may be superior to conservative therapy but it remains unclear for which subgroups of CSM patients (i.e., mJOA strata).

12.6.2 Rigorous vs Nonrigorous Conservative Treatment

Interestingly, in the aforementioned study by Yoshimatsu et al,[19] the authors further divided the conservative cohort. One group received "rigorous" therapy, consisting of continuous cervical traction for 3 to 4 hours daily for 1 to 3 months, immobilization with cervical orthosis during nontraction hours, and drug and thermal therapies which continued after the traction period. Nonrigorous care included 12 patients who refused treatment of any kind, and 20 patients whose treatment was undefined. Among patients receiving rigorous nonoperative treatment, 38% improved, compared to only 6% in those who had nonrigorous care. These results suggest that rigorous nonoperative treatment is associated with better outcomes than nonrigorous or no treatment. This conclusion is limited by the selection bias of the study design.

12.6.3 Anterior versus Posterior Approach

It is well established that surgical decompression of the cervical spinal cord is an effective treatment for CSM which can halt the progression of symptoms or even promote meaningful recovery in a significant portion of patients.[30,32] However, it is still unclear which surgical approach may provide the most effective clinical outcome combined with the lowest complication rate. This is partially due to differences in multiple variables within CSM patients (anterior versus posterior compression, focal versus diffuse disease, etc.) and differences in surgical techniques. In an effort to answer these questions, a number of recent studies have attempted to evaluate the effectiveness and safety of the anterior and posterior approaches.

A meta-analysis by Liu et al[33] summarized the results of 11 of these studies. Eight studies reported the postoperative JOA scores and found them to be significantly higher in the anterior group, suggesting greater efficacy of anterior surgery. However, subgroup analysis revealed that this difference was no longer present when analyzing patients who underwent surgery for 3 or more spinal levels. Nine of the studies reported recovery rates to assess the degree of neurological function improvement and found no significant difference between the groups. Nine studies also reported complication rates between the two groups and found a higher overall postoperative complication rate in the anterior group. In the anterior group, there was a higher rate of complications related to graft placement, instrumentation, and surgical approach (pseudoarthrosis, adjacent level deterioration, dysphagia, esophageal fistula), while there were higher rates of postoperative C5 radiculopathy, axial neck pain, and cervical kyphosis in the posterior group. These types of complications occurred more frequently in multilevel (three or more) surgeries. Reoperation rates were significantly higher in the anterior group (8.1%) compared to the posterior group (0.9%), while blood loss and operative time were also found to be significantly higher in the anterior corpectomy group (ACDF was not compared given high heterogeneity). Another meta-analysis by Luo et al[34] found nearly identical results for JOA scores, recovery rates, and surgical complications.

The authors drew a number of conclusions from their meta-analysis. First, anterior decompression is more effective in improving postoperative neural function for patients with less than 3 compressed levels. Second, anterior decompression and laminoplasty provide similar long-term effectiveness. Third, anterior surgery is associated with higher rates of postoperative complications and surgical morbidity, particularly when treating three or more levels. Finally, laminoplasty has a higher rate of postoperative axial neck pain and kyphosis, and thus should not be used alone in the treatment of CSM with preoperative kyphosis or instability.

12.6.4 Laminoplasty vs. Laminectomy and Fusion

Within the category of posterior surgical approaches for CSM, the two most commonly used procedures include laminoplasty and laminectomy with instrumented fusion. These procedures are typically utilized in the situation of diffuse, multilevel cervical spondylosis with spinal cord compression, and both techniques decompress the spinal cord by expanding the available space. However, the procedures have considerable differences. Laminoplasty involves temporary removal of the lamina to allow resection of ligamentous elements, followed by replacement of the lamina, resulting in expansion of the spinal canal while preserving the bony lamina. This technique avoids complications associated with fusion and preserves motion but is contraindicated in cases of cervical kyphosis or instability. Laminectomy with fusion involves complete removal of the lamina and associated ligaments to completely decompress the spinal cord, followed by placement of instrumentation to provide stability and avoid postlaminectomy kyphosis. Both procedures are generally thought to be effective, and there are strong proponents of each. However, it is still unclear which procedure might be more safe and effective.

A recent systematic review by Yoon et al[35] sought to determine the safety and efficacy of laminoplasty compared with laminectomy and fusion, along with any predictors of outcomes for each procedure. Their search found four retrospective cohort studies comparing the two posterior procedures. Two studies reported severity of myelopathy as estimated by JOA scores; one of these included patients with OPLL, while the other included patients with CSM. The latter found no difference in long-term change in mJOA scores between either group. Two other studies of patients with multilevel CSM reported the severity of myelopathy as measured by Nurick scores; both

studies reported no difference in long-term outcomes between the treatment groups. All four studies reported pain score measures; in all cases there was no significant difference in pain outcomes between the laminoplasty and laminectomy-fusion groups. Three studies reported reoperation rates, with two of the studies finding higher rates in the laminectomy-fusion group (15% vs. 0%, 27% vs. 13%). The other study found similar rates of reoperation (5% vs. 4%). In general, there was a slightly higher infection rate in the laminectomy-fusion group compared to the laminoplasty group. Two studies reported deep infection in 8% and 1% of laminectomy-fusion cases, while there were no reported cases of infection in laminoplasty cases. A third study reported a 15% infection rate in the laminectomy-fusion group and only a 7% rate in the laminoplasty group. One study reported the rate of neurologic deterioration, with a 16% rate in the laminoplasty group versus 0% in the laminectomy-fusion group. The same study reported a higher rate of C5 palsy in the laminectomy-fusion group (14%) compared to the laminoplasty group (8%). Only one study reported rates of postprocedure kyphosis and found the rate to be higher (15%) in the laminectomy-fusion group compared with 0% in the laminoplasty group. Ultimately, the authors concluded there is insufficient evidence to make a recommendation regarding the differential safety and efficacy of the two procedures.

A more recent prospective, multi-center cohort study by Fehlings et al[36] reported outcomes of 266 patients who underwent laminoplasty (n=100) or laminectomy with fusion (n=166). Ultimately, the authors concluded that both procedures are effective at improving clinical disease severity, functional status, and quality of life in patients with multilevel degenerative cervical myelopathy. In their unadjusted analysis, patients who underwent laminoplasty achieved greater improvements on the mJOA at 24-month follow-up than those who received laminectomy with fusion; however, these differences were insignificant following adjustment for relevant confounders.

In summary, both laminoplasty and laminectomy with fusion appear to be effective in treating patients with multilevel CSM. However, there is insufficient evidence to suggest overall superiority of either procedure in terms of efficacy or safety. Surgeons should consider each case on an individual basis and select the most appropriate procedure based on patient characteristics and individual expertise. Laminoplasty is contraindicated in cases of instability in which case laminectomy and fusion is recommended.

12.6.5 Anterior Discectomy vs. Corpectomy vs. Hybrid

Anterior surgical techniques for the treatment of multilevel CSM include multilevel discectomies, corpectomies, and a combination of the two. The potential advantages of discectomy include less intraoperative blood loss, greater potential to correct sagittal alignment, and the ability to achieve segmental fixation. On the other hand, possible advantages of corpectomy include the potential for more complete decompression, especially in significant stenosis directly behind the vertebral body, and fewer bone to graft interfaces with greater chance for fusion. Still, there is considerable debate over which procedure provides the safest and most effective long-term outcomes. In similar fashion to posterior procedures, numerous studies have attempted to compare the efficacy and safety of various anterior techniques.

A systematic review by Shamji et al[37] summarized the results of 10 of these studies, ultimately comparing outcomes between three study groups: multiple discectomies vs. single or multiple corpectomy; multiple discectomies vs. discectomy-corpectomy hybrid; and multiple corpectomies vs. discectomy-corpectomy hybrid.

Discectomy vs. Corpectomy

Three studies compared the change in Neck Disability Index (NDI) scores between discectomy and corpectomy; all three studies reported greater improvement after discectomy than after corpectomy. This difference was statistically significant in two of the studies. Similarly, six studies reported the difference in JOA scores, with four of the six finding a greater improvement after discectomy (though this difference was only statistically significant in one study). One study reported a statistically greater improvement with corpectomy, while one study reported no difference in the mean score change. Two studies reported Visual Analogue Scale (VAS) scores, with one study favoring discectomy and the other study reporting virtually identical score changes. Five studies reported the change in sagittal alignment, with all five reporting a greater change in the discectomy group (statistically significant in four of them).

Discectomy vs. Discectomy-Corpectomy Hybrid

Two studies reported pre- and postoperative NDI scores comparing discectomy to discectomy-corpectomy hybrid; both studies found a greater improvement after discectomy. The same two studies also reported greater improvement in JOA scores and in sagittal alignment after discectomy. These effects were all statistically significant.

Corpectomy vs. Discectomy-Corpectomy Hybrid

When evaluating change in NDI scores comparing corpectomy to the hybrid procedure, two studies reported a greater effect with the hybrid procedure, while one study reported greater improvement with corpectomy alone. In all studies, the effect was statistically significant. Four studies reported change in JOA scores, with all four finding a greater improvement after corpectomy alone. This effect was statistically significant in two of the studies, while the other two studies were smaller and likely underpowered. Three studies reported on change in sagittal alignment; two studies reported a significantly greater improvement after the hybrid procedure, while the other demonstrated a small effect favoring corpectomy (this was not statistically significant).

Comparative Safety of Anterior Procedures for Multilevel CSM

Complication rates were reported between at least one of the above comparative surgical groups for pseudoarthrosis, C5

palsy, infection, and dysphagia. Three studies reported pseudoarthrosis rates, with all of them finding a higher rate in the discectomy group. Only one study reported pseudoarthrosis rates after hybrid procedure and found no events. Four studies reported C5 palsy rates, generally finding a higher rate in the corpectomy group than for discectomy or hybrid. Only one study reported any statistically significant difference, finding a 3.9% rate for discectomy, 8.3% rate for hybrid, and 11.5% rate for corpectomy. Infection rates were quite low across all groups, with no events in the discectomy group, a 0 to2.6% rate in the corpectomy group, and a 0 to1.4% rate in the hybrid group. Dysphagia rates were reported in four studies, none of which found any statistically significant difference. Rates of dysphagia for discectomy ranged from 5.8 to11.6%; for corpectomy, 2.3 to20%; and for hybrid, 5.2 to9.7%.

In summary, all three anterior approaches provide patients with significant improvements in clinical outcomes of NDI, JOA, and VAS, as well as radiographical improvement in sagittal alignment. All are reasonable approaches with acceptable risk of complications and may be used in the appropriate patient. Beyond this, the authors were able to make a number of recommendations based on the evidence. First, when pathoanatomically appropriate with minimal retro-vertebral disease, multiple discectomy is recommended over corpectomy or hybrid procedures. Second, when significant retro-vertebral disease is present, it is recommended that a discectomy-corpectomy hybrid procedure be utilized over multi-level corpectomy alone, if possible.

12.7 Conclusion

Cervical spondylotic myelopathy is a complex disease with potentially devastating consequences. It is the leading cause of spinal cord dysfunction in the aging population, which is ever increasing in size. Cervical degenerative changes are nearly ubiquitous throughout patients over the age of 65, but only a fraction of patients will develop resulting spinal cord dysfunction. CSM generally is a progressive process affected by repetitive static, dynamic, and histopathologic changes over time. However, we still lack an understanding of which patients will progress to neurologic deterioration. Treatment for CSM is aimed at halting the progression of spinal cord dysfunction and includes surgical and nonsurgical measures. The clinical decision-making process should be tailored to each individual case, considering the patient's degree and location of spinal cord compression (ventral vs. dorsal, single vs. multi-level); disease severity (i.e. mJOA score) on presentation, and clinician/patient preference. In general, patients with asymptomatic or mild CSM may be managed nonoperatively, as a proportion of these patients will not decline neurologically (and some may even improve). Patients with moderate to severe CSM generally should be offered surgical treatment to halt the disease process and provide the best chance for neurologic improvement. Surgery may be approached anteriorly, posteriorly, or via combination of both. Anterior approaches include anterior discectomy and fusion (ACDF), total disc arthroplasty, anterior corpectomy, and discectomy/corpectomy hybrid procedures. Posterior surgery involves laminectomy for spinal cord decompression and either laminoplasty or instrumented fusion for fixation of the affected levels. Combination anterior-posterior surgery has the highest complication rates and is ideally reserved for severe, circumferential, multilevel disease or significant cervical deformity.

Key References

[1] Furlan JC, Kalsi-Ryan S, Kailaya-Vasan A, Massicotte EM, Fehlings MG. Functional and clinical outcomes following surgical treatment in patients with cervical spondylotic myelopathy: a prospective study of 81 cases. J Neurosurg Spine. 2011; 14(3):348–355

[2] Tetreault L, Goldstein CL, Arnold P, et al. Degenerative Cervical Myelopathy: A Spectrum of Related Disorders Affecting the Aging Spine. Neurosurgery. 2015; 77 Suppl 4:S51–S67

[3] Kadaňka Z, Bednařík J, Novotný O, Urbánek I, Dušek L. Cervical spondylotic myelopathy: conservative versus surgical treatment after 10 years. Eur Spine J. 2011; 20(9):1533–1538

[4] Shamji MF, Massicotte EM, Traynelis VC, Norvell DC, Hermsmeyer JT, Fehlings MG. Comparison of anterior surgical options for the treatment of multilevel cervical spondylotic myelopathy: a systematic review. Spine. 2013; 38(22) Suppl 1:S195–S209

References

[1] Wu J-C, Ko C-C, Yen Y-S, et al. Epidemiology of cervical spondylotic myelopathy and its risk of causing spinal cord injury: a national cohort study. Neurosurg Focus. 2013; 35(1):E10

[2] Kalsi-Ryan S, Karadimas SK, Fehlings MG. Cervical spondylotic myelopathy: the clinical phenomenon and the current pathobiology of an increasingly prevalent and devastating disorder. Neuroscientist. 2013; 19(4):409–421

[3] Tetreault L, Kopjar B, Nouri A, et al. The modified Japanese Orthopaedic Association scale: establishing criteria for mild, moderate and severe impairment in patients with degenerative cervical myelopathy. Eur Spine J. 2017; 26(1):78–84

[4] Gore DR, Sepic SB, Gardner GM. Roentgenographic findings of the cervical spine in asymptomatic people. Spine. 1986; 11(6):521–524

[5] Boden SD, McCowin PR, Davis DO, Dina TS, Mark AS, Wiesel S. Abnormal magnetic-resonance scans of the cervical spine in asymptomatic subjects. A prospective investigation. J Bone Joint Surg Am. 1990; 72(8):1178–1184

[6] Ernst CW, Stadnik TW, Peeters E, Breucq C, Osteaux MJC. Prevalence of annular tears and disc herniations on MR images of the cervical spine in symptom free volunteers. Eur J Radiol. 2005; 55(3):409–414

[7] Nakashima H, Yukawa Y, Suda K, Yamagata M, Ueta T, Kato F. Abnormal findings on magnetic resonance images of the cervical spines in 1211 asymptomatic subjects. Spine. 2015; 40(6):392–398

[8] Kato F, Yukawa Y, Suda K, Yamagata M, Ueta T. Normal morphology, age-related changes and abnormal findings of the cervical spine. Part II: Magnetic resonance imaging of over 1,200 asymptomatic subjects. Eur Spine J. 2012; 21(8):1499–1507

[9] Nouri A, Tetreault L, Singh A, Karadimas SK, Fehlings MG. Degenerative Cervical Myelopathy: Epidemiology, Genetics, and Pathogenesis. Spine. 2015; 40 (12):E675–E693

[10] Tetreault L, Goldstein CL, Arnold P, et al. Degenerative Cervical Myelopathy: A Spectrum of Related Disorders Affecting the Aging Spine. Neurosurgery. 2015; 77 Suppl 4:S51–S67

[11] Moore AP, Blumhardt LD. A prospective survey of the causes of non-traumatic spastic paraparesis and tetraparesis in 585 patients. Spinal Cord. 1997; 35(6): 361–367

[12] Northover JR, Wild JB, Braybrooke J, Blanco J. The epidemiology of cervical spondylotic myelopathy. Skeletal Radiol. 2012; 41(12):1543–1546

[13] New PW, Cripps RA, Bonne Lee B. Global maps of non-traumatic spinal cord injury epidemiology: towards a living data repository. Spinal Cord. 2014; 52 (2):97–109

[14] Boogaarts HD, Bartels RHMA. Prevalence of cervical spondylotic myelopathy. Eur Spine J. 2015; 24 Suppl 2:139–141

[15] Bednarik J, Kadanka Z, Dusek L, et al. Presymptomatic spondylotic cervical myelopathy: an updated predictive model. Eur Spine J. 2008; 17(3):421–431

[16] Sumi M, Miyamoto H, Suzuki T, Kaneyama S, Kanatani T, Uno K. Prospective cohort study of mild cervical spondylotic myelopathy without surgical treatment. J Neurosurg Spine. 2012; 16(1):8–14

[17] Oshima Y, Seichi A, Takeshita K, et al. Natural course and prognostic factors in patients with mild cervical spondylotic myelopathy with increased signal intensity on T2-weighted magnetic resonance imaging. Spine. 2012; 37(22): 1909–1913

[18] Shimomura T, Sumi M, Nishida K, et al. Prognostic factors for deterioration of patients with cervical spondylotic myelopathy after nonsurgical treatment. Spine. 2007; 32(22):2474–2479

[19] Yoshimatsu H, Nagata K, Goto H, et al. Conservative treatment for cervical spondylotic myelopathy. prediction of treatment effects by multivariate analysis. Spine J. 2001; 1(4):269–273

[20] Kadaňka Z, Bednařík J, Novotný O, Urbánek I, Dušek L. Cervical spondylotic myelopathy: conservative versus surgical treatment after 10 years. Eur Spine J. 2011; 20(9):1533–1538

[21] Karadimas SK, Erwin WM, Ely CG, Dettori JR, Fehlings MG. Pathophysiology and natural history of cervical spondylotic myelopathy. Spine. 2013; 38(22) Suppl 1:S21–S36

[22] White AA, III, Panjabi MM. Biomechanical considerations in the surgical management of cervical spondylotic myelopathy. Spine. 1988; 13(7):856–860

[23] Baptiste DC, Fehlings MG. Pathophysiology of cervical myelopathy. Spine J. 2006; 6(6) Suppl:190S–197S

[24] Breig A, Turnbull I, Hassler O. Effects of mechanical stresses on the spinal cord in cervical spondylosis. A study on fresh cadaver material. J Neurosurg. 1966; 25(1):45–56

[25] Ferguson RJ, Caplan LR. Cervical spondylitic myelopathy. Neurol Clin. 1985; 3 (2):373–382

[26] Karadimas SK, Gatzounis G, Fehlings MG. Pathobiology of cervical spondylotic myelopathy. Eur Spine J. 2015; 24 Suppl 2:132–138

[27] Karadimas S, Moon ES, Fehlings MG. 101 The Sodium Channel/Gluatamate Blocker Riluzole is Complementary to Decompression in a Preclinical Experimental Model of Cervical Spondylotic Myelopathy (CSM). Neurosurgery. 2012; 71(2):E543

[28] Yu WR, Liu T, Kiehl T-R, Fehlings MG. Human neuropathological and animal model evidence supporting a role for Fas-mediated apoptosis and inflammation in cervical spondylotic myelopathy. Brain. 2011; 134(Pt 5): 1277–1292

[29] Kadanka Z, Mares M, Bednaník J, et al. Approaches to spondylotic cervical myelopathy: conservative versus surgical results in a 3-year follow-up study. Spine. 2002; 27(20):2205–2210, discussion 2210–2211

[30] Sampath P, Bendebba M, Davis JD, Ducker TB. Outcome of patients treated for cervical myelopathy. A prospective, multicenter study with independent clinical review. Spine. 2000; 25(6):670–676

[31] Kadanka Z, Mares M, Bednarík J, et al. Predictive factors for spondylotic cervical myelopathy treated conservatively or surgically. Eur J Neurol. 2005; 12(1): 55–63

[32] Furlan JC, Kalsi-Ryan S, Kailaya-Vasan A, Massicotte EM, Fehlings MG. Functional and clinical outcomes following surgical treatment in patients with cervical spondylotic myelopathy: a prospective study of 81 cases. J Neurosurg Spine. 2011; 14(3):348–355

[33] Liu X, Wang H, Zhou Z, Jin A. Anterior decompression and fusion versus posterior laminoplasty for multilevel cervical compressive myelopathy. Orthopedics. 2014; 37(2):e117–e122

[34] Luo J, Cao K, Huang S, et al. Comparison of anterior approach versus posterior approach for the treatment of multilevel cervical spondylotic myelopathy. Eur Spine J. 2015; 24(8):1621–1630

[35] Yoon ST, Hashimoto RE, Raich A, Shaffrey CI, Rhee JM, Riew KD. Outcomes after laminoplasty compared with laminectomy and fusion in patients with cervical myelopathy: a systematic review. Spine. 2013; 38(22) Suppl 1:S183–S194

[36] Fehlings MG, Santaguida C, Tetreault L, et al. Laminectomy and fusion versus laminoplasty for the treatment of degenerative cervical myelopathy: results from the AOSpine North America and International prospective multicenter studies. Spine J. 2017; 17(1):102–108

[37] Shamji MF, Massicotte EM, Traynelis VC, Norvell DC, Hermsmeyer JT, Fehlings MG. Comparison of anterior surgical options for the treatment of multilevel cervical spondylotic myelopathy: a systematic review. Spine. 2013; 38(22) Suppl 1:S195–S209

13 Cervical Deformity

Swetha J. Sundar, Bryan S. Lee, Dominic W. Pelle, and Michael P. Steinmetz

Abstract

Cervical deformity is a common pathology in the aging population. Various structures in the cervical spine contribute significantly to overall cervical spine stability. Whether it is due to degenerative disease, inflammatory conditions, or iatrogenic causes, cervical deformity can induce pain and/or neurologic deficits and limit functional status and health-related quality of life. An accurate diagnosis of symptomatic cervical deformity using the clinical exam and radiographic evaluations is critical in guiding the surgical decision-making process. The goals of clinical assessment are to determine the etiology of the patient's symptoms and determine whether surgical management is indicated. Surgery is an option for symptomatic relief and prevention of disease progression after medical management fails. The goals of surgery should be based on the patient's specific symptoms, such as radiculopathy, myelopathy, neck pain, or functional deficits due to deformity. Preoperative images should be carefully evaluated, because radiographic correction of cervical alignment has been shown to be predictive of postoperative outcomes. Anterior or posterior approaches can be performed based on the location of the pathology, extent of the disease, and the degree of the kyphosis that needs to be corrected. A combined anterior and posterior approach is necessary in cases of rigid or incompletely reducible deformity. However, combined approaches, while providing the greater amount of deformity correction, also carry higher complication rates. Risks and benefits must always be discussed with the patient when opting for surgical management of cervical deformity.

Keywords: Cervical deformity, cervical sagittal alignment, cervical sagittal balance, health-related quality of life

Key Points

- Cervical deformity is a common pathology in the aging population.
- An accurate diagnosis of symptomatic cervical deformity using the clinical exam and radiographic evaluations is critical in guiding the surgical decision-making process.
- Preoperative images should be thoroughly evaluated, as radiographic correction of cervical alignment has been shown to be predictive of postoperative outcomes.
- Anterior or posterior approaches can be performed based on the location of the pathology, extent of the disease, and degree of kyphosis that needs to be corrected.
- Risks and benefits must always be discussed with the patient when considering surgical management.

13.1 Epidemiology

Cervical spondylosis is an extremely common condition of the aging cervical spine.[1] However, the prevalence of cervical deformity in the general population is less well known. A recent study demonstrates that 53% of patients previously diagnosed with degenerative thoracolumbar deformity have cervical deformity.[2] But observation would suggest that clinically symptomatic patients are less common. Unfortunately, the prevalence of patients with cervical deformity who are clinically symptomatic is not known.

Cervical deformity contributing to spinal imbalance presents a unique diagnostic and therapeutic challenge in the context of the aging spine. Whether it is due to degenerative disease; inflammatory conditions; or postsurgical, sagittal cervical kyphotic deformity, it can induce pain and/or neurologic deficits, thereby limiting functional status and health-related quality of life (HRQOL). This chapter considers the etiological and biomechanical factors that contribute to cervical spinal imbalance. Additionally, the evaluation and treatment of these patients with emphasis on surgical planning is discussed.

13.2 Biomechanical Considerations

The cervical spine is responsible for maintaining the weight of the head, performing multiplanar movement through its flexibility, housing the spinal cord as well as its exiting nerve roots, and allowing for passage of the vertebral arteries into the skull base. Physiologic cervical lordosis is counteracted by the kyphotic thoracic spine; the horizontal slope of T1 corresponds to the subaxial lordosis necessary to maintain the head's center of gravity in balance.[3,4] The head serves as an axial load, producing a bending moment through the cervical spine. The bony anatomy, musculature and ligamentous structures provide support of the head; without these structures, studies have demonstrated that the cervical spine would fail at one-fifth of the weight of the human head. Deviation from normal alignments, as is seen in patients with cervical deformity, causes increased loading forces on the cervical spine, leading to a cycle of progressive deformity and placement of large amounts of stress on paraspinal musculature.[5,6]

Cervical facet joints and their capsule contribute significantly to the overall cervical spine stability, as demonstrated in multiple cadaveric studies. They are oriented at about 45°in the coronal plane and about 80 °in the sagittal plane, which allows for a large range of motion in flexion and extension, but simultaneously limits translation and lateral bending.[7] Studies have demonstrated that surgical resection of 50% or more of the facet joint leads to instability in the sagittal plane.[8]

Significant increases in flexion-extension motion following multilevel cervical laminectomy have been demonstrated where there is removal of posterior bony and ligamentous elements. The same study showed 80% reduction in motion after the decompressed cervical spine underwent facet wiring for stabilization, further illustrating the extent of stability offered by the facet joints.[9]

Ligamentous structures also provide stability and resist forces, which help maintain the posture and function of the cervical spine. The anterior longitudinal ligament (ALL) and posterior longitudinal ligament (PLL) are fibrous bands extending from C2 down to the sacrum, anteriorly and posteriorly to the vertebral bodies, respectively. Because, unlike the ALL, the PLL narrows over vertebral bodies and widens at the intervertebral disc spaces, the ALL offers twice the strength.[10]

The ligamentum flavum has some amount of strain at baseline so that it does not buckle or generate force on the cord during neck extension. The weight of the head creates a compressive force on the anterior aspects of the cervical spine and a tensile force on the posterior aspects. The anterior elements of the spine, including the vertebral body and the disc, transmit about 35% of the total load, while the posterior elements, including the pedicles, facet joints, lamina, spinous process, and posterior ligamentous structures, transmit approximately 65% of the load. By comparison, in the lumbar spine, the anterior elements transmit about 80% of the load.[11] This can be attributed to the differing functions of the cervical and lumbar spines; the cervical spine needs to bear a large amount of force posteriorly in order to provide mobility and functional range of motion. As the posterior elements of the cervical spine become compromised, the anterior elements are forced to take on increasing amounts of load, causing stress on paraspinal musculature, leading to a cycle of progressive deformity through a positive feedback loop.[11,12,13,14]

13.2.1 Etiology and Pathomechanics

Cervical spine deformity is most often due to iatrogenic causes.[14,15] Sagittal plane kyphosis primarily occurs after a decompressive laminectomy without fusion. When the posterior arch is removed as part of a decompressive laminectomy, including disruption of the interspinous ligaments, laminae, and facets, the end result is a loss of stability. The anterior elements are required to bear more of the load, and cervical paraspinal muscles also undergo an increase in their load-bearing role, often leading to constant contraction and contributing to symptoms of neck pain, stiffness, and fatigue. This redistribution of biomechanical forces occurs in order to maintain the upright position of the head and overall spinal balance.[16]

Kyphotic deformity can lead to myelopathy due to increased tension on the spinal cord in the cranial-caudal axis. The cord becomes tethered due to stress on the cervical nerve roots and the dentate ligaments. Eventually, the cord becomes compressed and there is a rise in intramedullary pressure, leading to neuronal damage and restriction of blood supply.[17]

Postsurgical cervical kyphosis is not exclusive to posterior approach operations. Iatrogenic kyphosis can also be a result of anterior decompression, typically due to a failure to restore proper cervical lordosis, or due to pseudarthrosis, which causes increased load-bearing forces on the anterior elements.[18,19,20]

Cervical deformity can also be caused by degenerative disease. As the nucleus pulpous of the intervertebral discs becomes desiccated and loses its elasticity, the force distribution on the discs is altered. The annulus fibrosis becomes more load bearing, overall disc height is reduced, and encroachment into the epidural canal may occur, providing a mechanism for myelopathy and/or radiculopathy.[10,21] The attachment of the posterior longitudinal ligament to the vertebral bodies is compromised as the PLL also bulges into the posterior canal. These

changes lead to progressive kyphotic deformity, laxity of the PLL, and overall cervical spinal imbalance.

Systemic inflammatory diseases, such as rheumatoid arthritis (RA) or ankylosing spondylitis (AS) can cause specific patterns of cervical spinal deformity. The autoimmune destruction of connective tissue leads to ligamentous compromise and bony erosion. The occiput–C1 and C1–2 joints are synovial and more affected in RA due to destruction and inflammation of the synovial cells. This can lead to atlantoaxial subluxation, multilevel subaxial instability, or migration of the odontoid process.[22] With AS, chronic inflammation leads to the formation of syndesmophytes, bridging osteophytes, ossification of joints, and eventually, bony fusion of the entire spinal column. Most typically, AS is associated with low back pain, loss of lumbar lordosis, and involvement of the sacroiliac joint. Additionally, disease progression in patients with AS can impact the global spinal alignments and the cervical sagittal balance, leading to loss of cervical lordosis, which causes chin-on-chest deformity and loss of horizontal gaze.[22,23]

Less common etiologies of cervical deformity include trauma, neoplasm, and infection. Cervical spinal deformity exists in the coronal plane as well, typically due to bony abnormalities, and is associated with several congenital disorders, such as congenital scoliosis and neuromuscular diseases seen in the pediatric population.

Clinical Assessment

The history and physical exam are critical in guiding the clinical decision-making process. The goals of clinical assessment are to determine the etiology of the patient's symptoms, determine optimal treatment strategies and whether surgical management is indicated, and establish the location and degree of correction necessary. Given the complexity of surgical treatment of cervical deformity, special consideration should be given to medical comorbidities. Patients with histories that include tobacco usage, diabetes, or chronic nonsteroidal anti-inflammatory drug (NSAID) use may need lifestyle modifications and/or medical optimization prior to consideration for surgical treatment. Additionally, special consideration should be given to the bone health of each patient, and appropriate treatment for osteoporosis or osteopenia should ensue.

Patients may present with a variety of complaints, such as, neck pain, myelopathy, radiculopathy, dysphagia, inability to maintain horizontal gaze, and, in severe cases, respiratory compromise. Often, patients will complain of axial neck pain. Obtaining detailed history about pain is critical in making accurate clinical diagnoses. It is important to determine whether the pain is truly mechanical, that is, repeatedly and reliably occurs with movement but is not present at rest. Pain can also be present due to compensation by paraspinal musculature in the interscapular, thoracic, and lumbar regions. Range of motion, both active and passive, must be assessed to establish whether the patient has a fixed or flexible deformity. Often, what is believed to be cervical deformity may actually be a compensatory mechanism due to the global spine misalignment from the thoracolumbar spine or hip pathology. It is critical to perform a thorough clinical assessment to ensure that patients are not recommended unnecessary surgery. Patients with a flexible deformity that exists when upright but corrects when lying supine need to be assessed for various nonsurgical neuromuscular conditions, such as amyotrophic lateral sclerosis (ALS), Parkinsonian disorders, or myopathies. Such evaluation should include electromyography (EMG) or nerve conduction studies (NCS) and referrals to neurology and physical therapy prior to the consideration of any surgical intervention.[24] Evaluation should include a full neurological exam to assess for the presence of myelopathy, radicular symptoms, or neurologic deficits, which may impact the goals of surgery. The apex of kyphotic deformity is at the highest risk for cord compression due to maximum tension on the cord.[17]

Radiographic Assessment

Radiographic assessment of the deformity is important in determining a treatment plan. Upright and dynamic (flexion-extension) radiographs, in addition to 36-inch standing scoliosis films (with visualization of the skull base and femoral heads), help assess whether deformity is fixed or flexible, and enables a look at local and global spinal alignment. When obtaining the standing scoliosis films, patients should stand with knees fully extended to obtain accurate representation of sagittal plane deformity. At our institution, patients are instructed to place hands in the contralateral supracla-

vicular fossa to ensure no postural supportive devices are used.

Several radiographic metrics have been established as objective measures of spinal balance. Assessment of these metrics is essential to surgical planning because they have been demonstrated to be predictive of patient HRQOL and complications. The Cobb angle can be measured from C1 to C2 (▶ Fig. 13.1) or C2 to C7 (▶ Fig. 13.2) Preoperative measurements can be used as comparison to intraoperative imaging to establish whether adequate deformity correction has been obtained. Global sagittal alignment is determined by the distance from the posterosuperior corner of S1 to the plumb line extending down from the center of C7, or the distance from the center of the femoral head to the plumb line extending down from the center of C2. This value should be less than 5 cm. Numerous studies have demonstrated correlation between HRQOL metrics and the degree of global sagittal alignment with the C2 or C7 plumb line.[4,25,26,27,28] Cervical sagittal vertical axis (SVA) looks at local alignment with a plumb line drawn from the center of the C2 vertebral body and calculating the distance from this line to the posterior superior corner of the C7 vertebral body from standing radiographs (▶ Fig. 13.3). This measure has also shown to predict postoperative outcomes in patients undergoing multilevel cervical fusion surgery.[28]

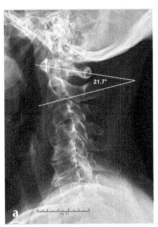 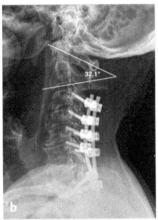

Fig. 13.1 (a) Preoperative lateral cervical radiograph showing C1–C2 lordosis; (b) Postoperative lateral cervical radiograph demonstrating improvement of C1–C2 lordosis

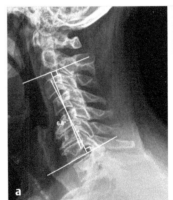 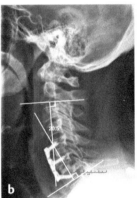

Fig. 13.2 (a) Preoperative lateral cervical radiograph showing C2–C7 Cobb angle; (b) Postoperative lateral cervical radiograph demonstrating improvement of C2–C7 lordosis

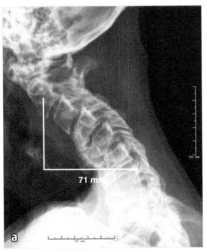 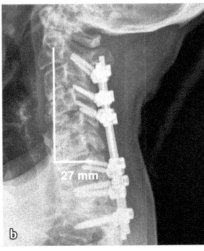

Fig. 13.3 (a) Preoperative lateral cervical radiograph showing C2–C7 sagittal vertical axis (SVA); (b) Postoperative lateral cervical radiograph demonstrating correction and improvement of C2–C7 SVA

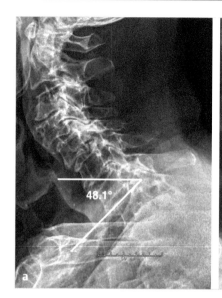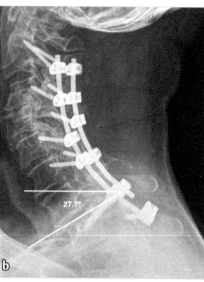

Fig. 13.4 (a) Preoperative lateral cervical radiograph showing T1 slope; **(b)** Postoperative lateral cervical radiograph demonstrating correction and improvement of T1 slope

The T1 slope, defined as the angle between the superior endplate of T1 and a horizontal line, can provide insight into the degree of cervical lordosis necessary to preserve sagittal balance (▶ Fig. 13.4). The chin brow vertical angle (CBVA) is a measure of cervical deformity that is useful in instances where patients have loss of horizontal gaze. The CBVA is the angle between the vertical and a line drawn between the glabella and anterior-most point of the chin. Improved outcomes (gait, activities of daily living) have been demonstrated when surgical intervention is focused on improving the CBVA and restoring horizontal gaze.[29]

Computed tomography (CT) is used to assess bony quality, osteophyte bridging, auto fusion or ankylosis of facet joints, which can determine the need for posterior osteotomies, landmarks, and sizing of instrumentation. Many patients who present with kyphotic deformity have histories of cervical spine surgery, and in such cases thin-slice CT can help assess prior fusion sites. Magnetic resonance imaging (MRI) is valuable in evaluating compression of neural structures such as cord injury/swelling, soft tissue compression, or presence of syrinx. Patients who cannot receive MRI may require CT myelogram. Depending on the degree of deformity and levels involved, computed tomography angiography (CTA) or magnetic resonance angiography (MRA) may be useful in assessing the course of vertebral arteries and other anomalous vascular structures for surgical planning.

13.3 Treatment Options

Generally, conservative treatments should be attempted before considering surgical intervention. These involve symptomatic treatments to target pain and include NSAIDs, muscle relaxants, steroid injections, bracing, and/or physical therapy. Cervical traction can be used to correct deformity either on its own, or as a preoperative intervention. If the deformity does not reduce after five days, it is unlikely to provide further reduction. Muscle relaxants and sedatives should be used in conjunction with traction.[30]

Surgery is usually considered when patients have neurologic compromise, instability, and/or deformity resulting in severe mechanical neck pain, and physical deformity leading to difficulty with ambulation, loss of horizontal gaze, dysphagia, or respiratory dysfunction, adversely impacting HRQOL.

Evaluation of the flexibility of the deformity with flexion-extension radiographs is important preoperatively. An anterior or posterior correction alone may suffice for a flexible deformity. However, if the deformity is rigid or involves ankylosis of the facet joints, a combined surgical approach may be necessary. The etiology of deformity is important to consider. For example, a bony tumor compromising the anterior column will require an anterior approach, while a flexible postlaminectomy kyphotic deformity may be best served with a posterior approach. The extent and quality of the kyphosis also impacts operative planning; focal kyphosis is more amenable to an anterior-alone approach, while longer-segment kyphosis may need posterior intervention.

The anterior-only approach can be used to correct deformity and place instrumentation to fixate the spine in the corrected position. It is most often utilized for rigid cervical kyphotic deformities when there is no ankylosis of the facet joints. The surgeon is able to directly visualize and decompress the anterior aspect of the spinal cord in addition to any anterior column reconstruction that may be necessary due to bony compromise.

Patients are kept supine in slight extension, and decompression is performed, including osteophytectomy, discectomy, and/or corpectomy. It is critical that the uncovertebral joints are released to obtain mobility. Deformity can segmentally be corrected by placing distraction pins in a convergent fashion to generate lordosis upon distraction of the pins. The patient may require gradual repositioning at this time. Lordotic cages can be used to promote fusion and provide additional deformity correction. Further lordosis can be obtained by contouring plates and using three-point bending to bring the middle-segment vertebral body up to the plate. Although an anterior approach is associated with decreased morbidity and mortality compared to combined approaches, the main drawback to this strategy is limited deformity correction.

The posterior-only approach is useful in cases of flexible cervical deformity where sagittal plane imbalance is due to insufficient posterior ligamentous structures or ossified posterior longitudinal ligament (OPLL); a posterior cervical fusion may suffice for correction. If adequate cervical alignment can be achieved with extension radiographs, there is consideration for a posterior approach using three-point skull fixation and extension positioning. Most typically, posterior alone approaches are used as a prophylactic measure after multilevel decompression to prevent the development of sagittal plane deformity as a result of ligamentous interruption, as seen in postlaminectomy kyphosis.

A combined posterior-anterior-posterior approach may be necessary in cases of rigid or incompletely reducible deformity with ankylosed facet joints.[31] Such an approach is frequently necessary in patients with AS. Generally speaking, a posterior-based facet release and osteotomy is completed first. Following this, anterior release, discectomy, and graft placement is undertaken. Finally, posterior instrumentation and deformity correction completes the surgery. This may be done in a staged fashion, with in-line cervical traction employed during each portion of the planned surgery, or, less typically, in one setting. In the setting of AS, posterior instrumentation is critical to prevent further deformity due to the large moment arms surrounding the fusion site.

In instances where osteotomy is necessary, if the degree of correction needed is less than 30°, posterior column osteotomies (facet resections) can be performed. There is a small increased risk of pseudarthrosis stemming from the need for multiple osteotomies to correct larger deformity. A flexible anterior column is needed for full closure of the osteotomy, necessitating either movement through the intervertebral disc, or, in cases with significant spondylosis, a combined anterior-posterior approach. The planned resections are completed through the facets with a high-speed burr down to the exiting nerve roots. Care must be taken to resect laterally through the lateral edge of the lateral masses, or remaining bone will pervent closure of the ostetomies. After all planned resections are completed, desired cervical alignment is achieved through extension positioning using three-point head fixation. Lateral radiographs are taken to ensure alignment goals have been met prior to placement of hardware. Alternatively, for larger deformity correction, a pedicle subtraction osteotomy (PSO) can be used. PSOs allow for up to 30°of correction without the need for an anterior-based procedure. PSOs allow for three-column correction and typically are completed in the lower cervical or upper thoracic segments, thereby correcting the overall position of the cervical spine. The downsides to performing a PSO are that it is technically demanding and has increased morbidity and perioperative complications. Surgeries involving osteotomies often have greater than average blood loss, so careful assessment of the patient's medical comorbidities is needed.

Multilevel fusion typically should not terminate at the cervicothoracic junction (CTJ). CTJ bears the high mechanical stresses between the mobile cervical spine and the relatively fixed thoracic spine. Moreover, it is a transitional zone between the cervical lordosis and thoracic kyphosis, further accentuating the high biomechanical forces.[32] As these special characteristics cause a predisposition for instrumentation failure and increased risk of revision surgery, fusion should be extended to

at least the T1 level.[33] In the cervical and thoracic spines respectively, lateral mass screws and pedicle screws are usually used. The use of pedicle screws may be considered in the cervical spine, despite the increase in difficulty and risk of damaging neurovascular structures, due to the potential benefits from increasing the load sharing across the disc space as well.

Multimodal intraoperative neuromonitoring is often used in deformity surgery. Both motor evoked potentials (MEPs, recording intermittently from corticospinal tracts) and somatosensory evoked potentials (SSEPs, recording continuously from dorsal columns) are used. Changes in the MEPs intraoperatively may guide deformity correction, such as timely reversal of reduction maneuvers. However, neuromonitoring changes should be interpreted in context and with a degree of suspicion. Studies have not reliably shown any changes to safety or outcomes with the use of intraoperative neuromonitoring.[23,34]

Additionally, the use of SSEPs alone should be avoided, as these readings can be misleading and insufficient. Studies have demonstrated that even in instances of normal recordings, patients can have significant deficits postoperatively.[35,36] The gold standard for assessing changes to neuromonitoring is the wake-up test; however, due to the complexity of these surgeries, oftenperformed with the patient in prone position, utilizing the wake-up test requires both time and an experienced anesthesiologist and may not always be an option intraoperatively.

Deformity surgery should always involve fluoroscopy, which allows for intraoperative adjustment of correction. Anesthetic considerations are also important during cervical deformity surgery. An experienced anesthesia team with expertise in spinal anesthesia is preferable. Depending upon the severity of myelopathy or the stability of the cervical spine, awake fiber-optic intubation may be required. Intraoperatively, the maintenance of mean arterial pressure to minimize any poor perfusion to the spinal cord is required. A preoperative huddle or meeting should be considered as a method whereby the details of the surgery and requirements of each member of the operating room team are checked and verified.

13.4 Pitfalls, Complications, and Avoidance

Surgery for deformity correction overall has higher rates of complications compared to all spine surgery due to larger exposures and increased operative time, which are further complicated by a history of prior surgery. Overall, there is a 25% rate of complications in patients treated for deformity.[37] Reported rates of major medical complications range from 3.1 to 44.4%, with 13.5% having neurological complications.[38]

Overall, there is a tradeoff between the degree of kyphotic correction and the rate of complications. Anterior-only approaches have lower complication rates (reported 22–33%) but decreased kyphotic correction and include complications secondary to exposure such as tracheostomy, esophageal injury, graft displacement/failure, vertebral artery injury, dysphagia, and vocal cord paralysis.[39,40,41] Posterior-only approaches carry the risk of postoperative C5 palsy, occurring in about 9.5% of cases.[42] Other complications include hematoma, durotomy, or pseudarthrosis. Posterior approaches also invoke more pain postoperatively in patients due to larger amounts of muscle dissection for exposure. Combined anterior-posterior approaches, while providing the greater amount of deformity correction, also carry higher complication rates, with rates of 32–44.4% reported in the literature.[17,43,44,45]

13.5 Outcomes

Studies have demonstrated correlation between sagittal alignment (both cervical and global) and improvements in pain, neurological symptoms, and HRQOL scores.[26,27,30,46,47,48,49,50] Although no randomized control trials assessing cervical deformity surgery are in the literature, several retrospective analyses provide some insight regarding outcomes. In a study by Simmons et al, patients with AS report increased satisfaction when horizontal gaze is restored.[29]

Grosso et al showed association between degree of kyphosis correction and neurological outcomes.[51] Although there is no difference demonstrated in the current literature between anterior and posterior approaches, both demonstrate significant improvements in pain and myelopathy scores with surgical deformity correction.[52]

Radiographic studies are able to quantify deformity correction from postoperative imaging. Anterior-only approaches have been shown to improve lordosis by 9 to 32°, with about 2° lost over 3-year follow up.[52,53] Meanwhile, posterior-only studies are able to improve lordosis by 6.5 to 54°.[52] The CBVA can be corrected 35 to 52°, and with PSO, there is a mean CBVA correction of 37°.

Outcomes data can be difficult to interpret for several reasons. Major cervical deformity surgeries are performed at lower volumes annually, even at major academic centers, when compared to less complex spine surgeries. The patients that make up this cohort have a heterogeneous set of indications, etiologies, alignment, and medical comorbidities, which make it difficult to draw reasonable conclusions when sample groups are small and have large variation.

13.6 Conclusions

Cervical deformity can be caused by degenerative disease, inflammatory disorders, or iatrogenic factors after spine surgery. Sagittal kyphotic deformity not only causes pathologically increased biomechanics forces on the anterior and posterior aspects of the cervical spinal elements, but also creates a cycle of progressive deformity. Thorough preoperative evaluation of imaging is essential because radiographic metrics such as cervical sagittal imbalance, increased T1 slope, and kyphosis have been correlated with adjacent segment disease, patient disability, and worse HRQOL. Determining whether cervical deformity is flexible or rigid is important in determining the surgical approach. In instances of flexible deformity, anterior- or posterior-only approaches can be considered. However, in cases of rigid deformity where facet joints are ankylosed, it is often times necessary to utilize a combined anterior-posterior approach. Cervical deformity surgery carries risk to the cord and is a complex case with significant perioperative risk, so thorough preoperative neurological evaluation of the patient and imaging are necessary, in addition to being prepared in the

operating room with necessary neuromonitoring and fluoroscopy. Such surgery has significant impact on patient pain, neurological function, and overall HRQOL, and it is a common treatment whose prevalence is only increasing as the aging population continues to grow.

Key References

[1] Scheer JK, Tang JA, Smith JS, et al. International Spine Study Group. Cervical spine alignment, sagittal deformity, and clinical implications: a review. J Neurosurg Spine. 2013; 19(2):141–159

[2] Tang JA, Scheer JK, Smith JS, et al. ISSG. The impact of standing regional cervical sagittal alignment on outcomes in posterior cervical fusion surgery. Neurosurgery. 2015; 76 Suppl 1:S14–S21, discussion S21

[3] Ames CP, Blondel B, Scheer JK, et al. Cervical radiographical alignment: comprehensive assessment techniques and potential importance in cervical myelopathy. Spine. 2013; 38(22) Suppl 1:S149–S160

[4] Steinmetz MP, Stewart TJ, Kager CD, Benzel EC, Vaccaro AR. Cervical deformity correction. Neurosurgery. 2007; 60(1) Supp1 1:S90–S97

[5] Grosso MJ, Hwang R, Mroz T, Benzel E, Steinmetz MP. Relationship between degree of focal kyphosis correction and neurological outcomes for patients undergoing cervical deformity correction surgery. J Neurosurg Spine. 2013; 18(6):537–544

[6] Grosso MJ, Hwang R, Krishnaney AA, Mroz TE, Benzel EC, Steinmetz MP. Complications and outcomes for surgical approaches to cervical kyphosis. J Spinal Disord Tech. 2015; 28(7):E385–E393

References

[1] Irvine DH, Foster JB, Newell DJ, Klukvin BN. Prevalence of cervical spondylosis in a general practice. Lancet. 1965; 1(7395):1089–1092

[2] Smith JS, Lafage V, Schwab FJ, et al. International Spine Study Group. Prevalence and type of cervical deformity among 470 adults with thoracolumbar deformity. Spine. 2014; 39(17):E1001–E1009

[3] Scheer JK, Tang JA, Smith JS, et al. International Spine Study Group. Cervical spine alignment, sagittal deformity, and clinical implications: a review. J Neurosurg Spine. 2013; 19(2):141–159

[4] Ames CP, Blondel B, Scheer JK, et al. Cervical radiographical alignment: comprehensive assessment techniques and potential importance in cervical myelopathy. Spine. 2013; 38(22) Suppl 1:S149–S160

[5] Panjabi MM, Cholewicki J, Nibu K, Grauer J, Babat LB, Dvorak J. Critical load of the human cervical spine: an in vitro experimental study. Clin Biomech (Bristol, Avon). 1998; 13(1):11–17

[6] Panjabi MM, Miura T, Cripton PA, Wang JL, Nain AS, DuBois C. Development of a system for in vitro neck muscle force replication in whole cervical spine experiments. Spine. 2001; 26(20):2214–2219

[7] Cusick JF, Yoganandan N, Pintar F, Myklebust J, Hussain H. Biomechanics of cervical spine facetectomy and fixation techniques. Spine. 1988; 13(7):808–812

[8] Zdeblick TA, Abitbol JJ, Kunz DN, McCabe RP, Garfin S. Cervical stability after sequential capsule resection. Spine. 1993; 18(14):2005–2008

[9] Goel VK, Clark CR, Harris KG, Schulte KR. Kinematics of the cervical spine: effects of multiple total laminectomy and facet wiring. J Orthop Res. 1988; 6(4):611–619

[10] White AA, III, Johnson RM, Panjabi MM, Southwick WO. Biomechanical analysis of clinical stability in the cervical spine. Clin Orthop Relat Res. 1975(109):85–96

[11] Pal GP, Sherk HH. The vertical stability of the cervical spine. Spine. 1988; 13(5):447–449

[12] Hardacker JW, Shuford RF, Capicotto PN, Pryor PW. Radiographic standing cervical segmental alignment in adult volunteers without neck symptoms. Spine. 1997; 22(13):1472–1480, discussion 1480

[13] Breig A. Biomechanics of the central nervous system. Stockholm: Almquist & Wiskell; 1960

[14] Albert TJ, Vacarro A. Postlaminectomy kyphosis. Spine. 1998; 23(24):2738–2745

[15] Lonstein JE. Post-laminectomy kyphosis. Clin Orthop Relat Res. 1977(128):93–100

[16] Herman JM, Sonntag VK. Cervical corpectomy and plate fixation for postlaminectomy kyphosis. J Neurosurg. 1994; 80(6):963–970

[17] Mummaneni PV, Deutsch H, Mummaneni VP. Cervicothoracic kyphosis. Neurosurg Clin N Am. 2006; 17(3):277–287, vi

[18] Zdeblick TA, Bohlman HH. Cervical kyphosis and myelopathy. Treatment by anterior corpectomy and strut-grafting. J Bone Joint Surg Am. 1989; 71(2):170–182

[19] Kaptain GJ, Simmons NE, Replogle RE, Pobereskin L. Incidence and outcome of kyphotic deformity following laminectomy for cervical spondylotic myelopathy. J Neurosurg. 2000; 93(2) Suppl:199–204

[20] Ryken TC, Heary RF, Matz PG, et al. Joint Section on Disorders of the Spine and Peripheral Nerves of the American Association of Neurological Surgeons and Congress of Neurological Surgeons. Cervical laminectomy for the treatment of cervical degenerative myelopathy. J Neurosurg Spine. 2009; 11(2):142–149

[21] Hunt WE. Cervical spondylosis: natural history and rare indications for surgical decompression. Clin Neurosurg. 1980; 27:466–480

[22] Katz J, Liang M. Differential diagnosis and conservative treatment of rheumatic disorders. In (eds). Philadelphia: Lippincott-Raven; 1991:699–718

[23] Hoh DJ, Khoueir P, Wang MY. Management of cervical deformity in ankylosing spondylitis. Neurosurg Focus. 2008; 24(1):E9

[24] Umapathi T, Chaudhry V, Cornblath D, Drachman D, Griffin J, Kuncl R. Head drop and camptocormia. J Neurol Neurosurg Psychiatry. 2002; 73(1):1–7

[25] Tang JA, Scheer JK, Smith JS, et al. ISSG. The impact of standing regional cervical sagittal alignment on outcomes in posterior cervical fusion surgery. Neurosurgery. 2015; 76 Suppl 1:S14–S21, discussion S21

[26] Mac-Thiong JM, Transfeldt EE, Mehbod AA, et al. Can c7 plumbline and gravity line predict health related quality of life in adult scoliosis? Spine. 2009; 34(15):E519–E527

[27] Bridwell KH, Baldus C, Berven S, et al. Changes in radiographic and clinical outcomes with primary treatment adult spinal deformity surgeries from two years to three- to five-years follow-up. Spine. 2010; 35(20):1849–1854

[28] Park MS, Kelly MP, Lee DH, Min WK, Rahman RK, Riew KD. Sagittal alignment as a predictor of clinical adjacent segment pathology requiring surgery after anterior cervical arthrodesis. Spine J. 2014; 14(7):1228–1234

[29] Simmons EDJ, DiStefano RJ, Zheng Y, Simmons EH. Thirty-six years experience of cervical extension osteotomy in ankylosing spondylitis: techniques and outcomes. Spine. 2006; 31(26):3006–3012

[30] Steinmetz MP, Stewart TJ, Kager CD, Benzel EC, Vaccaro AR. Cervical deformity correction. Neurosurgery. 2007; 60(1) Suppl 1:S90–S97

[31] Wang VY, Aryan H, Ames CP. A novel anterior technique for simultaneous single-stage anterior and posterior cervical release for fixed kyphosis. J Neurosurg Spine. 2008; 8(6):594–599

[32] Benzel EC. American Association of Neurological Surgeons: Biomechanics of spine stabilization. Rolling Meadows, Ill.: American Association of Neurological Surgeons; 2001

[33] Schroeder GD, Kepler CK, Kurd MF, et al. Is It Necessary to Extend a Multilevel Posterior Cervical Decompression and Fusion to the Upper Thoracic Spine? Spine. 2016; 41(23):1845–1849

[34] Resnick DK, Anderson PA, Kaiser MG, et al. Joint Section on Disorders of the Spine and Peripheral Nerves of the American Association of Neurological Surgeons and Congress of Neurological Surgeons. Electrophysiological monitoring during surgery for cervical degenerative myelopathy and radiculopathy. J Neurosurg Spine. 2009; 11(2):245–252

[35] Ben-David B, Haller G, Taylor P. Anterior spinal fusion complicated by paraplegia. A case report of a false-negative somatosensory-evoked potential. Spine. 1987; 12(6):536–539

[36] Lesser RP, Raudzens P, Lüders H, et al. Postoperative neurological deficits may occur despite unchanged intraoperative somatosensory evoked potentials. Ann Neurol. 1986; 19(1):22–25

[37] Grosso MJ, Hwang R, Krishnaney AA, Mroz TE, Benzel EC, Steinmetz MP. Complications and outcomes for surgical approaches to cervical kyphosis. J Spinal Disord Tech. 2015; 28(7):E385–E393

[38] Etame AB, Wang AC, Than KD, La Marca F, Park P. Outcomes after surgery for cervical spine deformity: review of the literature. Neurosurg Focus. 2010; 28(3):E14

[39] Han K, Lu C, Li J, et al. Surgical treatment of cervical kyphosis. Eur Spine J. 2011; 20(4):523–536

[40] Eleraky MA, Llanos C, Sonntag VKH. Cervical corpectomy: report of 185 cases and review of the literature. J Neurosurg. 1999; 90(1) Suppl:35–41

[41] Mayr MT, Subach BR, Comey CH, Rodts GE, Haid RW, Jr. Cervical spinal stenosis: outcome after anterior corpectomy, allograft reconstruction, and instrumentation. J Neurosurg. 2002; 96(1) Suppl:10–16

[42] Nassr A, Eck JC, Ponnappan RK, Zanoun RR, Donaldson WF, III, Kang JD. The incidence of C5 palsy after multilevel cervical decompression procedures: a review of 750 consecutive cases. Spine. 2012; 37(3):174–178

[43] Mummaneni PV, Dhall SS, Rodts GE, Haid RW. Circumferential fusion for cervical kyphotic deformity. J Neurosurg Spine. 2008; 9(6):515–521

[44] Schultz KD, Jr, McLaughlin MR, Haid RW, Jr, Comey CH, Rodts GE, Jr, Alexander J. Single-stage anterior-posterior decompression and stabilization for complex cervical spine disorders. J Neurosurg. 2000; 93(2) Suppl:214–221

[45] McMaster MJ. Osteotomy of the cervical spine in ankylosing spondylitis. J Bone Joint Surg Br. 1997; 79(2):197–203

[46] Villavicencio AT, Babuska JM, Ashton A, et al. Prospective, randomized, double-blind clinical study evaluating the correlation of clinical outcomes and cervical sagittal alignment. Neurosurgery. 2011; 68(5):1309–1316, discussion 1316

[47] Guérin P, Obeid I, Gille O, et al. Sagittal alignment after single cervical disc arthroplasty. J Spinal Disord Tech. 2012; 25(1):10–16

[48] Baba H, Maezawa Y, Furusawa N, Imura S, Tomita K. Flexibility and alignment of the cervical spine after laminoplasty for spondylotic myelopathy. A radiographic study. Int Orthop. 1995; 19(2):116–121

[49] Suda K, Abumi K, Ito M, Shono Y, Kaneda K, Fujiya M. Local kyphosis reduces surgical outcomes of expansive open-door laminoplasty for cervical spondylotic myelopathy. Spine. 2003; 28(12):1258–1262

[50] Tokala DP, Lam KS, Freeman BJ, Webb JK. C7 decancellisation closing wedge osteotomy for the correction of fixed cervico-thoracic kyphosis. Eur Spine J. 2007; 16(9):1471–1478

[51] Grosso MJ, Hwang R, Mroz T, Benzel E, Steinmetz MP. Relationship between degree of focal kyphosis correction and neurological outcomes for patients undergoing cervical deformity correction surgery. J Neurosurg Spine. 2013; 18(6):537–544

[52] Cabraja M, Abbushi A, Koeppen D, Kroppenstedt S, Woiciechowsky C. Comparison between anterior and posterior decompression with instrumentation for cervical spondylotic myelopathy: sagittal alignment and clinical outcome. Neurosurg Focus. 2010; 28(3):E15–E19

[53] Nottmeier EW, Deen HG, Patel N, Birch B. Cervical kyphotic deformity correction using 360-degree reconstruction. J Spinal Disord Tech. 2009; 22(6):385–391

14 Lumbar Stenosis with Neurogenic Claudication

Ahmed A. AlBayar and Ajit A. Krishnaney

Abstract

Lumbar stenosis with neurogenic claudication is a common problem in older patients and is the most common reason for spine surgery in patients over the age of 65 in the United States. The diagnosis is based on clinical presentation and evidence of lumbar stenosis on either CT or MR imaging. A variety of treatment options are available including medications, physical therapy, epidural injections, and surgical decompression either with or without fusion. Of these, surgical intervention may be the most effective in appropriately selected older adults who suffer from lumbar spinal stenosis with neurogenic claudication.

Keywords: Lumbar spinal stenosis, neurgenic claudication, lumbar fusion, elderly

Key Points

- Lumbar spinal stenosis is predominantly a disorder of the aging population and is a common radiological finding that is usually appreciated whether patients are symptomatic or not. The subsequent mechanical compression and vascular insufficiency on the lumbar nerve roots contribute to the set of symptoms known as neurogenic claudication.
- It is the most common reason for spine surgery in persons older than 65 years in the United States.[1]
- Symptomatic lumbar spinal stenosis (LSS) can cause a dramatic change in a patient's life. It is associated with a significant negative effect on quality of life and sometimes leads to an unbearable level of disability and pain symptoms.
- The majority of cases of lumbar stenosis are due to age-related degeneration of intervertebral disks and facet joints. This necessarily means that as the population ages, there is a consequent increase in the incidence and prevalence of LSS. Furthermore, this increase may result in increased social and economic burdens.
- Management of such a common and disabling condition can employ several options: nonsurgical, surgical, and combinations of both. The selection of the management strategy depends on several factors that should be kept in mind during evaluation by clinicians.

14.1 Epidemiology

A diagnosis of symptomatic lumbar spinal stenosis (LSS) is made if the patient has radiographic evidence of lumbar stenosis and symptoms of neurogenic claudication or lumbar radiculopathy. Neurogenic claudication presents with pain and dysfunction that starts proximally in the back and buttocks and then progresses distally into the limbs. In some cases, in a dermatomal distribution. Symptoms of neurogenic claudication are of moderate sensitivity but are highly specific to LSS. Patients usually report numbness, weakness, or discomfort radiating from the spine to the buttocks and legs while standing or walking for prolonged distances. Although radiating back and leg pain is a major characteristic of neurogenic claudication, some patients might present with neurologic deficit such as paresthesia or lower extremity weakness. Neurogenic claudication is characterized by an insidious onset and gradual progressive course over months to years. Lumbar stenosis may also present with radiculopathy that may be unilateral or bilateral, resulting in mechanical, motor, reflex, and sensory signs related to the involved levels. The symptoms of neurogenic claudication are typically exaggerated, with extension of the lumbar spine while walking or standing because spine lordosis further narrows the spinal canal. Conversely, symptoms are typically relieved by sitting or flexing the lumbar spine. Noticeable relief at rest may be reported with activities that involve a bending position (e.g., leaning on a shopping cart, lumbar flexion while riding a bicycle). This relief tends to decrease as the condition progresses. Bladder dysfunction in the form of urinary incontinence is commonly reported in the geriatric population, with noticeable improvement after decompression surgeries.[2]

Although LSS is a common diagnosis in the elderly, there is a paucity of literature discussing its incidence and prevalence in different populations. In one study, LSS reached five cases per 100,000 individuals, four times more than cervical spine stenosis.[3] In another study, it was found that 14% of patients complaining of low back pain and seeking specialist care have spinal stenosis.[1] In one study, when evaluated by imaging techniques, there was a degree of spinal stenosis in 80% of the patients above 70 years old.[4] In another study, the prevalence of symptomatic LSS and its association with physical performance using MRI in a population-based cohort was 9.3% overall (10.1% in men and 8.9% in women) In addition, a 6-minute walking time at a maximal pace compared to normal pace walking was a more sensitive test to recognize symptomatic LSS.[5]

The age of onset of symptoms of lumbar stenosis crudely indicates the etiology of the stenosis, as patients with congenital stenosis tend to become symptomatic at younger ages, in the third to fifth decades of life. More commonly, LSS often becomes symptomatic in the mid-sixties and seventies.[6] In one study, absolute lumbar stenosis, defined as a spinal canal diameter of less than 10 mm, has a prevalence as high as 19.4% in the 60–69 year age group.[7]

The main contraindications to surgical decompression of LSS are misdiagnosis and the inability of the patient to benefit from surgical intervention. Symptomatic LSS rarely occurs in isolation. The same degenerative and pathologic processes that cause spinal stenosis may also cause other masquerading pathology. Therefore, great care must be taken to identify other diagnoses with history, clinical examination and ancillary testing that would limit or negate the benefit of surgical intervention. The most common are: vascular claudication, hip and knee osteoarthritis, and medical comorbidities.

The most common diagnostic mimic of neurogenic claudication is vascular claudication. Vascular claudication typically presents in the distal lower extremities and progresses proximally with activity. Typically, the patient will achieve relief at rest standing still. The patient typically will not describe relief by bending forward or leaning on a shopping cart. Other clinical features that distinguish vascular from neurogenic claudication are skin pallor, decreased skin temperature, loss of hair on the legs, and diminished or absent peripheral pulses.

14.1.1 Diagnostic Studies

Before considering invasive therapies for symptomatic lumbar stenosis, confirmation of the presence of LSS and the involved levels is necessary. Imaging modalities such as magnetic resonance imaging, computed tomography and myelography may be useful in the diagnosis and treatment planning of these patients. In cases where vascular claudication is suspected, vascular imaging should be obtained.

14.1.2 Magnetic Resonance Imaging

MRI is considered the best tool to assess for lumbar stenosis. With MRI one is able to visualize soft tissue abnormalities such as ligamentum flavum hypertrophy, disc herniations or protrusions and facet joint compromise. It also can help identify nerve roots and intrinsic cord abnormalities, edema, and demyelination. LSS is most easily seen on T2-weighted images and presents as effacement of CSF signal on T2-weighted sequences. MRI also enables surgeons to accurately localize lesions via simultaneous sagittal, para-sagittal and axial views. (▶ Fig. 14.1) The use of MRI is contraindicated in patients with many types of implants, including cardiac pacemakers, deep brain stimulators, and spinal cord and peripheral nerve stimulators. The presence of these implants is relatively more common in the geriatric population. The presence of these devices should be ascertained and MR-compatibility confirmed prior to ordering the imaging study. It is important to associate the patients' presenting symptoms with the MRI findings. In one study, only one-third of patients older than 60 years with disc herniation (36%) and spinal stenosis (21%) were symptomatic.[8]

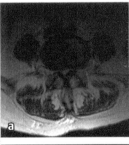
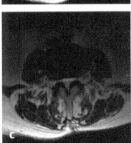
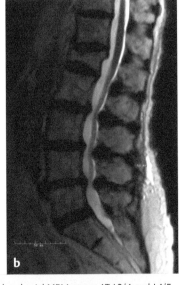

Fig. 14.1 T2-weighted sagittal and axial MRI images AT L3/4 and L4/5 of an 88-year-old woman with neurogenic claudication showing the classic findings of central, lateral recess and foraminal stenosis.

14.1.3 Computed Tomography

CT scan can be useful to demonstrate ossified and calcified structures such as hypertrophied ligaments, facet arthropathy, fractures of the pars, or vertebral bodies. While CT may be used to assess for central and foraminal stenosis, it has been largely supplanted by MRI. However, in cases where significant distortion/metallic artifact is present (as in cases of prior instrumented fusion), CT may provide better visualization than MRI. The sensitivity of detecting neural compression with CT can be increased by the addition of intrathecal contrast (CT myelography). In cases where a patient is unable to obtain an MRI or where significant metallic artifact is present, CT myelography is the modality of choice for diagnosing LSS.

14.1.4 X-ray

Anterior posterior radiographs can demonstrate lateral osteophytes, presence of spondylosis, bony anomalies, and the presence of instability or deformity. Global sagittal and coronal balance may be best assessed via scoliosis X-rays.

14.2 Biomechanical Considerations

LSS can be attributed to several anatomical findings. As a consequence of the degeneration of disks, ventral compression can be caused by centrally located herniated discs or disc bulges. The degenerative process leads to loss of disk height that forces infoldings of the ligamentum flavum and formation of spurs, osteophytes or, in rare occasions, a consequent hypertrophic posterior longitudinal ligament. The subsequent mechanical compression and vascular insufficiency in the lumbar nerve roots and cauda equina contribute to the set of symptoms known as neurogenic claudication. The symptoms of neurogenic claudication are typically exaggerated with extension of the lumbar spine such as with walking or standing due to increased spine lordosis resulting in further narrowing of the spinal canal. Conversely, symptoms are typically relieved by sitting or flexing the lumbar spine.

14.3 Treatment Options

Treatment of symptomatic LSS employs an array of both surgical and conservative options, including physical therapy, membrane stabilizers, analgesics and pain interventions. Commonly, many patients with symptoms of variable severities that are not associated with neurologic deficits are initially treated conservatively. Special consideration should be given to medical treatment in the elderly population, not only to primarily treat the symptoms of LSS, but also to optimize the medical perioperative care for associated comorbidities—cardiac, pulmonary, renal, and endocrine—to achieve the best outcomes.[9] The spine surgeon should give special attention to patient's bone health, given the high prevalence of bone disease in the elderly population.[9]

Understanding the natural history of LSS is a key to managing patients due to the variable severities of presenting symptoms. Although LSS in the elderly is primarily due to degenerative changes in the spine, this fact does not anticipate an inevitable worsening of the symptoms. In fact, according to the North American Spine Society (NASS) guidelines, the natural history of one-third to one-half of mild-to-moderate LSS patients was favorable.[10] In addition, other reviews reported improvement in one-third of the cases as well as no change of severity during 8 years of follow-up, making the rapid progression of pain or disabilities in such patients seem to be rare.[11] Similarly, another study reported no dramatic progression in LSS symptoms in 60% of patients, despite MRI-confirmed progressive stenosis of the spinal canal.[12]

14.3.1 Surgical Management

The natural history of LSS shows that the course of symptom progression is gradual and occurs over years. It is unusual to encounter a patient who has a rapid deterioration in symptoms, and it may indicate an association with other pathology, such as tumors, compression fractures, or disc herniaitons. Therefore, surgery is almost always elective and planned after discussing the severity of symptoms and the expected outcomes of surgery with the patient.[13] Although there is no high-quality evidence of its effects, a trial of nonoperative treatment options is usually performed prior to considering surgical intervention.[1,14] Several studies have compared surgery to other nonoperative management. The Spine Patient Outcomes Research Trial (SPORT) demonstrated an early significant benefit of surgery over nonoperative treatment. However, this advantage decreased over time to provide no difference in 6-year and 8-year follow-up.[15] The conclusions drawn were considered low quality because of the high rate of crossover from the conservative treatment group to surgery.

The goal of surgery is to decompress the nerve roots that are trapped within the stenotic spinal canal, which gives a chance for pain relief and functional recovery in cases with neural deficits. The decompression surgeries have many surgical approaches and techniques that vary depending on the level,

extent, and severity of the stenosis as well as of the associated conditions. It also depends on the surgeon's preference and the patient's history with spine surgery.

These techniques involve unilateral and bilateral laminectomy and bilateral decompression through unilateral laminectomy, in addition to different methods of laminoplasty and minimally invasive surgery. However, current evidence does not prefer any of the surgical approaches.[16] A systematic review in 2015 compared the effects of three of the new approaches—unilateral laminotomy for bilateral decompression, bilateral laminotomy, and split-spinous process laminotomy—to conventional laminectomy. The results showed similarity in outcomes of functional disability, perceived recovery, and leg pain after all approaches, although the evidence was low to very low quality. It highlighted the poor methodology of the currently available studies of these new approaches and the lack of long-term outcomes data.[17] In another as-treated analysis of SPORT, predominant leg pain patients improved significantly more with surgery than predominant LBP patients, who still improved significantly more with surgery than with nonoperative treatment.[18]

Spinal fusion in LSS patient with decompression surgery has been a major controversy in the surgical management of LSS. It has been recommended for patients with associated degenerative spondylolisthesis, recurrent stenosis despite decompression, instability or deformity.[13] (▶ Fig. 14.2) According to one retrospective cohort, the rate of complex lumbar fusion surgeries in the elderly has increased 15-fold (from 1.3 to 19.9 per 100,000 beneficiaries) compared to decompression alone or simple fusion surgeries. This increase was associated with an increase in the rate of major complications, 30-day mortality, costs, and resource use compared to decompression alone.[19] In another retrospective cohort, posterior lumbar interbody fusion (PLIF) was compared to decompressive laminectomy and flavectomy without fusion (DLF) in elderly patients (> 75 years old). It showed a statistically significant decrease in LBP and lower recurrence after PLIF versus DLF. Moreover, the study concluded

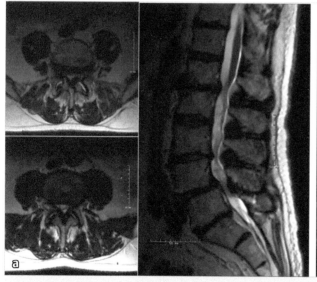
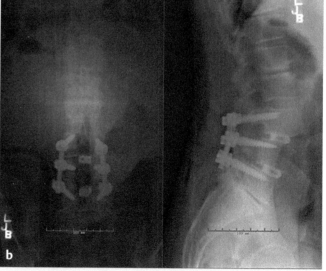

Fig. 14.2 T2 weighted MRI with sagittal and axial cuts with severe central, lateral recess, and foraminal stenosis in a 75-year-old male with neurogenic claudication and mechanical back pain **(a)**. Note grade 1 spondylolisthesis at L4–5. He underwent L3–4 and L4–5 decompression and instrumented fusion with TLIF **(b)** with complete resolution of his claudication and mechanical back pain.

that lumbar surgery is safe and justifiable even in elderly patients > 75 years old and recommended lumbar fusion surgery in patients with predominant back pain.[20] A clinical practice guideline update on 2013 recommended that "in the absence of deformity or instability, lumbar fusion has not been shown to improve outcomes in patients with isolated stenosis, and is not recommended"[10]. According to NASS guidelines, in the absence of instability or deformity, decompression alone is recommended for patients with prominent leg symptoms.[21]

Use of intraspinous spacers as an alternative to lumbar decompression has been advocated in the literature. Patients whose symptoms improve with forward flexion and have single-level stenosis are considered candidates for this procedure. Placement of the spacer between the spinous processes of the stenotic level forces the spine into focal kyphosis, thereby enlarging the diameter of the canal. While initial studies showed improvement in claudicant symptoms, symptom relief may not be as durable as conventional decompressive surgery, with high failure rates in medium- to long-term follow up.[22]

14.4 Benefit and Risks

When considering surgical intervention for symptomatic lumbar stenosis, a critical appraisal of the risks and benefits of surgery is mandatory. The benefits of surgical intervention in the appropriately selected patient, as described above, include improved posture, improved ambulatory distance, and reduced pain and discomfort. The risks of surgery can be divided into two general catagories: risks related to having surgery and risks related to the specific operation. Surgical risks include perioperative cardiovascular events, pulmonary events, venous thromboembolism, and, in older adults, cognitive impairment. Risks specific to lumbar decompression include injury to the neural elements, durotomy, postoperative pseudomeningocele, postoperative epidural hematoma, iatrogenic instability, and postoperative wound infection. If a fusion is performed, additional risks include pseudoarthrosis, hardware failure/fracture, and iatrogenic deformity.

14.5 Pitfalls, Complications and Avoidance

While the presentation and basic treatment paradigms for the management of symptomatic lumbar stenosis are not age specific, the increased incidence of medical comorbidities, challenges with mobility, presence of frailty, cognitive decline, and complex social situations must be assessed prior to embarking on a treatment plan. In general, medical management has a lower risk profile than surgical intervention and should be considered first. However, in patients whom symptoms do not improve, surgery should be considered.

Frailty and advanced patient age correlate with increased risk of postoperative morbidity and poor outcome. They have also been associated with increased cost of care in the immediate postoperative period.[23,24] Despite the risk of comorbidity, in at least one study the most frail patients achieved the biggest improvement in self-reported outcome measures (ODI).[24] Therefore, if the risks of surgery can be effectively mitigated, surgery in even the frail elderly could be considered.[25]

Strategies for risk reduction include rehabilitation, nutritional optimization, and comanagement perioperatively with a geriatrician.[26]

Prior to surgical intervention, social factors must be assessed to optimize recovery and reduce the risk of readmission. Patients with poor mobility, those who live alone or have declining cognitive function, may require placement in a skilled nursing facility postoperatively. This possibility should be discussed with the patient and his/her family prior to surgical intervention. End-of-life issues, such as durable power of attorney for health care and do-not-resuscitate orders should be addressed.

When fusion is being considered, the patient's bone quality needs to be assessed. Relative osteopenia/osteoporosis rates are high in the elderly. Achieving good fixation can be challenging in these cases, as can be seen by the higher rates of hardware failure and proximal junctional kyphosis in the frail and elderly.[24] Bone health should be assessed and optimized prior to surgical intervention to minimize this risk whenever possible. Strategies to improve fixation and outcomes of fusion surgery include cement augmentation, partial correction of deformity, and focal fusion without deformity correction in select cases. (▶ Fig. 14.3)

14.6 Outcomes/Evidence

There is a lack of consensus on either conservative or surgical treatments. This can be explained by the paucity of high-quality randomized trials investigating the efficacy of the various conservative treatment options that are being utilized.[1] A systematic review of LSS confirmed with MRI and presenting with neurogenic claudication concluded that there is no significant evidence supporting any type of conservative treatment.[27] Moreover, there was a lack of clear description of nonsurgical treatment protocols, which makes treatment outcomes analysis difficult.[1]

Most patients with LSS and neurogenic claudication are treated with a course of conservative treatment before surgical intervention.[27] In the elderly population, patients commonly present with other severe comorbidities which may make surgery a risky choice.[28,29] Such cases are usually treated by multimodality pain centers.[30] If conservative measures fail and surgery is considered, patients must be selected carefully based on the imaging findings and the expected outcomes based on their overall health.

Few randomized controlled trials have studied the conservative (nonoperative) strategies of LSS treatment. A systematic review of nonoperative interventions in imaging-confirmed symptomatic LSS patients failed to conclude a sufficient evidence to recommend any nonoperative strategy. Those strategies included calcitonin, prostaglandins, gabapentin, methylcobalamin, epidural steroid injections, exercise, and multimodal nonoperative treatment. It also noted that the lack of clearly defined descriptions of these protocols is preventing data pooling and analysis for better testing of the outcomes.[27]

Pharmacologic treatments of LSS include drugs such as NSAIDs, acetaminophen, gabapentin, prostaglandins, and vitamin B1. However, the only available evidence is of low to very low quality provided by single-center small trials.[27,31]

Several studies have suggested that NSAIDs do not offer more relief than acetaminophen.[32] Prostaglandins are theorized to

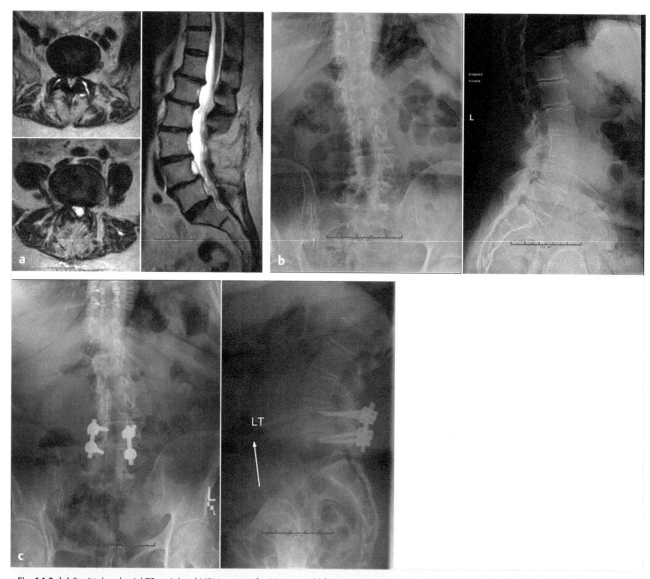

Fig. 14.3 **(a)** Sagittal and axial T2-weighted MRI images of a 78-year-oold female with neurogenic claudication and radiculopathy. Note the recurrent lateral recess stenosis at L4–5, where there has been a prior decompressive laminectomy. There is also grade 1 spondylolisthesis at the L4–5 level as well as severe stenosis at L5-S1. **(b)** AP and lateral standing radiographs of the same patient again demonstrating the L4–5 spondylolisthesis (Lat) seen on the MRI as well as a coronal degenerative deformity (AP). **(c)** Postoperative AP and lateral standing radiographs showing a focal instrumented fusion at L4–5 without attempt at deformity correction after L5-S1 and revision L4–5 lumbar decompression. The patient had complete resolution of her claudicant and radicular symptoms.

enhance blood supply to the nerve roots, but a single-center small trial did not offer more than a low- to very low-quality evidence of symptom relief.[33]

In a retrospective cohort study, quality of life (QOL) of LSS patients with concordant neurogenic claudication was evaluated after treatment with membrane-stabilizing agents (MSAs) (701 patients) vs. conservative treatment without MSAs (2,104 patients). The results suggested better QOL for the patients treated with MSAs compared to the other group.[34] A recent retrospective cohort, by the same institution, sought to create a prediction model for MSAs posttreatment outcomes. It concluded that greatest effects of MSAs will be in those with worse QOL, those with less depression, those who are married, and in patients with high socioeconomic state.[35]

Another randomized controlled trial compared a group of patients receiving the standard medical care (therapeutic exercise, lumbosacral closet with steel bracing, and NSAIDS) against a group that received gabapentin in addition to the standard medical treatment. Gabapentin resulted in improvements in walking distance, pain scores, and sensory deficit recovery.[36]

In the past, calcitonin was suggested to cause improvement of symptoms, but a recent meta-analysis showed no better effect than acetaminophen or placebo.[37]

Opioids have been used for pain control, but their role in the long-term control of symptoms is unclear.[1] A randomized, double-blinded crossover trial tested the efficacy of oxymorphone and propoxyphene/acetaminophen in LSS with neurogenic claudication. The study failed to demonstrate a benefit from the tested opioids.[38] Corticosteroids are often used in LSS conservative management schemes although there is still no high-quality evidence of their efficacy in LSS.[1]

Physiotherapy is commonly utilized in the nonoperative treatment of LSS. It includes exercise that can be for increasing flexibility, core strengthening, or aerobic conditioning to increase exercise tolerance. Bracing, corsets and lumbar semi-rigid orthosis have been utilized in some cases. Other pain-relieving methods such as applying heat or ice, electric stimulation, massage or ultrasonic waves, as well as spine manipulation and postural instructions, are often included in medical management programs.[1] In a systematic review of nonoperative treatment options, there was low-quality evidence from a single trial that exercise is of short-term benefit for leg pain and function compared to no treatment.[27] In another systematic review of physical therapy trials in LSS treatment, it could not be concluded which physical therapy treatment was superior for LSS. It also found low-quality evidence suggesting that physical therapy modalities such as ultrasound, Transcutaneous Electrical Nerve Stimulation (TENS), and heat packs have no additional effect to exercise. Moreover, surgery leads to better long-term (2-year) outcomes for pain and disability but not for walking distance.[39] In a secondary analysis of the SPORT study, the relationship between physical therapy and the long-term prognosis for LSS patients was evaluated. It concluded that physical therapy was associated with a reduced likelihood of patients' receiving surgery within 1 year.[40]

Epidural steroid injections are commonly used to treat symptoms of LSS, in spite of the variability of the results of the trials. In one meta-analysis that included eight trials involving patients with symptomatic LSS, epidural corticosteroid injections did not have a clear effect on spinal stenosis.[41] Another meta-analysis in 2015 that included 10 randomized controlled trials demonstrated a minimal evidence that epidural steroid injections have better effects than Lidocaine alone. It also demonstrated a fair amount of short-term and long-term benefits in LSS patients.[42] The steroid injections are performed utilizing three main approaches in the lumbar spine—caudal, interlaminar and transforaminal—but the literature discussing the superiority of one approach over another is sporadic.[43]

In an analysis of two randomized controlled trials for both caudal and interlaminar injections in the management of pain and disability of central LSS, results at 2 year follow up showed significant improvement with caudal and interlaminar epidural approaches, either with local anesthetic only, or with steroids at 2 years. In addition, the interlaminar approach provided significantly better results than the caudal injection in that management setting.[43] It is commonly believed that epidural steroid injections are primarily helpful only for short-term pain relief and disability improvement. Notably, other trials also concluded that pain sensitivity in patients with LSS has no effect on the degree of pain relief after epidural steroid injections.[44,45] It is important to mention that epidural injections in general bear a risk of introducing infections to the CNS. This should be kept in mind when making the decision to proceed with injections in the aging population, where there may be a higher incidence of depressed immunity.[35]

Among the other treatments that have some popularity is spinal manipulation. It is commonly used to treat chronic low back pain, although until recently it was considered contraindicated for confirmed LSS.[46] Recent studies showed very low-quality evidence that flexion distraction manipulation could be beneficial for LSS.[22,31,47] Acupuncture is another common treatment, although there is limited evidence that it is beneficial for LSS.[23]

A systematic review in 2014 evaluated the effectiveness of spine surgery for symptomatic LSS in the elderly and the safety of surgery in the same population, with emphasis on the incidence of perioperative complications. The results showed significant overall improvement of pain and disability.[24] Moreover, the rate of perioperative complication such as durotomy, wound infection, and general mortality was infrequent. It also showed less favorable complication rates and outcomes for obese and diabetic patients.[24] Another systematic review in 2011 that included five studies on a total of 918 patients compared the effectiveness of surgery vs. conservative treatment. In all five trials, surgery showed superiority in pain relief, disability, and quality of life, although not for walking ability. The advantage of surgery was noticeable at 3 to 6 months and remained for up to 2 to 4 years, but the differences tended to be smaller by the end of that period.[30] Another randomized controlled trial involved 94 patients and compared outcomes of nonoperative management of 44 patients vs. decompression surgery for 50 patients, of which 10 had additional fusions. It concluded that surgery achieved better pain relief and less overall disability than nonoperative management over 2 years of follow-up.[25] Moreover, using a design of a randomized trial concurrently with an observational cohort study, SPORT provided 4-year results that compared surgery to nonoperative care in LSS. It showed clinically significant advantages of surgery that were maintained for 4 years. These advantages included significantly less bodily pain and Oswestry Disability Index (ODI) scores.[26]

On the other hand, a case series compared outcomes using ODI and the surgeon's clinical assessment of nonoperative treatment of 54 matched pairs of patients with LSS vs. laminectomy. It concluded no statistically significant difference in outcomes between them.[48] In addition, in another nonrandomized cohort of patients with LSS, decompression (54 patients) and decompression with fusion for degenerative spondylolisthesis (42 patients) were compared to nonoperative treatment (29 patients). Both surgical interventions groups showed better outcomes and scored better on Roland Morris Disability Questionnaires for outcomes assessment.[49]

Conclusion

Lumbar stenosis with neurogenic claudication is prevalent in the aging population. In cases where medical management of the patient's symptoms fail, surgical decompression with or without fusion may be indicated. If risks are appropriately assessed and mitigated, older adults can derive significant benefit from indicated surgery.

Key References

[1] Gerhardt J, Bette S, Janssen I, Gempt J, Meyer B, Ryang YM. Is eighty the new sixty? Outcomes and complications after lumbar decompression surgery in elderly patients over 80 years of age. World Neurosurg. 2018; 112:e555–e560

[2] Reid DBC, Daniels AH, Ailon T, et al. International Spine Study Group. Frailty and health-related quality of life improvement following adult spinal deformity surgery. World Neurosurg. 2018; 112:e548–e554

[3] Battié MC, Jones CA, Schopflocher DP, Hu RW. Health-related quality of life and comorbidities associated with lumbar spinal stenosis. Spine J. 2012; 12 (3):189–195

References

[1] Lurie J, Tomkins-Lane C. Management of lumbar spinal stenosis. BMJ. 2016; 352:h6234

[2] Battié MC, Jones CA, Schopflocher DP, Hu RW. Health-related quality of life and comorbidities associated with lumbar spinal stenosis. Spine J. 2012; 12 (3):189–195

[3] Siebert E, Prüss H, Klingebiel R, Failli V, Einhäupl KM, Schwab JM. Lumbar spinal stenosis: syndrome, diagnostics and treatment. Nat Rev Neurol. 2009; 5 (7):392–403

[4] Sasaki K. Magnetic resonance imaging findings of the lumbar root pathway in patients over 50 years old. Eur Spine J. 1995; 4(2):71–76–Accessed October 17, –2018

[5] Ishimoto Y, Yoshimura N, Muraki S, et al. Prevalence of symptomatic lumbar spinal stenosis and its association with physical performance in a population-based cohort in Japan: the Wakayama Spine Study. Osteoarthritis Cartilage. 2012; 20(10):1103–1108

[6] Fraser JF, Huang RC, Girardi FP, Cammisa FP, Jr. Pathogenesis, presentation, and treatment of lumbar spinal stenosis associated with coronal or sagittal spinal deformities. Neurosurg Focus. 2003; 14(1):e6–Accessed October 17, 2018

[7] Kalichman L, Cole R, Kim DH, et al. Spinal stenosis prevalence and association with symptoms: the Framingham Study. Spine J. 2009; 9(7):545–550

[8] Epstein NE. Surgical management of lumbar stenosis: decompression and indications for fusion. Neurosurg Focus. 1997; 3(2):e1–, discussion 1, e4–Accessed October 17, 2018

[9] Choma TJ, Rechtine GR, McGuire RA, Jr, Brodke DS. Treating the Aging Spine. J Am Acad Orthop Surg. 2015; 23(12):e91–e100

[10] Kreiner DS, Shaffer WO, Baisden JL, et al. North American Spine Society. An evidence-based clinical guideline for the diagnosis and treatment of degenerative lumbar spinal stenosis (update). Spine J. 2013; 13(7):734–743

[11] Benoist M. The natural history of lumbar degenerative spinal stenosis. Joint Bone Spine. 2002; 69(5):450–457–Accessed November 3, 2017

[12] Haig AJ, Tong HC, Yamakawa KSJ, et al. Predictors of pain and function in persons with spinal stenosis, low back pain, and no back pain. Spine. 2006; 31 (25):2950–2957

[13] Sengupta DK, Herkowitz HN. Lumbar spinal stenosis. Treatment strategies and indications for surgery. Orthop Clin North Am. 2003; 34(2):281–295–Accessed November 17, 2017

[14] Backstrom KM, Whitman JM, Flynn TW. Lumbar spinal stenosis-diagnosis and management of the aging spine. Man Ther. 2011; 16(4):308–317

[15] Lurie JD, Tosteson TD, Tosteson ANA, et al. Surgical versus nonoperative treatment for lumbar disc herniation: eight-year results for the spine patient outcomes research trial. Spine. 2014; 39(1):3–16

[16] Jacobs WCH, Rubinstein SM, Koes B, van Tulder MW, Peul WC. Evidence for surgery in degenerative lumbar spine disorders. Best Pract Res Clin Rheumatol. 2013; 27(5):673–684

[17] Overdevest GM, Jacobs W, Vleggeert-Lankamp C, Thomé C, Gunzburg R, Peul W. Effectiveness of posterior decompression techniques compared with conventional laminectomy for lumbar stenosis. Overdevest GM, ed. Cochrane database Syst Rev. 2015;24(3):CD010036

[18] Pearson A, Blood E, Lurie J, et al. Predominant leg pain is associated with better surgical outcomes in degenerative spondylolisthesis and spinal stenosis: results from the Spine Patient Outcomes Research Trial (SPORT). Spine. 2011; 36(3):219–229

[19] Deyo RA, Mirza SK, Martin BI, Kreuter W, Goodman DC, Jarvik JG. Trends, major medical complications, and charges associated with surgery for lumbar spinal stenosis in older adults. JAMA. 2010; 303(13):1259–1265

[20] Lee C-H, Hyun S-J, Kim K-J, Jahng T-A, Kim H-J. Decompression only versus fusion surgery for lumbar stenosis in elderly patients over 75 years old: which is reasonable? Neurol Med Chir (Tokyo). 2013; 53(12):870–874

[21] Resnick DK, Watters WC, III, Mummaneni PV, et al. Guideline update for the performance of fusion procedures for degenerative disease of the lumbar spine. Part 10: lumbar fusion for stenosis without spondylolisthesis. J Neurosurg Spine. 2014; 21(1):62–66

[22] Cambron JA, Schneider M, Dexheimer JM, et al. A pilot randomized controlled trial of flexion-distraction dosage for chiropractic treatment of lumbar spinal stenosis. J Manipulative Physiol Ther. 2014; 37(6):396–406

[23] Kim KH, Kim T-H, Lee BR, et al. Acupuncture for lumbar spinal stenosis: a systematic review and meta-analysis. Complement Ther Med. 2013; 21(5):535–556

[24] Shamji MF, Mroz T, Hsu W, Chutkan N. Management of degenerative lumbar spinal stenosis in the elderly. Neurosurgery. 2015; 77(4) Suppl 4: S68–S74

[25] Malmivaara A, Slätis P, Heliövaara M, et al. Finnish Lumbar Spinal Research Group. Surgical or nonoperative treatment for lumbar spinal stenosis? A randomized controlled trial. Spine. 2007; 32(1):1–8

[26] Weinstein JN, Lurie JD, Tosteson TD, et al. Surgical versus nonoperative treatment for lumbar disc herniation: four-year results for the Spine Patient Outcomes Research Trial (SPORT). Spine. 2008; 33(25):2789–2800

[27] Ammendolia C, Stuber K, de Bruin LK, et al. Nonoperative treatment of lumbar spinal stenosis with neurogenic claudication: a systematic review. Spine. 2012; 37(10):E609–E616

[28] Djurasovic M, Glassman SD, Carreon LY, Dimar JR, II. Contemporary management of symptomatic lumbar spinal stenosis. Orthop Clin North Am. 2010; 41(2):183–191

[29] Szpalski M, Gunzburg R. Lumbar spinal stenosis in the elderly: an overview. Eur Spine J. 2003; 12 Suppl 2:S170–S175

[30] Kovacs FM, Urrútia G, Alarcón JD. Surgery versus conservative treatment for symptomatic lumbar spinal stenosis: a systematic review of randomized controlled trials. Spine. 2011; 36(20):E1335–E1351

[31] Schneider M, Ammendolia C, Murphy D, et al. Comparison of non-surgical treatment methods for patients with lumbar spinal stenosis: protocol for a randomized controlled trial. Chiropr Man Therap. 2014; 22(1): 19

[32] Roelofs PD, Deyo RA, Koes BW, Scholten RJ, van Tulder MW. Non-steroidal anti-inflammatory drugs for low back pain. In: Roelofs PD, ed. Cochrane Database of Systematic Reviews. Chichester, UK: John Wiley & Sons, Ltd; 2008: CD000396. doi:10.1002/14651858.CD000396.pub3

[33] Yoshihara H. Prostaglandin E1 Treatment for Lumbar Spinal Canal Stenosis: Review of the Literature. Pain Pract. 2016; 16(2):245–256

[34] Bansal S, Lubelski D, Thompson NR, et al. Membrane-Stabilizing Agents Improve Quality-of-Life Outcomes for Patients with Lumbar Stenosis. Global Spine J. 2016; 6(2):139–146

[35] Lubelski D, Thompson NR, Agrawal B, et al. Prediction of quality of life improvements in patients with lumbar stenosis following use of membrane stabilizing agents. Clin Neurol Neurosurg. 2015; 139:234–240

[36] Yaksi A, Ozgönenel L, Ozgönenel B. The efficiency of gabapentin therapy in patients with lumbar spinal stenosis. Spine. 2007; 32(9):939–942

[37] Podichetty VK, Varley ES, Lieberman I. Calcitonin treatment in lumbar spinal stenosis: a meta-analysis. Spine. 2011; 36(5):E357–E364

[38] Markman JD, Gewandter JS, Frazer ME, et al. A Randomized, Double-blind, Placebo-Controlled Crossover Trial of Oxymorphone Hydrochloride and Propoxyphene/Acetaminophen Combination for the Treatment of Neurogenic Claudication Associated With Lumbar Spinal Stenosis. Spine. 2015; 40(10): 684–691

[39] Macedo LG, Hum A, Kuleba L, et al. Physical therapy interventions for degenerative lumbar spinal stenosis: a systematic review. Phys Ther. 2013; 93(12): 1646–1660

[40] Fritz JM, Lurie JD, Zhao W, et al. Associations between physical therapy and long-term outcomes for individuals with lumbar spinal stenosis in the SPORT study. Spine J. 2014; 14(8):1611–1621

[41] Chou R, Hashimoto R, Friedly J, et al. Epidural Corticosteroid Injections for Radiculopathy and Spinal Stenosis: A Systematic Review and Meta-analysis. Ann Intern Med. 2015; 163(5):373–381

[42] Liu K, Liu P, Liu R, Wu X, Cai M. Steroid for epidural injection in spinal stenosis: a systematic review and meta-analysis. Drug Des Devel Ther. 2015; 9: 707–716

[43] Manchikanti L, Singh V, Pampati V, Falco FJ, Hirsch JA. Comparison of the efficacy of caudal, interlaminar, and transforaminal epidural injections in managing lumbar disc herniation: is one method superior to the other? Korean J Pain. 2015; 28(1):11–21

[44] Park C-H, Lee S-H. Correlation between severity of lumbar spinal stenosis and lumbar epidural steroid injection. Pain Med. 2014; 15(4):556–561

[45] Kim H-J, Yeom JS, Lee JW, et al. The influence of pain sensitivity on the treatment outcome of transforaminal epidural steroid injection in patients with lumbar spinal stenosis. Pain Pract. 2014; 14(5):405–412

[46] Fritz JM, Delitto A, Welch WC, Erhard RE. Lumbar spinal stenosis: a review of current concepts in evaluation, management, and outcome measurements. Arch Phys Med Rehabil. 1998; 79(6):700–708

[47] Stuber K, Sajko S, Kristmanson K. Chiropractic treatment of lumbar spinal stenosis: a review of the literature. J Chiropr Med. 2009; 8(2):77–85

[48] Herno A, Airaksinen O, Saari T, Luukkonen M. Lumbar spinal stenosis: a matched-pair study of operated and non-operated patients. Br J Neurosurg. 1996; 10(5):461–465

[49] Athiviraham A, Yen D. Is spinal stenosis better treated surgically or nonsurgically? Clin Orthop Relat Res. 2007; 458(458):90–93

15 Lumbar Spondylolisthesis

Sharad Rajpal and Sigita Burneikiene

Abstract

Symptomatic lumbar degenerative disease is a growing problem, and degenerative spondylolisthesis (DS) is one of the most common conditions for which surgery is performed. Spine surgeons are increasingly being challenged to evaluate the risk-to-benefit ratio of spine surgery carefully, but the literature specifically dedicated to the aging patient is sparse. This chapter reviews the epidemiology, clinical presentation, and biomechanical aspects of the disease. Conservative and various surgical treatment options including decompression and fusion surgeries are discussed, with special consideration of benefits, risks, and clinical outcomes in aging patients. In summary, age alone should not be considered a contraindication to surgical intervention; older adults who are optimized perioperatively can and should expect successful outcomes similar to their younger counterparts.

Keywords: Aging population, decompression, degenerative spondylolisthesis, spinal fusion.

Key Points

- Conservative treatment is typically the first treatment of choice in patients with degenerative spondylolisthesis
- Decompression may be a more appropriate treatment option due to shorter operative times and reduced blood loss, but there is increased risk associated with instability
- Instrumented fusion may have improved fusion rates and results in better long-term clinical outcomes in properly selected patients
- A comprehensive preoperative assessment, elimination of modifiable risk factors, and optimization of preventative measures and postoperative care can help to minimize or avoid complications in the aging patient population.

15.1 Epidemiology

Degenerative spondylolisthesis (DS) is a common problem in older adults. DS is one of the most common conditions for which surgery is performed in the United States.[1,2] Life expectancy in Western countries has been increasing over the past several consecutive decades.[3] It is estimated that spondylolisthesis has a prevalence of about 20 to 25% among women, and 4 to 8% among men in the United States.[4,5,6] In those over the age of 65 years, the prevalence is reported to be 29% among women[4] and 31% among men.[7] He et al[8] found a prevalence of lumbar spondylolisthesis of 19.1% in Chinese men and 25.0% in Chinese women aged 65 years and older. Only a single vertebral level was involved 96% of the time, with the degree of slip ranging from 5 to 28% among those diagnosed with spondylolisthesis. Progression of existing spondylolisthesis over a 5-year period was observed in 12% of patients, with new onset of spondylolisthesis occurring among 12% without the condition at baseline. The authors found that the prevalence of spondyl-

olisthesis did not vary by height, BMI, smoking history, diabetes, or heart disease. However, men with spondylolisthesis more often reported higher levels of physical activity or walking daily for exercise than men without spondylolisthesis. Similar results were reported by Wang et al,[9] where they found that spondylolisthesis progressed in 13.0% and 16.5% of men and women, respectively, and appeared de novo in 12.4% and 12.7% of men and women, respectively, at the 4-year follow-up on patients 65 years and older. In their epidemiologic study among older men, Denard et al[7] observed that the prevalence of back pain, back pain severity, and being bothered by back pain in the past year were not different among men with or without radiographic DS. Compared to their counterparts, however, men were more likely to report neurogenic symptoms in the last year and to have experienced recent limitations in performing activities requiring lower extremity function.

Clinical presentation of DS consists of intermitted low back pain, radiculopathy, and neurogenic claudication,[10] the latter being the most common symptom, reported by up to 82% of patients seeking surgical treatment.[11] Cauda equina syndrome is less common, but requires immediate medical attention and is reported in 3% of patients with spondylolisthesis.[12]

The literature on the natural history of DS is limited. Matsunaga et al[13] published a prospective study which evaluated a total of 145 conservatively-managed patients for a minimum of 10 years. The progression of spondylolisthesis was observed in 34% of patients, but the authors noted that as the intervertebral disc space decreased, the patients reported improvement in low back pain. A total of 84 out of 110 (76%) patients remained free of neurological symptoms for the entire follow-up time. Although 29 out of 35 (83%) patients who had neurological symptoms experienced significant deterioration, this was not correlated with progression of spondylolisthesis.

15.2 Biomechanical Considerations

Spondylolisthesis is defined as a forward translation, or slip, of one vertebral body in relation to the adjacent caudal vertebral body (▶ Fig. 15.1a, b). Although spondylolisthesis can occur at any level in the spine, L4-L5 has been reported as the most common level.[7,14] According to the Wiltse[15] classification system, spondylolisthesis is often divided into one of six distinct categories defined by cause:

- Type I: congenital/dysplastic: due to agenesis of the superior articulating facet
- Type II: isthmic (spondylolytic): due to a pars interarticularis defect
- Type III: degenerative: chronic instability secondary to articular degeneration
- Type IV: traumatic: caused by a fracture or dislocation not involving the pars
- Type V: pathologic: caused by a malignancy, infection, or other abnormal bone
- Type VI: postsurgical (iatrogenic)

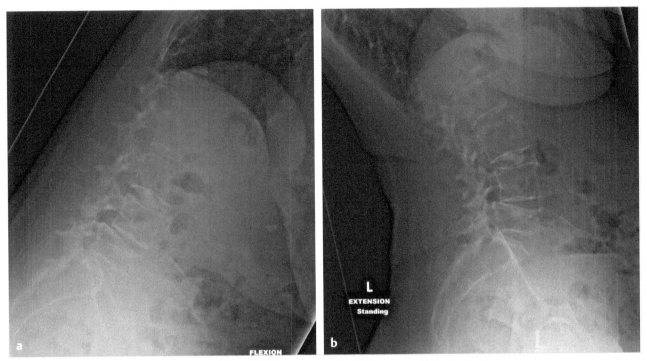

Fig. 15.1 Stable spondylolisthesis. Grade I spondylolisthesis at L4-L5 on flexion **(a)** and extension **(b)** radiographs.

A common method of grading spondylolisthesis is by the severity of the slip, as defined by how far one vertebral body has migrated in relation to the adjacent vertebral body. The most common classification system is known as the Meyerding Grading System[16] and is defined by the severity of the slippage: Grade I: 1–25%; Grade II: 26–50%; Grade III: 51–75%; Grade IV: 76–100%; Grade V (also known as spondyloptosis): > 100%, with one vertebral body completely over the adjacent vertebral body. Further, radiographic instability is defined as translational motion of one segment by more than 3 mm in the lumbar spine (5 mm at L5-S1) or angulation by more than 10° on flexion-extension radiographs.[17] ▶ Fig. 15.2 depicts a case of mobile spondylolisthesis and facet joint degenerative changes at the segment of radiographic instability.

The exact cause of DS is still not well understood, but it is believed to be caused by disc degeneration and subsequent disc height loss, followed by degeneration of the facet joints and hypertrophy of the ligament flavum, resulting in instability and subluxation of the superior vertebra. The further degeneration processes may actually lead to secondary stabilization and auto-fusion of the spinal segment as facet arthrosis, osteophytes, and ossification of the intervertebral ligaments develop.[13,18] Multiple studies investigating the role of the facet joints in DS development report that it occurs more often in patients with sagittal orientation and a greater angle of the L4-L5 facet joints,[19,20,21] as the diminished anterior restraint results in anterior slippage of the vertebra. Love et al, however, argued that the sagittal orientation of the facet joints was the result of arthritic remodeling in older patients rather than the primary cause of DS.[22]

Iatrogenic spondylolisthesis has been observed in patients after spinal fusion at the level above or below the fusion due to increased stress and accelerated degeneration. Iatrogenic spondylolisthesis can also be due to decompression procedures when a large extent of bone is removed, especially if a greater amount of the facet joints is removed. The study by Fox et al[23] found that preoperative anterior spondylolisthesis in patients undergoing decompression surgery for spinal stenosis was the single most important factor predicting postoperative radiological instability. Moelleken et al recommended limiting excision to one-third of each facet during decompression or adding fusion with instrumentation in patients with spondylolisthesis when a more extensive decompression is required.[24]

15.3 Treatment Options

15.3.1 Nonsurgical Treatment Options

The indications for surgical treatment of DS have been reviewed by Herkowitz et al[25] and include: a) persistent or recurrent back and/or leg pain or neurogenic claudication, with significant reduction of quality of life, despite a reasonable trial of nonoperative treatment (a minimum of 3 months), b) progressive neurologic deficit, and/or c) bladder or bowel symptoms. Nonoperative interventions, however, are typically the first treatment of choice in patients with DS. Frymoyer[26] suggested the following treatment protocol: a) nonsteroidal anti-inflammatory drugs (NSAIDs); b) encouragement of aerobic conditioning; c) weight reduction, and d) management of osteoporosis. In the elderly population, however, there should be careful monitoring for gastrointestinal complaints and melena when administering NSAIDs and acetaminophen or cardiovascular complaints when prescribing COX-2 inhibitors.[27]

Physical therapy (PT) is another very common conservative treatment modality for symptoms associated with DS, which helps teach patients methods of pain relief via activity

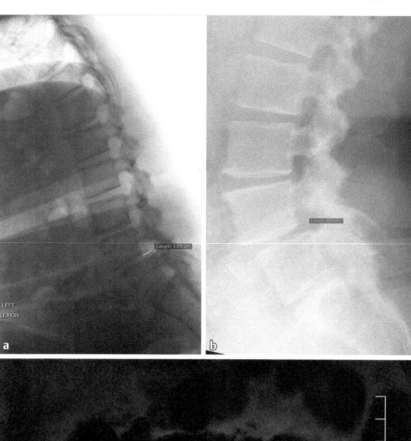

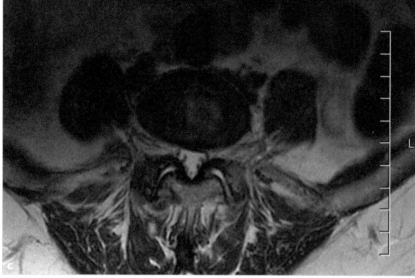

Fig. 15.2 Mobile spondylolisthesis. On standing upright lumbar X-rays flexion **(a)** and extension **(b)** views, the patient develops a 4.5-mm anterolisthesis of L4 in relation to L5, demonstrating a mobile spondylolisthesis. Axial MRI T2 through the L4–5 facet joint **(c)** demonstrates T2 signal changes in the facet joint (widened facet joint capsule).

modification and exercise. Other alternative treatment modalities, such as ultrasound, electrical stimulation, and dry needling can also be used. Finally, if patients fail a reasonable course of PT (4–6 weeks), then they may benefit in the short term from a course of epidural steroid injections.[10] There is little empiric evidence to support many of the common nonsurgical interventions for symptomatic elderly patients with DS; it generally is agreed, however, that nonoperative treatment should be attempted in most cases before surgical intervention is pursued.[27,28] Of the nonoperative options, none is known to be superior to the others, and all could have a role in the treatment of symptomatic patients. It is important to understand that for many patients, nonsurgical treatments may be used in combination or sequentially, and their use may change depending on the severity of symptoms and their change with time.[27]

15.3.2 Surgical Treatment Options

Surgery is often considered when a patient fails to respond to nonoperative modalities, develops neurologic deficits, or when the patient's symptoms are debilitating.

Surgical treatment of DS fulfills two primary objectives: decompression of the neural elements and stabilization, if indicated. The first objective is to decompress the neural structures in order to relieve spinal stenosis and neurogenic claudication symptoms. A laminectomy with or without lateral recess and foraminal decompression is one option. A laminotomy preserving the vertebral arch is another method to achieve a decompression. The second objective is internal stabilization via fusion. A fusion is performed to prevent any further slip from developing between the vertebrae as well as stabilizing the associated degenerative disc and arthritic facets, often times for improving back pain and preventing possible instability. Traditional factors favoring fusion include: improved spine stability, minimization of long-term back pain from the operated degenerative levels, and concern for recurrent leg pain from progression of the spondylolisthesis in the absence of fusion.[29] Decompression and fusion is becoming the most common surgical technique for the management of DS.[30] Fusion options for DS are variable and can include a noninstrumented or an instrumented posterolateral fusion (PLF), in addition to an interbody fusion via various approaches: anterior lumbar interbody fusion (ALIF), lateral interbody fusion (LIF), posterior lumbar interbody fusion (PLIF), and transforaminal lumbar interbody fusion (TLIF). Other surgical options for patients may include a minimally invasive decompression with or without fusion, dynamic stabilization, and interspinous spacers.

15.3.3 Benefits and Risks

The benefit of surgical intervention in patients with lumbar DS is twofold. One, the neural elements are decompressed, which can improve neurologic morbidity. Two, the spondylolisthesis can be stabilized to improve mechanical back pain or prevent progressive instability. Decompression compared with instrumented fusion may be a more appropriate treatment option in the aging patient population due to shorter operative times and reduced blood loss, but there is increased risk of developing instability. The risks and benefits of each specific surgical approach are further elucidated in an excellent summary by Eismont et al. [31] The Spine Patient Outcomes Research Trial (SPORT) demonstrated that surgery was superior to nonoperative care for the management of lumbar DS, though this study was not focused on the aging population.[1] Rihn et al[32] evaluated the effectiveness of surgery for lumbar stenosis and DS in the octogenarian population. They found that surgery offered a significant benefit over nonoperative treatment in patients at least 80 years of age ($p < 0.05$), with no significant increases in the complication and mortality rates compared with younger patients ($p > 0.05$).

Proceeding with any type of surgical intervention in the aging population involves several concerns, including an increased risk for complications such as pseudoarthrosis, hardware failure, or loosening secondary to poor bone quality, as well as an increased number and severity of comorbidities, with a resultant higher rate of perioperative morbidity.[31] In their analysis of a subset of Medicare patients treated for lumbar spinal stenosis and/or spondylolisthesis via fusion, Ong et al[33] found that older patients may require more extensive postoperative care and may be more predisposed to certain types of surgical complications. Becker et al[34] retrospectively evaluated 195 patients over the age of 70 who underwent spinal fusion with pedicle screws and rod instrumentation with or without intervertebral cages and reported a 14.7% major complication rate and 18.9% minor complication rate. Benz et al[35] reviewed 68 patients aged 70 years and older who underwent lumbar decompression with or without fusion and reported a 40% total complication rate: 12% major and 28% minor complication rates, respectively. The early mortality rate was 1.4% in their series. The authors noted that arthrodesis with or without instrumentation was significantly associated with complications. Carreon

et al[36] found complications in 78 patients in their series of 98 patients over the age of 65 years undergoing posterior decompression and fusion for degenerative disease of the spine. Twenty-one patients had at least one major complication, and 69 had at least one minor complication. The most common major complication was wound infection (10%), while urinary tract infection was the most common minor complication (34%). Complication rates increased significantly with older age, increased blood loss, longer operative time, and the number of arthrodesis levels. In their series of 166 patients aged 65 years or older undergoing lumbar decompression and fusion with (n = 75) or without (n = 91) instrumentation, Cassinelli et al[37] reported a 3% major complication rate and 30.7 and 31.9% minor complication rates in patients undergoing decompression with or without fusion, respectively. The authors also noted that decompression associated with fusion of four or more segments significantly increased the occurrence of major complications. Hayashi et al[38] compared the perioperative complication rates between patients under and over the age of 80 years undergoing surgery for lumbar degenerative disease. They found major complications in 16% of patients in the ≥ 80 group and 9% of patients in the < 80 group. Medical complications occurred in 21% of patients in the ≥ 80 group and 16% of patients in the < 80 group. Likewise, surgery-specific complications occurred in 37% of patients in the ≥ 80 group and 19% of patients in the < 80 group. Although the incidence of complications was not significantly different between the two groups, patients in the ≥ 80 group had a higher tendency towards complications. Balabaud et al[21] was one of the first to evaluate the morbidity and mortality of spine surgery in patients 80 years of age or older in a large cohort. Patients underwent a posterior decompression with or without spinal instrumentation. The purpose of their study was to determine whether preoperative and perioperative factors correlated with morbidity and mortality. After a diagnosis of spinal stenosis, DS was the second most common diagnosis in 45 of their 121 patients. For DS and/or preoperative assessed instability, an instrumented fusion or dynamic stabilization was always performed. They found an average hospital stay of 11.3 ± 8.1 days (range, 7–71 days), and significantly increased average blood loss with instrumentation (538 vs. 280 ml, $p < 0.0001$). Average operative time was 103 ± 38 min, and, again, increased significantly with instrumentation (131.2 vs. 84 min, $p = 0.003$). Fusion occurred in 30 out of 37 patients (81%) after a minimum of 1 year. With regard to complications, they found major complications in 16 of 121 patients (13%), with the most common ones being from wound infection (4%), followed by epidural hematoma and neurologic deficit (3.3% each) and either new onset of cardiac arrhythmia or pneumonia and respiratory distress (2.4% each). Less than 2% of patients developed any of the following: congestive heart failure, thromboembolic disease, renal failure, pulmonary embolus, or syndrome of inappropriate antidiuretic hormone (SIADH). Minor complications occurred in 29.7% of patients, and most commonly was confusion (13%), urinary retention (8%), and urinary tract infection (5%). Other minor complications (less than 2.5% each) included ileus, hyponatremia, hypokalemia, digestive tract infection, and morphine intoxication. Although their 4% wound infection rates were similar to those reported in the literature, the authors discovered that the infecting organism appeared unique to the elderly population, which was primarily due to gram-negative bacteria: *E coli* (two patients) and *E faecalis* (two patients), with only one patient suffering from *S aureus. S aureus* tends to be the more causative agent for infections within a younger population. This indicates that wound infections in the elderly are more commonly caused by the urinary tract or fecal organisms.

Lieber et al[39] studied postoperative complications and compared patients > 80 years old (n = 227) with a typical age cohort 45–65 years old (n = 2248) undergoing a single-level lumbar fusion for spondylolisthesis. They found a difference in the preoperative characteristics and comorbidities between the younger and older age cohorts. The older patient cohort had more preoperative comorbidities, including a lack of independent functional health status before surgery ($p < 0.001$), severe chronic obstructive pulmonary disease ($p < 0.020$), and hypertension requiring medication ($p < 0.001$). They also found a significantly greater morbidity among the > 80 years old cohort regarding urinary tract infection ($p = 0.008$) and intraoperative and postoperative transfusions ($p < 0.001$). Interestingly, there was significantly greater morbidity among the younger cohort regarding cardiac arrest requiring cardiopulmonary resuscitation ($p = 0.043$). Oldridge et al[40] identified 80–85 years as a threshold for a dramatic increase in morbidity and mortality.

Raffo and Lauermann[41] reported on their series of 20 patients aged 80 years or older undergoing lumbar spine surgery. They reported a 35% major complication rate with no mortalities. Ragab et al[42] reviewed the outcomes of patients over the age of 70 years who underwent surgery for spinal stenosis. They found a minor and major complication rate of 8% and 2%, respectively. Takahashi et al[43] found an overall complication rate of 34.3% in patients 70 years and older undergoing TLIF procedures for spondylolisthesis. Vitaz et al[44] reported on 65 patients with lumbar stenosis at least 75 years of age who underwent lumbar decompression with and without spinal fusion and reported a 10% major complication rate and 27% minor complication rate—this in comparison to a major complication rate of 7.7% and minor complication rate of 11.5% reported by Wang et al[45] in their series of 26 patients 85 years and older undergoing lumbar spine surgery. They found that operative time of longer than 180 minutes (p=0.0134) was associated with complications.

In the study by Glassman et al[46] of 85 patients over the age of 65 years undergoing lumbar spine surgery, complications occurred in 27 patients (31.8%). Complications included seven incidental durotomies, five ileus, four wound infections, three urinary tract infections, three mental confusions, and five others. This was compared to a rate of 11 (11.8%) complications in patients aged younger than 65 years (p = 0.001). Fourteen patients (16.5%) over the age of 65 years underwent a subsequent revision, compared with 17.2% in the under 65 years group (p= 0.90). Revision procedures were a repair of nonunion in three patients, an adjacent-level fusion in 10 patients, and a repeat decompression in one patient in the older population. Sansur et al reviewed 10,242 adults with DS and isthmic spondylolisthesis (IS) from the morbidity and mortality index of the Scoliosis Research Society.[47] The rate of total complications for treatment of DS and IS was 9.2% in 7.9% of total patients studied. On univariate analysis, the complication rate was significantly higher in patients with high-grade spondylolisthesis, with a diagnosis of DS, and in older patients. The

surgical approach and history of previous surgery were not significantly correlated with increased complication rates. On multivariate analysis, only the grade of spondylolisthesis was significantly associated with the occurrence of complications.

Minimally Invasive Surgery

Rosen et al[48] reviewed their outcomes of minimally invasive (MI) lumbar decompression on patients at least 75 years of age and reported a 1% major complication rate and a 30% minor complication rate. Rodgers et al[49] found complication rates, blood loss/transfusion rate, and hospital stay to be significantly ($p < 0.0001$) lower following MI interbody fusion compared to open PLIF in patients 80 years. Lee et al[50] reported overall clinical success in 88.9% of patients, with a low rate of complications (7.4%) at a minimum follow-up of 36 months. The authors performed MI-TLIFs in patients aged 65 years and older and found significant improvements in Visual Analog Scale (VAG) and Oswestry Disability Index (ODI) scores ($p = 0.001$), with a pseudoarthrosis and adjacent segment disease rate of 22.2% and 44.4%, respectively. There were no reoperations in their series, and clinical outcome measures were successful in all patients without a solid fusion.

15.4 Pitfalls, Complications, and Avoidance

Surgical treatment is effective in improving the quality of life in the aging patient population, but due to significant comorbidities and an increased risk of complications, treatment of DS requires not only careful selection of surgical approach but also careful management of potential complications and adaptation of preventative measures in order to minimize them.[51]

15.4.1 Identify Instability

Care should be taken to identify patients who are unstable preoperatively or may be rendered unstable by the decompression to avoid iatrogenic progression of the spondylolisthesis leading to reoperation. Sengupta and Herkowitz[52] determined the indications for performing fusion with instrumentation based on preoperative and intraoperative factors. The authors recommended instrumented fusion in the following clinical situations: a) to prevent progression of listhesis if the preoperative disc height is > 2 mm; b) when correction of deformity is performed with presence of kyphosis; c) to assure that fusion is achieved when instability is > 5 mm; d) listhesis of > 50%; e) when revision decompression is performed and requires additional facetectomy; f) listhetic or symptomatic adjacent segment degeneration is present; g) bilateral facet excision of > 50%; h) reduction of listhesis is performed and disc height is restored. Blumenthal et al[53] reported a 37.5% reoperation rate at a mean follow-up of 3.6 years for pain caused by instability at the index level following decompression only for Grade I lumbar spondylolisthesis. Similar reoperation rates (34%) were confirmed by Ghogawala et al[54] for patients undergoing decompression alone to address instability, but the authors also reported 14% revision surgery rates in the fusion group due to symptomatic adjacent-level degeneration. Appropriate selection of patients that would benefit from fusion can help avoid the need for revision surgery due to instability.

15.4.2 Identify and Optimize Comorbidities

Multiple reports in the literature discuss prevention of general medical and organ-specific complications associated with the surgical care of older patients. It is important to identify patients at high risk of postoperative events and to maintain perioperative hemodynamic stability and normothermia, as well as to provide adequate fluid replacement and effective pain control. A study by Rajpal et al[51] identified perioperative medical complications and mortality rates specific to octogenarians undergoing elective spinal surgeries. A comprehensive geriatric preoperative assessment, elimination of modifiable risk factors, and optimization of preventative measures and postoperative care can help to minimize or avoid complications in this patient population. Balabaud et al[55] questioned whether preoperative comorbidities increased complication rates. In their study, they did not find such a relationship. The published literature also does not appear to be clear. While some studies found no correlation,[35,36,42] other studies found that the number of comorbidities increased complication rates.[40,41,56,57]

15.5 Outcomes and Evidence

Surgical outcomes of DS treatment, including morbidity and mortality rates, have been extensively studied in the literature. The biggest challenge in assessing the literature is the very limited number of publications dedicated specifically to the surgical treatment for DS in older adults. This chapter, therefore, reviews the literature devoted to lumbar spine surgery in the elderly with a variety of diagnoses, since many authors summarize their results for a spectrum of diagnoses.

Greenfield et al[58] evaluated the outcome and efficacy of instrumented arthrodesis in 38 patients aged 60 years and older. The mean age in their study was 73.8 years (range, 60–90 years). Based on the authors' method of evaluation of fusion, the fusion rate was 92%. Functional gains of 50% or more were reported by 71% of the respondents. Results of excellent/good, fair, and poor were reported in 57%, 26%, and 17% of patients, respectively. They concluded that despite the increase in age, comorbidity, and the associated risk of perioperative complications in this population, an outcome comparable with that of younger patients was reported. Hayashi et al[38] reviewed 96 patients ≥ 70 years old who underwent PLIF and compared the clinical outcomes of two patient groups: a ≥ 80 group (n = 19) and a < 80 group (n = 77). They found the rate of bony union in the ≥ 80 group to be 73.7%, which was significantly lower than that of the < 80 group (94.8%). Considering their data, the authors concluded that age was one of the possible risk factors of nonunion.

Glassman et al[46] evaluated clinical outcomes based on modern standardized Health-Related Quality of Life (HRQOL) measures in patients over 65 years of age treated by lumbar decompression and fusion surgery. Spondylolisthesis was the most common indication for surgery in 36.5% of their patients studied. They found a mean improvement of 6.2 points in SF-36 Physical Component Summary (PCS) and 5.8 points in SF-36 Mental Component Summary (MCS) scores. They also reported a mean 16.4-, 3.1-, and 2.7-point reduction in ODI, back pain, and leg pain numeric rating scale (NRS) scores, respectively. SF-36 subscale scores showed improvement for all parameters except general health, where there was a small but statistically significant decline. There was no difference in outcomes two years postoperatively based on the occurrence of perioperative complications. The patients undergoing a primary lumbar surgical procedure had consistently better outcomes than the patients undergoing a revision procedure. The results of their study "support the efficacy of lumbar decompression and fusion in selected patients over 65 years of age".

A more recent paper by Ghogawala et al[54] analyzed the effectiveness of instrumented fusion in addition to decompression in a prospective study that enrolled patients with the mean age of 67 years (range, 50–80) with stable grade I degenerative spondylolisthesis. A total of 66 patients were randomized to undergo either decompression alone or decompression with posterolateral instrumented fusion at a single level. An additional 40 patients were included in an observation group, as they declined to be randomized. At the 2-year follow-up, there was a significantly greater improvement of the SF-36 PCS scores in the patients who had fusion than in those who had decompression alone, a difference which was sustained at the 4-year follow-up. However, there were no statistically significant differences between the groups in disability related to back pain scores. To address the subsequent instability, a total of 14% of patients in the fusion group had reoperations at the adjacent level, compared with 34% in the decompression-alone group. The authors also noted that due to significantly longer operative times and increased blood loss, fusion surgery might not be appropriate for older patients.

Conversely, Forsth et al[59] did not find any statistically significant differences in clinical outcomes in a study that included a total of 135 patients with lumbar spinal stenosis and spondylolisthesis who were randomized to undergo decompression with fusion (n=67) or decompression alone (n=68). The average age of patients was 67/68 ± 7 years. The ODI, European Quality of Life – 5 Dimensions (EQ-5D), Zurich Claudication Questionnaire (ZCQ), VAS, patient satisfaction scores and the results of the 6-minute walk test were all comparable at 2- or 5-year follow-ups.

15.6 Conclusion

The rising life expectancy and quality-of-life expectations of patients place increasing demands on spine surgeons to consider both nonoperative and operative treatment options for lumbar DS. The literature on surgical treatment for degenerative conditions in the elderly is growing, but for DS specifically, the literature is sparse. Although nonoperative interventions are clearly favored for patients overall, in those circumstances when patients are no longer responding to nonoperative interventions, surgery needs to be carefully weighed against the medical comorbidities. Age alone should not be considered a contraindication to surgical intervention; elderly patients who are optimized perioperatively can and should expect successful outcomes like their younger counterparts.

Key References

[1] Weinstein JN, Lurie JD, Tosteson TD, et al. Surgical versus nonsurgical treatment for lumbar degenerative spondylolisthesis. N Engl J Med. 2007; 356 (22):2257–2270

[2] Balabaud L, Pitel S, Caux I, et al. Lumbar spine surgery in patients 80 years of age or older: morbidity and mortality. Eur J Orthop Surg Traumatol. 2015; 25 Suppl 1:S205–S212

[3] Eismont FJ, Norton RP, Hirsch BP. Surgical management of lumbar degenerative spondylolisthesis. J Am Acad Orthop Surg. 2014; 22(4):203–213

[4] Ghogawala Z, Dziura J, Butler WE, et al. Laminectomy plus Fusion versus Laminectomy Alone for Lumbar Spondylolisthesis. N Engl J Med. 2016; 374(15): 1424–1434

[5] Lieber BA, Chiang V, Prabhu AV, et al. Postoperative Complications for Elderly Patients After Single-Level Lumbar Fusions for Spondylolisthesis. World Neurosurg. 2016; 91:149–153

References

[1] Weinstein JN, Lurie JD, Tosteson TD, et al. Surgical versus nonsurgical treatment for lumbar degenerative spondylolisthesis. N Engl J Med. 2007; 356 (22):2257–2270

[2] Deyo RA, Gray DT, Kreuter W, Mirza S, Martin BI. United States trends in lumbar fusion surgery for degenerative conditions. Spine. 2005; 30(12):1441–1445, discussion 1446–1447

[3] Arias E, Heron M, Xu J. United States Life Tables, 2012. Natl Vital Stat Rep. 2016; 65(8):1–65

[4] Vogt MT, Rubin D, Valentin RS, et al. The Study of Osteoporotic Fractures. Lumbar olisthesis and lower back symptoms in elderly white women. Spine. 1998; 23(23):2640–2647

[5] Kauppila LI, Eustace S, Kiel DP, Felson DT, Wright AM. Degenerative displacement of lumbar vertebrae. A 25-year follow-up study in Framingham. Spine. 1998; 23(17):1868–1873, discussion 1873–1874

[6] Kalichman L, Kim DH, Li L, Guermazi A, Berkin V, Hunter DJ. Spondylolysis and spondylolisthesis: prevalence and association with low back pain in the adult community-based population. Spine. 2009; 34(2):199–205

[7] Denard PJ, Holton KF, Miller J, et al. Osteoporotic Fractures in Men (MrOS) Study Group. Lumbar spondylolisthesis among elderly men: prevalence, correlates, and progression. Spine. 2010; 35(10):1072–1078

[8] He LC, Wang YX, Gong JS, et al. Prevalence and risk factors of lumbar spondylolisthesis in elderly Chinese men and women. Eur Radiol. 2014; 24(2):441–448

[9] Wáng YX, Deng M, Griffith JF, et al. Lumbar Spondylolisthesis Progression and De Novo Spondylolisthesis in Elderly Chinese Men and Women: A Year-4 Follow-up Study. Spine. 2016; 41(13):1096–1103

[10] Vibert BT, Sliva CD, Herkowitz HN. Treatment of instability and spondylolisthesis: surgical versus nonsurgical treatment. Clin Orthop Relat Res. 2006; 443(443):222–227

[11] Frymoyer JW. Degenerative spondylolisthesis. St Louis: Mosby Year Book; 1992

[12] Kostuik JP, Harrington I, Alexander D, Rand W, Evans D. Cauda equina syndrome and lumbar disc herniation. J Bone Joint Surg Am. 1986; 68(3):386–391

[13] Matsunaga S, Ijiri K, Hayashi K. Nonsurgically managed patients with degenerative spondylolisthesis: a 10- to 18-year follow-up study. J Neurosurg. 2000; 93(2) Suppl:194–198

[14] Rosenberg NJ. Degenerative spondylolisthesis. Predisposing factors. J Bone Joint Surg Am. 1975; 57(4):467–474

[15] Wiltse LL, Winter RB. Terminology and measurement of spondylolisthesis. J Bone Joint Surg Am. 1983; 65(6):768–772

[16] Meyerding HW. Spondylolisthesis. Surg Gynecol Obstet. 1932; 54:371–379

[17] White AA, Pajjabi MM. Clinical Biomechanics of the Spine. Philadelphia: Lippincott; 1978

[18] Kirkaldy-Willis WH, Farfan HF. Instability of the lumbar spine. Clin Orthop Relat Res. 1982(165):110–123

[19] Grobler LJ, Robertson PA, Novotny JE, Pope MH. Etiology of spondylolisthesis. Assessment of the role played by lumbar facet joint morphology. Spine. 1993; 18(1):80–91

[20] Toyone T, Ozawa T, Kamikawa K, et al. Facet joint orientation difference between cephalad and caudad portions: a possible cause of degenerative spondylolisthesis. Spine. 2009; 34(21):2259–2262

[21] Kalichman L, Suri P, Guermazi A, Li L, Hunter DJ. Facet orientation and tropism: associations with facet joint osteoarthritis and degeneratives. Spine. 2009; 34(16):E579–E585

[22] Love TW, Fagan AB, Fraser RD. Degenerative spondylolisthesis. Developmental or acquired? J Bone Joint Surg Br. 1999; 81(4):670–674

[23] Fox MW, Onofrio BM, Onofrio BM, Hanssen AD. Clinical outcomes and radiological instability following decompressive lumbar laminectomy for degenerative spinal stenosis: a comparison of patients undergoing concomitant arthrodesis versus decompression alone. J Neurosurg. 1996; 85(5):793–802

[24] Moelleken AGZ, Cooper P. Iatrogenic Deformities of the Spine. The Practice of Neurosurgery: Williams & Wilkins; 1996:2593–2607

[25] Herkowitz HN. Spine update. Degenerative lumbar spondylolisthesis. Spine. 1995; 20(9):1084–1090

[26] Frymoyer JW. Degenerative Spondylolisthesis: Diagnosis and Treatment. J Am Acad Orthop Surg. 1994; 2(1):9–15

[27] Kalichman L, Hunter DJ. Diagnosis and conservative management of degenerative lumbar spondylolisthesis. Eur Spine J. 2008; 17(3):327–335

[28] McNeely ML, Torrance G, Magee DJ. A systematic review of physiotherapy for spondylolysis and spondylolisthesis. Man Ther. 2003; 8(2):80–91

[29] Abdu WA, Lurie JD, Spratt KF, et al. Degenerative spondylolisthesis: does fusion method influence outcome? Four-year results of the spine patient outcomes research trial. Spine. 2009; 34(21):2351–2360

[30] Deyo RA, Mirza SK, Martin BI, Kreuter W, Goodman DC, Jarvik JG. Trends, major medical complications, and charges associated with surgery for lumbar spinal stenosis in older adults. JAMA. 2010; 303(13):1259–1265

[31] Eismont FJ, Norton RP, Hirsch BP. Surgical management of lumbar degenerative spondylolisthesis. J Am Acad Orthop Surg. 2014; 22(4):203–213

[32] Rihn JA, Hilibrand AS, Zhao W, et al. Effectiveness of surgery for lumbar stenosis and degenerative spondylolisthesis in the octogenarian population: analysis of the Spine Patient Outcomes Research Trial (SPORT) data. J Bone Joint Surg Am. 2015; 97(3):177–185

[33] Ong KL, Auerbach JD, Lau E, Schmier J, Ochoa JA. Perioperative outcomes, complications, and costs associated with lumbar spinal fusion in older patients with spinal stenosis and spondylolisthesis. Neurosurg Focus. 2014; 36(6):E5

[34] Becker P, Bretschneider W, Tuschel A, Ogon M. Life quality after instrumented lumbar fusion in the elderly. Spine. 2010; 35(15):1478–1481

[35] Benz RJ, Ibrahim ZG, Afshar P, Garfin SR. Predicting complications in elderly patients undergoing lumbar decompression. Clin Orthop Relat Res. 2001 (384):116–121

[36] Carreon LY, Puno RM, Dimar JR, II, Glassman SD, Johnson JR. Perioperative complications of posterior lumbar decompression and arthrodesis in older adults. J Bone Joint Surg Am. 2003; 85-A(11):2089–2092

[37] Cassinelli EH, Eubanks J, Vogt M, Furey C, Yoo J, Bohlman HH. Risk factors for the development of perioperative complications in elderly patients undergoing lumbar decompression and arthrodesis for spinal stenosis: an analysis of 166 patients. Spine. 2007; 32(2):230–235

[38] Hayashi K, Matsumura A, Konishi S, Kato M, Namikawa T, Nakamura H. Clinical Outcomes of Posterior Lumbar Interbody Fusion for Patients 80 Years of Age and Older with Lumbar Degenerative Disease: Minimum 2 Years' Follow-Up. Global Spine J. 2016; 6(7):665–672

[39] Lieber BA, Chiang V, Prabhu AV, et al. Postoperative Complications for Elderly Patients After Single-Level Lumbar Fusions for Spondylolisthesis. World Neurosurg. 2016; 91:149–153

[40] Oldridge NB, Yuan Z, Stoll JE, Rimm AR. Lumbar spine surgery and mortality among Medicare beneficiaries, 1986. Am J Public Health. 1994; 84(8):1292–1298

[41] Raffo CS, Lauerman WC. Predicting morbidity and mortality of lumbar spine arthrodesis in patients in their ninth decade. Spine. 2006; 31(1):99–103

[42] Ragab AA, Fye MA, Bohlman HH. Surgery of the lumbar spine for spinal stenosis in 118 patients 70 years of age or older. Spine. 2003; 28(4):348–353

[43] Takahashi T, Hanakita J, Minami M, et al. Clinical outcomes and adverse events following transforaminal interbody fusion for lumbar degenerative spondylolisthesis in elderly patients. Neurol Med Chir (Tokyo). 2011; 51(12): 829–835

[44] Vitaz TW, Raque GH, Shields CB, Glassman SD. Surgical treatment of lumbar spinal stenosis in patients older than 75 years of age. J Neurosurg. 1999; 91 (2) Suppl:181–185

[45] Wang MY, Widi G, Levi AD. The safety profile of lumbar spinal surgery in elderly patients 85 years and older. Neurosurg Focus. 2015; 39(4):E3

[46] Glassman SD, Carreon LY, Dimar JR, Campbell MJ, Puno RM, Johnson JR. Clinical outcomes in older patients after posterolateral lumbar fusion. Spine J. 2007; 7(5):547–551

[47] Sansur CA, Reames DL, Smith JS, et al. Morbidity and mortality in the surgical treatment of 10,242 adults with spondylolisthesis. J Neurosurg Spine. 2010; 13(5):589–593

[48] Rosen DS, O'Toole JE, Eichholz KM, et al. Minimally invasive lumbar spinal decompression in the elderly: outcomes of 50 patients aged 75 years and older. Neurosurgery. 2007; 60(3):503–509, discussion 509–510

[49] Rodgers WB, Gerber EJ, Rodgers JA. Lumbar fusion in octogenarians: the promise of minimally invasive surgery. Spine. 2010; 35(26) Suppl:S355–S360

[50] Lee DY, Jung TG, Lee SH. Single-level instrumented mini-open transforaminal lumbar interbody fusion in elderly patients. J Neurosurg Spine. 2008; 9(2): 137–144

[51] Rajpal S, Lee Nelson E, Villavicencio AT, et al. Medical complications and mortality in octogenarians undergoing elective spinal fusion surgeries. Acta Neurochir (Wien). 2017

[52] Sengupta DK, Herkowitz HN. Degenerative spondylolisthesis: review of current trends and controversies. Spine. 2005; 30(6) Suppl:S71–S81

[53] Blumenthal C, Curran J, Benzel EC, et al. Radiographic predictors of delayed instability following decompression without fusion for degenerative grade I lumbar spondylolisthesis. J Neurosurg Spine. 2013; 18(4):340–346

[54] Ghogawala Z, Dziura J, Butler WE, et al. Laminectomy plus Fusion versus Laminectomy Alone for Lumbar Spondylolisthesis. N Engl J Med. 2016; 374(15): 1424–1434

[55] Balabaud L, Pitel S, Caux I, et al. Lumbar spine surgery in patients 80 years of age or older: morbidity and mortality. Eur J Orthop Surg Traumatol. 2015; 25 Suppl 1:S205–S212

[56] Li G, Patil CG, Lad SP, Ho C, Tian W, Boakye M. Effects of age and comorbidities on complication rates and adverse outcomes after lumbar laminectomy in elderly patients. Spine. 2008; 33(11):1250–1255

[57] Deyo RA, Cherkin DC, Loeser JD, Bigos SJ, Ciol MA. Morbidity and mortality in association with operations on the lumbar spine. The influence of age, diagnosis, and procedure. J Bone Joint Surg Am. 1992; 74(4):536–543

[58] Greenfield RT, III, Capen DA, Thomas JC, Jr, et al. Pedicle screw fixation for arthrodesis of the lumbosacral spine in the elderly. An outcome study. Spine. 1998; 23(13):1470–1475

[59] Försth P, Ólafsson G, Carlsson T, et al. A Randomized, Controlled Trial of Fusion Surgery for Lumbar Spinal Stenosis. N Engl J Med. 2016; 374(15): 1413–1423

16 Sagittal Plane Malalignment and Degenerative Scoliosis in the Aging Spine

Casey Slattery, Kushagra Verma, Samantha Sokol, and Sigurd Berven

Abstract

Degenerative deformity in the aging spine has become a prevalent issue in medicine due to the increasing aging population. This chapter describes the etiology and biomechanics of degenerative scoliosis, as well as appropriate goals and strategies for managing spinal deformity. Treatment options discussed include nonoperative management, limited decompression, focal stabilization, and deformity correction. The reader will then learn the benefits and risks of surgery associated with degenerative scoliosis. Surgical considerations to avoid complications described in this chapter include the use of multiple surgeons and tranexamic acid to reduce blood loss. Another common complication discussed is proximal junctional kyphosis. Understanding the aging spine and the importance of sagittal balance correction in degenerative scoliosis will help providers execute decisions for management and surgical considerations for our aging population.

Keywords: Sagittal plane malalignment, degenerative, scoliosis, elderly, aging, spine deformity, nonoperative management, surgery

Key Points

- Sagittal alignment is a key component in the evaluation and treatment of deformity in scoliosis.
- The primary goal for management of these patients is to relieve pain, improve function, halt curve progression, and perhaps improve cosmetic appearance.
- Nonoperative management should be considered for all patients. If nonoperative modalities fail, surgery may be considered with careful patient selection and attention to modifiable risk factors.
- Implementing a shared decision-making model among providers can decrease unnecessary surgeries.
- Once the patient and their providers have agreed that the benefits of surgery outweigh the risks, careful surgical planning is necessary to optimize surgical outcomes and reduce risks.
- Surgical risks highlighted in this chapter include proximal junctional kyphosis and blood loss, with evaluation of research and guidelines to minimize these risks.
- Understanding the changes that occur in the aging spine will help surgeons and other providers execute decisions for management and surgical considerations for our aging population.

16.1 Epidemiology

In the aging population, one of the most prevalent causes of spinal deformity is degenerative (de novo) scoliosis.[1] The reported incidence of adult degenerative scoliosis varies greatly, with reports reaching 64 to 68% in the elderly,[2] and is most commonly seen in patients older than 40 years of age.[3]

The disease process is not entirely understood, but it is widely believed to be a result of accumulative degenerative changes that result from an aging spine. These changes include asymmetric disc degeneration, dehydration, and collapse along with ligament laxity and facet joint degeneration, leading to spinal column laxity.[1] Asymmetric degeneration, along with the subsequent unequal loading of the spinal column, initiates a dynamic and possibly synergistic pattern of curve progression and 3-dimensional deformity.[4] Vertebral column fractures due to osteoporosis, an all-but-inevitable consequence of aging, is a major risk factor for development of sagittal plane deformity. Iatrogenic spinal deformity as a result of lumbar fusion and simple decompression (laminectomy) can lead to a loss of lumbar lordosis (LL) known as flat back syndrome. This is a significant risk factor for sagittal malalignment and further spinal deformity in the aging spine. In those with degenerative scoliosis, the spinal curvature tends to progress at a rate of 1–6° per year with an average of 3° per year.[5]

The clinical presentation of adult-onset degenerative scoliosis varies widely, with back and leg pain being the most commonly reported complaints in spinal deformity. Aside from pain and deformity, patients will often present with a previous spinal surgery history or have failed nonoperative management. An appropriate physical exam will include a full neurologic exam and assessment of deformity in supine, sitting, standing, and ambulatory positions.

Back pain has been reported in 40 to 90% of patients with degenerative scoliosis,[4] with an etiology that is often multifactorial. Back pain can be attributed to muscle fatigue, likely due to a compensatory mechanism to malalignment as a result of degenerative disk disease. Facet arthropathy is also a common pain generator in the aging spine.[5] The amount of back pain patients experience is not directly related to the size of the curvature; however, apical rotation and sagittal imbalance can exacerbate back pain.[6]

Leg pain usually presents as radiating pain or intermittent claudication as a result of spinal stenosis, which is observed in around 90% of degenerative scoliosis.[7,8,9] Foraminal stenosis is more likely to affect the nerve roots on the concave side of the curve as a result of compression, although neurological symptoms may develop on the convex side as a result of the overstretching of nerve roots.

In the aging patient, it is important to assess quality of life, as aging patients are more likely to have comorbidities such as depression.[10,11,12,13] Measuring a patient's health-related quality of life (HRQOL) can give a base line of a patient's health and the resulting degree of satisfaction following surgery.

Comorbid conditions that are common in the aging include diabetes and osteoporosis. Uncontrolled diabetes has been linked to poor wound healing and a higher risk of infection.[14] A hemoglobin A1c over 8 has shown a significantly slower wound-healing rate in diabetic patients.[15] A dual-energy X-ray absorptiometry (DEXA) scan should also be considered in the aging, as they are at an increased risk of osteoporosis. Asymptomatic women > 65 years old and men > 70 years old, along with any symptomatic patients should be tested. Other patients for whom a DEXA scan should be considered are those with known endocrine or medical conditions affecting bone mineral density and risk factors such as cigarette and glucocorticoid use, a low BMI, estrogen deficiency, loss of height, or history of amenorrhea. Obesity and smoking have also shown a correlation with lower back pain, which should also be addressed in this population.[16]

Radiographic imaging is required to properly evaluate patients with degenerative scoliosis. Standing frontal (anterior-posterior (AP) or posterior-anterior (PA)) and sagittal (lateral) whole spine, along with supine (nonweight-bearing) imaging characterize the deformity and give information on the flexibility of the deformity. As previously mentioned, a full-body sagittal radiograph is also useful to evaluate compensatory mechanisms.

Adult degenerative scoliosis (ADS) is fundamentally defined as an abnormal curvature of the spine with a coronal deviation greater than 10°. However, characterizing scoliosis is far more difficult. Although some studies have reported characteristic parameters, there has been no large-scaled studies or comprehensive description of ADS, which is essential to understanding and treatment of ADS.[2] A number of studies in recent years have looked at asymptomatic patient spines in relation to age to develop baseline parameters.[17,18,19] Among the most important radiographic parameters of interest in degenerative scoliosis include pelvic incidence (PI), lumbar lordosis (LL), pelvic incidence minus lumbar lordosis (PI-LL), pelvic tilt (PT), sacral slope (SS), sagittal vertical axis (SVA) (▶ Fig. 16.1), coronal Cobb angle, number of segments involved, apex rotation, and thoracic kyphosis (TK) (▶ Fig. 16.2). Among all radiographic measurements associated with degenerative scoliosis, the most concerning characteristics are global imbalance in the sagittal and coronal planes, measured with lateral and AP/PA films respectively.

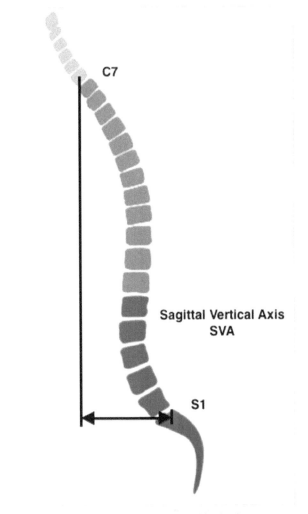

Fig. 16.1 Sagittal Vertical Axis (SVA) is measured by the distance between a vertical line through the geometric center of C7 and the dorsal/rostral corner of the sacrum

16.2 Biomechanical Considerations

Sagittal malalignment plays a role in most, if not all spinal pathologies. Depending on age, the spine will also have a differing range of what is considered normal, making the benefit of analyzing sagittal alignment not strictly limited to patients with deformity.[18] The literature clearly shows that sagittal alignment is also the radiographic parameter most highly correlated with adverse health status outcomes and quality of life.[6,18,20,21]

Sagittal alignment is determined by measuring the distance between a vertical line through the geometric center of C7, also known as the plumb line (C7PL) and the dorsal/rostral corner of the sacrum.[22] This difference, known as SVA, changes significantly with age and is also affected by the patient's positioning and pelvic rotation (▶ Fig. 16.1). An increase in the SVA is associated with increased pain and disability.[23] The SVA does not capture the whole picture of sagittal alignment however. Research has shown that the pelvis is a key regulator for sagittal alignment, and its associated parameters (pelvic tilt and pelvic

incidence minus lumbar lordosis specifically) also show a strong correlation between pain and disability.[24]

As a patient develops sagittal plane malalignment, their bodies recruit mechanisms to compensate. This tends to start in the flexible part of the altered levels and eventually progresses distally to affect the hip and lower extremities.[25] One of the main drivers of sagittal alignment deterioration is the loss of LL as a result of spinal degeneration.[26] To counter their forward translation of their center of mass they straighten the thoracic region, causing muscle exertion.[27] This is usually followed by posterior translation and retroversion of the pelvis, along with flexion of the knees.[25] These compensatory mechanisms are important to evaluate, as they can mask an abnormal SVA if they are not taken into account.

The PT and PI-LL should also be taken into account for a comprehensive analysis on sagittal alignment (▶ Fig. 16.2).[18] A high PT reflects a compensatory mechanism that can reduce the apparent global sagittal alignment.[24] Patients with greater PT often need larger corrections (osteotomies) to reduce the risk of postoperative failures.[23] PT assesses the degree of retroversion

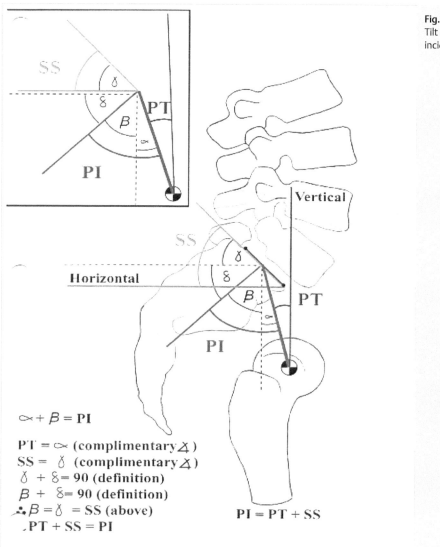

Fig. 16.2 Illustration of Sacral Slope (SS), Pelvic Tilt (PT), and Pelvic Incidence (PI). Pelvic incidence is calculated by PT + SS.

by measuring the angle between the line from midpoint on the sacral end plate to the axis of the femoral head and the vertical axis through the femoral head.

Measuring the PI-LL is important for surgical planning for patients with a small LL relative to their PI to emphasize proper postoperative LL alignment.[23] The LL is the measurement of the sagittal Cobb angle between the superior endplate of S1 and the superior endplate of L1. PI is the angle between the midpoint perpendicular axis of the sagittal end plate and a line from the midpoint of the sagittal end point to the axis of the femoral head. Diebo et al has shown that PT, PI-LL, and SVA all normally increase in the aging spine and the alignment goals should be individualized to the patient.[18] Although not commonly practiced, a full body radiograph is better than a full spinal image to visualize a patient's alignment and all compensatory mechanisms utilized to maintain an erect posture.[18]

In the aging population with spinal deformity, surgery aims to correct sagittal parameters (▶ Fig. 16.3) more than coronal parameters to relieve associated pain and disability. Coronal curves (▶ Fig. 16.4a, b) and imbalance can also cause back pain and impaired functioning but is more commonly associated with an unsatisfactory appearance.[20] Biomechanical considerations must include both sagittal and coronal parameters during surgical correction to achieve the highest possible HRQOL.

16.2.1 Classifying Scoliosis

Classification systems are useful tools that allow effective comparison and communication and provide a framework for evidence-based approaches to better understand management and prognosis.[22] In regard to spinal deformity, there are a number of systems with differing degrees of complexity. Simpler classification systems tend to be of more use in clinical practice but lack many of the deformity's characteristics, and vice versa for more complicated systems.

The most commonly used system is the SRS-Schwab classification system that was designed based on clinical relevance,[23] as the curve types and sagittal modifiers in this system were

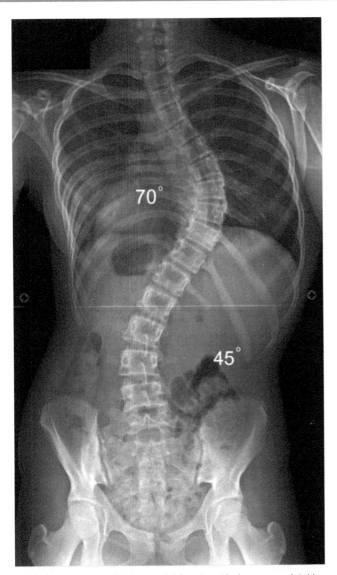

Fig. 16.3 Case example of coronal deformity with the measured Cobb angle. The Cobb angle is perpendicular lines from the superior end plate and inferior end plate of the cephalad and caudal end vertebrae, respectively, of the maximally tilted vertebrae.

16.3 Treatment Options

16.3.1 Nonoperative Management

DS is a progressive disease that takes years before it significantly impacts a patient's quality of life. Nonoperative treatment is the mainstay of treatment to obviate the risks of spinal deformity surgery. The primary goals of both nonsurgical and surgical treatment are the same: to relieve pain, improve function, halt curve progression, and perhaps to improve cosmetic appearance.[22] Even patients with relatively limited disability based on HRQOL measures may benefit from a focused nonoperative treatment regimen.[31]

In the case of DS, there is a lack of evidence-based research specific for nonoperative management. In 2010, Glassman et al studied HRQOL outcomes in ADS with the following modalities: physical therapy, exercise, injections, chiropractic care, and pain management. This study showed no significant benefit based on change in HRQOL measures over a 2-year observation period, but it was unclear if the disease progression slowed as a result of treatment.[31] Patients with ADS, regardless of the quantity and severity of their symptoms, use a significant amount of resources aside from surgery to try and manage their disease.[31,32]

16.3.2 Shared Decision-Making

Most degenerative spinal conditions are managed by a single surgeon.[33] In spinal deformity cases, there is a growing trend to utilize multidisciplinary spine conferences to identify patients most likely to benefit from surgical treatment. Shared decision-making with physiatrists, anesthesia pain specialists, and other nonsurgical providers has demonstrated benefits in the literature while decreasing the amount of unnecessary surgeries.[33] Even a second opinion from another spinal surgeon has shown a decrease in surgical rates.[34] A study by Yanamadala et al showed that when 100 degenerative spinal patients were referred to a multidisciplinary spine center for surgery, 58 of them were instead recommended nonoperative management.[33] Nonoperative interventions commonly employed include physical therapy, epidural steroid injections, weight loss, smoking cessation, and spinal cord stimulation. The long-term benefits of these nonoperative treatments, however, remains debatable.

16.3.3 When is Surgery Appropriate

Surgical management of spinal deformity requires diligent planning and careful patient selection. Spinal deformity surgery is often associated with prolonged recovery times, higher complication rates, and significant cost.

The most common indication for surgery in ADS is radiculopathy, neurogenic claudication, or myelopathy refractory to nonoperative procedures and progressive deficit.[7,8] Radiating pain in ADS is mostly due to foraminal stenosis. Back pain, although common in ADS is rarely an indication for surgery alone,[7] as is the case with progression of scoliosis without any other symptoms.[8] That being said, following surgery, resolution of back pain is 6 times, and leg pain 3 times, more likely to improve compared to nonoperative treatment.[35] Scheer et al also found that patients with sagittal malalignment and more severe symptoms showed a better improvement in pain and Oswestry

found to be closely related with quality of life in the initial study.[23] Other classification systems for adult spinal deformity include the Aebi[28] and the Berjano and Lamartina[29] systems. The classification designed by Aebi et al grouped deformity based on etiology, which proved simple to use, but surgical planning and treatment decisions had some difficulty using this system.[23] Berjano and Lamartina's classification system was designed to assist surgeons with operative planning.[29] The rationale behind this system was to identify selected fusions as to avoid full curve fusion to reduce surgical risk while maintaining a larger range of motion and reducing the risk of junctional disease and decompensation. With the addition of a more recent system, the Comprehensive Spinal Osteotomy classification allows easy communication regarding the varying degrees of bony resections performed in deformity surgery.[30]

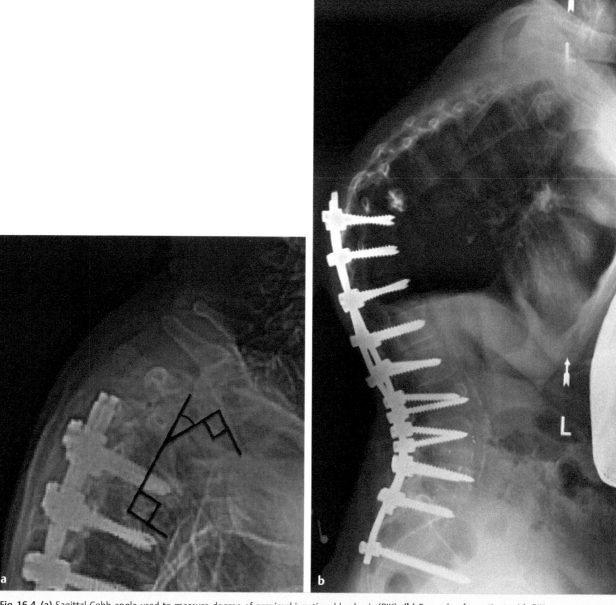

Fig. 16.4 **(a)** Sagittal Cobb angle used to measure degree of proximal junctional kyphosis (PJK). **(b)** Example of a patient with PJK.

Disability Index (ODI) scores postoperatively.[10,35,36] Other surgical indications include compression of neural structures causing bowel/bladder dysfunction or gait disturbances, instability, flat back deformities, iatrogenic deformities, or pain from progressive degenerative deformity.

Radiographic parameters are useful in characterizing the severity of the deformity but do not always predict resolution of clinical symptoms once corrected. Measurements that favor surgical correction include a pelvic tilt > 20°, a sagittal vertical axis > 5 cm, and coronal imbalance > 4 cm.[37]

A study in 2016 by Chen et al sought to answer the question of the appropriateness of surgical intervention.[38] They

conducted a systematically relevant literature review and ran a panel of experts through 260 clinical scenarios. Their results, although subjective, found that surgery is generally appropriate when patients with degenerative scoliosis have at least moderate symptoms and a progressive or larger deformity, sagittal plane imbalance, or moderate stenosis.[38] They also concluded that surgery was generally inappropriate for mild symptoms and smaller deformities, without moderate stenosis or sagittal imbalance, particularly in patients with multiple comorbidities and advanced age.[38]

There is no clear consensus on when surgery is appropriate for ADS, given its complexity. A decision must be made between the surgeon and patient regarding the symptom severities, degree of stenosis, degree of deformity, risk factors, and any other additional factors to decide whether the benefits of surgery outweigh the risks. Discussion of complex deformities with a multidisciplinary conference may help to identify patients best suited to surgical intervention.

16.3.4 Mental Well-Being Assessments

Aside from assessing pain, physical symptoms, and the degree of deformity, it is also necessary to evaluate a patient's overall well-being. In the aging population, this becomes critical, as degenerative scoliosis and sagittal malalignment can negatively impact the patient's quality of life. This assessment can be accomplished with different methods to calculate an HRQOL. To measure someone's HRQOL, various tools such as Scoliosis Research Society-22 Patient Questionnaire (SRS-22)[39] instrument, ODI,[40] and the Medical Outcomes Form Short Form–12 (SF-12) are used to better understand someone's physical, mental, emotional, and social functioning in relation to their quality of life. Improvements in disability scoring systems are a major priority both in the clinical setting and in research to further improve how degenerative scoliosis is managed in the future. Additional work has been done to better understand the psychosocial effects of spinal deformity, and pretreating patients with counseling and therapy may help patients prior to surgery.

16.3.5 Surgical Strategy

Decision-making with spine deformity is often challenging, particularly with relation to curve correction and level selection. Research has shown that alignment goals need to be age specific due to degenerative changes in the aging.[41] It was once believed that the best practice involved overcorrection to mitigate the loss of correction that occurs in the aging, as alignment deterioration is more common.[42] However, this practice is likely harmful, as less strict alignment goals have been shown to reach population HRQOL.[41] Overcorrection can also lead to complications such as proximal junctional kyphosis.[41] When aging patients receive appropriate correction of LL, they also have modest changes in proximal thoracic kyphosis and improvements in PT and SVA.[43] With age-adjusted alignment goals, patients may have better clinical outcomes and quality of life.[44] With this in mind, there are essentially three broad strategies to consider for treating degenerative scoliosis patients: limited decompression, focal stabilization and deformity correction.

16.3.6 Limited Decompression

For a subset of patients who present with predominantly radicular symptoms from isolated foraminal stenosis, Minimally invasive surgery (MIS) approaches have offered potential options to reduce morbidity in patients with smaller spinal deformities.[45] MIS offers less soft-tissue dissection and easier recovery than open posterior approaches.

Aging patients with degenerative scoliosis may benefit from a minimally invasive laminectomy with or without a foraminotomy. This procedure may allow for symptomatic relief of radicular symptoms while avoiding the risks of a large open fusion.[45]

These patients must also be carefully selected, as back pain and sagittal imbalance remain largely unchanged. A potential side effect from this procedure is recurrent radiculopathy and mechanical instability, requiring fusion with posterior multilevel pedicle screw placement.

16.3.7 Focal Stabilization

Focal fusion is often the treatment of choice for single- or two-level degenerative disease. In these scenarios, patients have stenosis with a spondylolisthesis or degenerative disc disease. For patients with mild or moderate deformity, a short fusion construct may be reasonable to restore alignment. For example, a patient with lumbar flat back with an L4-L5 spondylolisthesis may be a candidate for an anterior lumbar interbody fusion of L4-L5 and L5-S1 followed by a posterior fusion L4-S1. Under this patient scenario, degenerative pathology is addressed, while restoring lordosis from L4-S1. Focal fusions can also be addressed with minimally invasive techniques.

Lateral interbody fusion (LIF) is a transpsoas approach that gains access to the anterior column of the spine without disrupting paraspinal musculature, reducing morbidity and postoperative pain. By avoiding the posterior tension band in this approach, it is also hypothesized to protect against adjacent segment disease (ASD).[46,47] This approach allows better access to the disc space than posterior approaches, allowing for large cage placement and improved fusion rates. With a resulting increase in disc height, this causes indirect neural decompression. It also negates a traditional anterior approach, reducing the risk to visceral organs. As a consequence, the approach has the potential to injure nerves in the lumbar plexus from the approach.

A meta-analysis by Dangelmajer et al in 2014 found no significant difference in complication rates of MIS vs. open approaches.[45] They did find a significant difference in the age of patients undergoing MIS vs. open surgeries, with older patients being better candidates for MIS due to their poor bone quality and comorbidities. With aging patients who have degenerative scoliosis, MIS has been shown to correct sagittal and predominantly coronal deformities, with the LIF showing the greatest change.[45]

16.3.8 Deformity Correction

Correcting deformity is almost exclusively done through a large posterior approach. With access to the vertebrae of interest, whose curves often include a large portion of the lumbar and thoracic spine, a large fusion construct can be built with appropriate osteotomies to allow proper manipulation.

Depending on the type,[30] an osteotomy (▶ Fig. 16.5) provides a certain amount of curvature correction to help balance the deformed spine. The first two types of osteotomies involve the facet joint. There are six Grades (1-6) that correlate with the degree of bone resection. The first is a partial facet excision, with removal of the inferior facet (Grade 1), and the second type involves both inferior and superior facet excision, along with removal of ligamentum flavum and possibly other posterior elements (Grade 2). Both types of facet osteotomies require a mobile anterior column and provide limited deformity correction.[30] A pedicle subtraction (Grade 3), also known as a closing

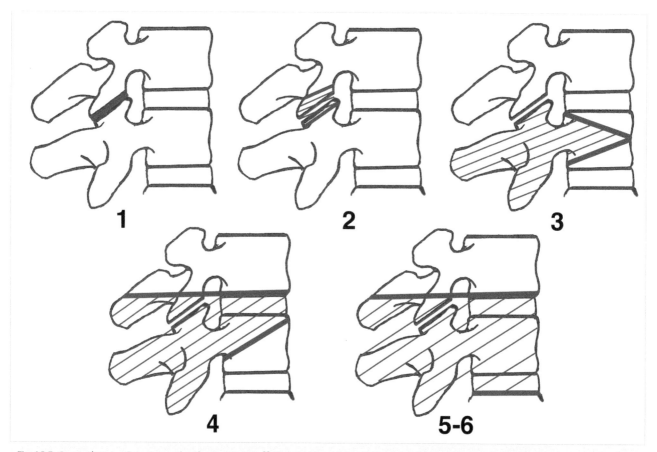

Fig. 16.5 Comprehensive Osteotomy Classification System.[30] **1)** Partial facet joint. **2)** Complete facet joint. **3)** Pedicle/partial body. **4)** Pedicle/partial body/disc. **5)** Complete vertebra and adjacent discs. **6)** Multiple vertebrae and adjacent discs.

wedge, is a resection of a wedge portion of the posterior vertebral body, including the pedicles, creating a hinge at the anterior column while sparing the disc. For a larger resection, grade 4 involves a wedge through the vertebral body that the endplate and a portion of one adjacent disc are removed, along with posterior elements with pedicles. With this type of resection, an anterior cage may be placed, particularly in cases with marked shortening.

In certain circumstances, severe inflexible deformities can be managed with a vertebral column resection (VCR). VCR (osteotomy grade 5 and 6)[30] is a powerful operative method, defined as an osteotomy involving the vertebral body, intervening discs, pedicles, and all of the dorsal elements to create a segmental defect requiring provisional instrumentation.[48,49] Once dorsal instrumentation is placed, the spine may be manipulated to achieve balance in both the sagittal and coronal planes while shortening the length of the spinal column if necessary.[22] An interbody graft may also be used to augment the anterior column and prevent unwanted shortening of the spine. This technically-difficult procedure has a high associated complication rate, extensive operative times, and significant blood loss.[48,50]

16.4 Benefits and Risks

Spinal deformity surgery is a potentially life-changing operation. The surgery usually provides more benefit than risk, but it is essential to understand both. Patients who fail conservative therapy, especially those with progressive decline in neurological functioning, intractable pain, significant disability, or deformity can have significant improvements in their quality of life after surgery.[51,52,53,54] Radiographic parameters that are most associated with disability and thus benefit after correction is the global sagittal alignment (SVA) and the spinopelvic parameters PT and PI-LL.[6,53,55] Studies continue to show a strong correlation between HRQOL and correction of previously mentioned radiographic parameters, particularly the SVA.[56] Yoshida et al found improvement in every category of the HRQOL questionnaires besides lifting and personal care at 1 year post-spinal deformity surgery, although these did improve at the 2-year postsurgery assessment.[56] Looking specifically at degenerative scoliosis, quality of life improved in all domains at 2-years post-surgery.

Determining the causes and rates of morbidity and mortality associated with each surgery is valuable for surgical planning, patient counseling, and efforts to improve patient care.[57] This is increasingly important in aging patients contemplating spinal deformity surgery.

Mortality in spinal surgery is rare, but the risk increases with a patient's age. In a study by Smith et al looking at the Scoliosis Research Society (SRS) Morbidity and Mortality Database, the authors found a mortality rate of one per 1,000 < 60-year-old patients, with an exponential increase in the aging. In patients older than 90, mortality is 34.4 per 1,000.[57] The majority of deaths in the aging degenerative scoliosis population came from respiratory/ pulmonary complications (28%), cardiac complications (22%), sepsis (16%), and stroke (9%).[57]

Morbidity in the aging spinal deformity population is common, with rates ranging from 11 to 35% in large-population database studies and showing an increase with age.[58,59] A meta-analysis in 2015 reported a complication rate of 55% in adult deformity surgery, although age and etiology was not specified.[52] In Sansur's study, the complications were broken down, with the majority of them being wound infections (37%), followed by dural tears (29%), neurologic complications (16%), and implant complications (13%).[59] Compared to the younger population, aging patients typically suffer from more postoperative complications due to poorer general health. With age, the spine has increased spondylosis in conjunction with poor bone quality, which reduces the likelihood of a successful fusion without major instrumentation problems.[52,60]

16.5 Pitfalls, Complications, and Avoidance

Several modifiable risk factors have been shown to correlate with worse surgical outcomes following spinal deformity surgery. These risk factors include an elevated BMI, smoking, narcotic use, and anxiety/depression.[11] Surgeons should optimize these risk factors to decrease surgical risk.

16.5.1 Multisurgeon

Due to technical complexity, extensive operating times, and high complication risks in surgery, many centers have implemented strategies involving two attending surgeons to improve efficiency and safety.[44,61] Using two surgeons for complex cases is not a novel concept, but there remains a paucity of literature on this as it relates to spinal deformity.[44,61,62,63] In a recent study by Gomez et al (2017) looking at one vs. two attending surgeons on ASD, they found no significant differences in length of stay, OR time, and EBL between the two cohorts, but did find a decrease in intraoperative complications.[44] However, a survey of 199 SRS membership surgeons found that they believe a second attending improves patient care, although most centers do not regularly practice this.[61] Further investigation into this approach is needed to better assess its utility. In another recent study, two-surgeon approaches led to a decrease in operative time, blood loss, and overall complication rate when compared to single-surgeon approaches.[62] This study was limited, however, by historical bias and surgeon-to-surgeon variation between groups.

16.5.2 Proximal Junctional Kyphosis

One of the most recognized complications in patients undergoing instrumented posterior fusion for spinal deformity is proximal junctional kyphosis (PJK). As with other complications, older age at the time of surgery has been a consistent risk factor for developing PJK.[41,64,65,66] The severity of sagittal plane deformity and the extent of operative sagittal plane realignment are also risk factors for this complication.[67] PJK is defined as abnormal kyphosis immediately above the uppermost

instrumented vertebrae (UIV) and is measured using the sagittal Cobb angle between the inferior endplate of UIV and the superior endplate of the second vertebrae above the UIV (**Fig. 16.4a**).[68]

The definition of PJK varies in the literature based on radiographic findings and clinical sequela, which includes pain, neurologic deficit, and impaired quality of life. Although the causes of PJK are not fully understood, age-related degeneration and deformity are believed to be main factors. Other potential causes include disruption of the posterior ligamentous complex, instrumentation failure, vertebral fractures, and facet violation.[68]

Several methods can be used to prevent the onset of PJK following fusion. Vertebroplasty, hook fixation, terminal rod contouring, and ligament augmentation can all be used in appropriately selected patients, individually or in combination. These techniques warrant further investigation but have some supporting data and compelling biomechanical rationale, especially in aging high-risk patients.[68]

16.5.3 Tranexamic Acid and Blood Loss

Given the complexity associated with spinal deformity surgery, excessive blood loss can lead to significant morbidity. To mitigate these losses, numerous methods may be employed. Techniques with established efficacy include acute normovolemic hemodilution, hemostatic agents, and intrathecal morphine.[69] Other factors that influence blood loss include surgical technique, use of MIS, appropriate patient positioning with the abdomen free, local and topical hemostatic agents, maintaining normothermia, red-blood-cell salvage, and controlled hypotension. Maintaining a mean arterial blood pressure of < 75 mm Hg also helps to mitigate blood loss.[70,71] Many of these techniques have limited data supporting a reduction in blood transfusion.[69]

More recently, administering antifibrinolytics prior to and during surgery has become a popular method of reducing blood loss, especially in orthopedics. Tranexamic acid (TXA) has shown to be safe and effective for use in spinal surgery. TXA is a synthetic analogue of the amino acid lysine and works by inhibiting fibrinolysis. The medication can be given orally, parentally, or topically with 100% bioavailability and a half-life of 1–3 hours.[72] There is no current standard of care regarding the dosage for TXA in spinal surgery. Recently, there have been two randomized control studies in adolescent scoliosis and adult deformity patients showing a reduction in blood loss with TXA as compared to saline with 10 mg/kg loading dose followed by 1 mg/kg maintenance per hour.[70,71]

16.6 Outcomes and Evidence

Although correcting spinal deformity remains a complex operation and has associated risks, current evidence shows the outcomes to be beneficial in the correct patients. Correcting coronal and sagittal parameters are important outcomes in measuring technical success, as discussed earlier, but HRQOL measures prove to be more important to the patient. HRQOL results are now being used for further research in spinal deformity correction and thus guide future patient management.

As previously stated, the parameters discussed in this chapter (SVA, PT, PI-LL) correlate with patient-reported outcomes

(HRQOL) and have shown the largest increase in quality of life once corrected compared to other parameters.[6,53,55] Correcting SVA continuous to show the most benefit in the literature and must be emphasized.[6,53] The amount of SVA negatively correlates with a patient's quality of life. Patients with a significant amount of global sagittal malalignment (> 120 mm) show the largest improvements in their HRQOL postsurgery.[53,56] A successful surgery will correct the deformity to an acceptable standard, improving cosmetic appearance; it will reduce pain and any neurologic issues as well as improve functioning, all of which are key components associated with a higher quality of life.

16.7 Conclusion

With a growing aging population and greater awareness of degenerative scoliosis, it is likely that the incidence of spinal deformity fusions will increase in the future.[52,58] Understanding the normative aging process in the spine and the management of scoliosis in this population is essential for proper patient selection and optimal surgical outcomes. With age, the spine naturally has reduced bone quality, increased spondylosis, and progressive sagittal deformity. Identifying appropriate surgical candidates and targeting an appropriate surgical treatment plan come with experience and perhaps with a multidisciplinary approach. Research has shown us the value in restoring sagittal balance to an age-specific normal parameter but has also demonstrated the potential pitfalls of overcorrection. Research in the field of adult spinal deformity is rapidly evolving.

Key References

[1] Bridwell KH, Anderson PA, Boden SD, Kim HJ, Vaccaro AR, Wang JC. What's New in Spine Surgery. J Bone Joint Surg Am. 2014; 96(12):1048–1054

[2] Schwab F, Lafage V, Farcy J-P, et al. Surgical rates and operative outcome analysis in thoracolumbar and lumbar major adult scoliosis: application of the new adult deformity classification. Spine. 2007; 32(24):2723–2730

[3] Schwab F, Ungar B, Blondel B, et al. Scoliosis Research Society-Schwab adult spinal deformity classification: a validation study. Spine. 2012; 37(12):1077–1082

[4] Schwab FJ, Blondel B, Bess S, et al. International Spine Study Group (ISSG). Radiographical spinopelvic parameters and disability in the setting of adult spinal deformity: a prospective multicenter analysis. Spine. 2013; 38(13): E803–E812

[5] Glassman SD, Bridwell K, Dimar JR, Horton W, Berven S, Schwab F. The impact of positive sagittal balance in adult spinal deformity. Spine. 2005; 30(18): 2024–2029

References

[1] Ailon T, Smith JS, Shaffrey CI, et al. Degenerative Spinal Deformity. Neurosurgery. 2015; 77 Suppl 4:S75–S91

[2] Yang C, Yang M, Chen Y, et al. Radiographic Parameters in Adult Degenerative Scoliosis and Different Parameters Between Sagittal Balanced and Imbalanced ADS Patients. Medicine (Baltimore). 2015; 94(29):e1198

[3] Silva FE, Lenke LG. Adult degenerative scoliosis: evaluation and management. Neurosurg Focus. 2010; 28(3):E1

[4] Wong E, Altaf F, Oh LJ, Gray RJ. Adult Degenerative Lumbar Scoliosis. Orthopedics. 2017; 40(6):e930–e939

[5] Ploumis A, Transfledt EE, Denis F. Degenerative lumbar scoliosis associated with spinal stenosis. Spine J. 2007; 7(4):428–436

[6] Glassman SD, Bridwell K, Dimar JR, Horton WC, Berven S, Schwab F. The impact of positive sagittal balance in adult spinal deformity. Spine. 2005; 30(18): 2024–2029

[7] Cho K-J, Kim Y-T, Shin S-H, Suk S-I. Surgical treatment of adult degenerative scoliosis. Asian Spine J. 2014; 8(3):371–381

[8] Di Silvestre M, Lolli F, Bakaloudis G. Degenerative lumbar scoliosis in elderly patients: dynamic stabilization without fusion versus posterior instrumented fusion. Spine J. 2014; 14(1):1–10

[9] Grubb SA, Lipscomb HJ, Suh PB. Results of surgical treatment of painful adult scoliosis. Spine. 1994; 19(14):1619–1627

[10] Bakhsheshian J, Scheer JK, Gum JL, et al. International Spine Study Group (ISSG). Comparison of Structural Disease Burden to Health-related Quality of Life Scores in 264 Adult Spinal Deformity Patients With 2-Year Follow-up: Novel Insights into Drivers of Disability. Clin Spine Surg. 2017; 30(2):E124–E131

[11] Smith JS, Shaffrey CI, Glassman SD, et al. Spinal Deformity Study Group. Clinical and radiographic parameters that distinguish between the best and worst outcomes of scoliosis surgery for adults. Eur Spine J. 2013; 22(2):402–410

[12] Khajavi K, Shen A, Lagina M, Hutchison A. Comparison of clinical outcomes following minimally invasive lateral interbody fusion stratified by preoperative diagnosis. Eur Spine J. 2015; 24 Suppl 3:322–330

[13] Parker SL, Shau DN, Mendenhall SK, McGirt MJ. Factors influencing 2-year health care costs in patients undergoing revision lumbar fusion procedures. J Neurosurg Spine. 2012; 16(4):323–328

[14] Meyer JS. Diabetes and wound healing. Crit Care Nurs Clin North Am. 1996; 8 (2):195–201

[15] Christman AL, Selvin E, Margolis DJ, Lazarus GS, Garza LA. Hemoglobin A1c predicts healing rate in diabetic wounds. J Invest Dermatol. 2011; 131(10): 2121–2127

[16] Bridwell KH, Anderson PA, Boden SD, Kim HJ, Vaccaro AR, Wang JC. What's New in Spine Surgery. J Bone Joint Surg Am. 2014; 96(12):1048–1054

[17] Iyer S, Lenke LG, Nemani VM, et al. Variations in Sagittal Alignment Parameters Based on Age: A Prospective Study of Asymptomatic Volunteers Using Full-Body Radiographs. Spine. 2016; 41(23):1826–1836

[18] Diebo BG, Varghese JJ, Lafage R, Schwab FJ, Lafage V. Sagittal alignment of the spine: What do you need to know? Clin Neurol Neurosurg. 2015; 139:295–301

[19] Schwab FJ, Lafage R, Liabaud B, et al. Does One Size Fit All? Defining Spinopelvic Alignment Thresholds Based on Age. Spine J. 2014; 14(11):S120–S121

[20] Bao H, Zhu F, Liu Z, et al. Coronal curvature and spinal imbalance in degenerative lumbar scoliosis: disc degeneration is associated. Spine. 2014; 39(24): E1441–E1447

[21] Schwab F, Lafage V, Farcy J-P, et al. Surgical rates and operative outcome analysis in thoracolumbar and lumbar major adult scoliosis: application of the new adult deformity classification. Spine. 2007; 32(24):2723–2730

[22] Steinmetz MP, Benzel EC. Benzel's Spine Surgery. Elsevier Health Sciences; 2016

[23] Schwab F, Ungar B, Blondel B, et al. Scoliosis Research Society-Schwab adult spinal deformity classification: a validation study. Spine. 2012; 37(12):1077–1082

[24] Lafage V, Schwab F, Patel A, Hawkinson N, Farcy J-P. Pelvic tilt and truncal inclination: two key radiographic parameters in the setting of adults with spinal deformity. Spine. 2009; 34(17):E599–E606

[25] Obeid I, Hauger O, Aunoble S, Bourghli A, Pellet N, Vital JM. Global analysis of sagittal spinal alignment in major deformities: correlation between lack of lumbar lordosis and flexion of the knee. Eur Spine J. 2011; 20(5) Suppl 5: 681–685

[26] Kim YB, Kim YJ, Ahn Y-J, et al. A comparative analysis of sagittal spinopelvic alignment between young and old men without localized disc degeneration. Eur Spine J. 2014; 23(7):1400–1406

[27] Aurouer N, Obeid I, Gille O, Pointillart V, Vital JM. Computerized preoperative planning for correction of sagittal deformity of the spine. Surg Radiol Anat. 2009; 31(10):781–792

[28] Aebi M. The adult scoliosis. Eur Spine J. 2005; 14(10):925–948

[29] Berjano P, Lamartina C. Classification of degenerative segment disease in adults with deformity of the lumbar or thoracolumbar spine. Eur Spine J. 2014; 23(9):1815–1824

[30] Schwab F, Blondel B, Chay E, et al. The Comprehensive Anatomical Spinal Osteotomy Classification. Neurosurgery. 2013; 1(November):•••

[31] Glassman SD, Carreon LY, Shaffrey CI, et al. The costs and benefits of nonoperative management for adult scoliosis. Spine. 2010; 35(5):578–582

[32] Glassman SD, Berven S, Kostuik J, Dimar JR, Horton WC, Bridwell K. Nonsurgical resource utilization in adult spinal deformity. Spine. 2006; 31(8):941–947

[33] Yanamadala V, Kim Y, Buchlak QD, et al. Multidisciplinary Evaluation Leads to the Decreased Utilization of Lumbar Spine Fusion: An Observational Cohort Pilot Study. Spine. 2017; 42(17):E1016–E1023

[34] Gamache FW. The value of "another" opinion for spinal surgery: A prospective 14-month study of one surgeon's experience. Surg Neurol Int. 2012; 3 Suppl 5:S350–S354

[35] Scheer JK, Smith JS, Clark AJ, et al. International Spine Study Group. Comprehensive study of back and leg pain improvements after adult spinal deformity surgery: analysis of 421 patients with 2-year follow-up and of the impact of the surgery on treatment satisfaction. J Neurosurg Spine. 2015; 22(5):540–553

[36] Smith JS, Shaffrey CI, Berven S, et al. Spinal Deformity Study Group. Improvement of back pain with operative and nonoperative treatment in adults with scoliosis. Neurosurgery. 2009; 65(1):86–93, discussion 93–94

[37] Ferrero E, Lafage R, Diebo BG, et al. Tridimensional Analysis of Rotatory Subluxation and Sagittal Spinopelvic Alignment in the Setting of Adult Spinal Deformity. Spine Deform. 2017; 5(4):255–264

[38] Chen PG-C, Daubs MD, Berven S, et al. Degenerative Lumbar Scoliosis Appropriateness Group. Surgery for Degenerative Lumbar Scoliosis: The Development of Appropriateness Criteria. Spine. 2016; 41(10):910–918

[39] Haher TR, Gorup JM, Shin TM, et al. Results of the Scoliosis Research Society instrument for evaluation of surgical outcome in adolescent idiopathic scoliosis. A multicenter study of 244 patients. Spine. 1999; 24(14):1435–1440

[40] Fairbank JC, Couper J, Davies JB, O'Brien JP. The Oswestry low back pain disability questionnaire. Physiotherapy. 1980; 66(8):271–273

[41] Lafage R, Schwab F, Glassman S, et al. International Spine Study Group. Age-Adjusted Alignment Goals Have the Potential to Reduce PJK. Spine. 2017; 42(17):1275–1282

[42] Cho K-J, Kim K-T, Kim W-J, et al. Pedicle subtraction osteotomy in elderly patients with degenerative sagittal imbalance. Spine. 2013; 38(24):E1561–E1566

[43] Lafage V, Ames C, Schwab F, et al. International Spine Study Group. Changes in thoracic kyphosis negatively impact sagittal alignment after lumbar pedicle subtraction osteotomy: a comprehensive radiographic analysis. Spine. 2012; 37(3):E180–E187

[44] Gomez JA, Lafage V, Scuiba DM, et al. International Spine Study Group. Adult Scoliosis Deformity Surgery: Comparison of Outcomes Between One Versus Two Attending Surgeons. Spine. 2017; 42(13):992–998

[45] Dangelmajer S, Zadnik PL, Rodriguez ST, Gokaslan ZL, Sciubba DM. Minimally invasive spine surgery for adult degenerative lumbar scoliosis. Neurosurg Focus. 2014; 36(5):E7

[46] Cheh G, Bridwell KH, Lenke LG, et al. Adjacent segment disease followinglumbar/thoracolumbar fusion with pedicle screw instrumentation: a minimum 5-year follow-up. Spine. 2007; 32(20):2253–2257

[47] Helgeson MD, Bevevino AJ, Hilibrand AS. Update on the evidence for adjacent segment degeneration and disease. Spine J. 2013; 13(3):342–351

[48] Yang C, Zheng Z, Liu H, Wang J, Kim YJ, Cho S. Posterior vertebral column resection in spinal deformity: a systematic review. Eur Spine J. 2016; 25(8):2368–2375

[49] Jeszenszky D, Haschtmann D, Kleinstück FS, et al. Posterior vertebral column resection in early onset spinal deformities. Eur Spine J. 2014; 23(1):198–208

[50] Lenke LG, Newton PO, Sucato DJ, et al. Complications after 147 consecutive vertebral column resections for severe pediatric spinal deformity: a multicenter analysis. Spine. 2013; 38(2):119–132

[51] Bridwell KH, Baldus C, Berven S, et al. Changes in radiographic and clinical outcomes with primary treatment adult spinal deformity surgeries from two years to three- to five-years follow-up. Spine. 2010; 35(20):1849–1854

[52] Sciubba DM, Yurter A, Smith JS, et al. International Spine Study Group (ISSG). A Comprehensive Review of Complication Rates After Surgery for Adult Deformity: A Reference for Informed Consent. Spine Deform. 2015; 3(6):575–594

[53] Blondel B, Schwab F, Ungar B, et al. Impact of magnitude and percentage of global sagittal plane correction on health-related quality of life at 2-years follow-up. Neurosurgery. 2012; 71(2):341–348, discussion 348

[54] Yadla S, Maltenfort MG, Ratliff JK, Harrop JS. Adult scoliosis surgery outcomes: a systematic review. Neurosurg Focus. 2010; 28(3):E3

[55] Schwab FJ, Blondel B, Bess S, et al. International Spine Study Group (ISSG). Radiographical spinopelvic parameters and disability in the setting of adult spinal deformity: a prospective multicenter analysis. Spine. 2013; 38(13):E803–E812

[56] Yoshida G, Boissiere L, Larrieu D, et al. ESSG, European Spine Study Group. Advantages and Disadvantages of Adult Spinal Deformity Surgery and Its Impact on Health-Related Quality of Life. Spine. 2017; 42(6):411–419

[57] Smith JS, Saulle D, Chen C-J, et al. Rates and causes of mortality associated with spine surgery based on 108,419 procedures: a review of the Scoliosis Research Society Morbidity and Mortality Database. Spine. 2012; 37(23):1975–1982

[58] Sing DC, Berven SH, Burch S, Metz LN. Increase in spinal deformity surgery in patients age 60 and older is not associated with increased complications. Spine J. 2017; 17(5):627–635

[59] Sansur CA, Smith JS, Coe JD, et al. Scoliosis research society morbidity and mortality of adult scoliosis surgery. Spine. 2011; 36(9):E593–E597

[60] Takahashi S, Delécrin J, Passuti N. Surgical treatment of idiopathic scoliosis in adults: an age-related analysis of outcome. Spine. 2002; 27(16):1742–1748

[61] Scheer JK, Sethi RK, Hey LA, et al. and the SRS Adult Spinal Deformity Committee. Results of the 2015 Scoliosis Research Society Survey on Single Versus Dual Attending Surgeon Approach for Adult Spinal Deformity Surgery. Spine. 2017; 42(12):932–942

[62] Ames CP, Barry JJ, Keshavarzi S, Dede O, Weber MH, Deviren V. Perioperative Outcomes and Complications of Pedicle Subtraction Osteotomy in Cases With Single Versus Two Attending Surgeons. Spine Deform. 2013; 1(1):51–58

[63] Gurtner GC, Robertson CS, Chung SC, Li AK. Two-team synchronous oesophagectomy. Br J Surg. 1994; 81(11):1620–1622

[64] Kim YJ, Bridwell KH, Lenke LG, Glattes CR, Rhim S, Cheh G. Proximal junctional kyphosis in adult spinal deformity after segmental posterior spinal instrumentation and fusion: minimum five-year follow-up. Spine. 2008; 33(20):2179–2184

[65] Kim HJ, Lenke LG, Shaffrey CI, Van Alstyne EM, Skelly AC. Proximal junctional kyphosis as a distinct form of adjacent segment pathology after spinal deformity surgery: a systematic review. Spine. 2012; 37(22) Suppl:S144–S164

[66] Kim HJ, Bridwell KH, Lenke LG, et al. Proximal junctional kyphosis results in inferior SRS pain subscores in adult deformity patients. Spine. 2013; 38(11):896–901

[67] Hart R, McCarthy I, O'brien M, et al. International Spine Study Group. Identification of decision criteria for revision surgery among patients with proximal junctional failure after surgical treatment of spinal deformity. Spine. 2013; 38(19):E1223–E1227

[68] Safaee MM, Osorio JA, Verma K, et al. Proximal Junctional Kyphosis Prevention Strategies: A Video Technique Guide. Oper Neurosurg (Hagerstown). 2017. doi:10.1093/ons/opx054

[69] Tse EYW, Cheung WY, Ng KFJ, Luk KDK. Reducing perioperative blood loss and allogeneic blood transfusion in patients undergoing major spine surgery. J Bone Joint Surg Am. 2011; 93(13):1268–1277

[70] Verma K, Errico T, Diefenbach C, et al. The relative efficacy of antifibrinolytics in adolescent idiopathic scoliosis: a prospective randomized trial. J Bone Joint Surg Am. 2014; 96(10):e80–e10

[71] Verma K, Kohan E, Ames CP, et al. A Comparison of Two Different Dosing Protocols for Tranexamic Acid in Posterior Spinal Fusion for Spinal Deformity: A Prospective, Randomized Trial. Int J Spine Surg. 2015; 9:65–69

[72] Verma K, Errico TJ, Vaz KM, Lonner BS. A prospective, randomized, double-blinded single-site control study comparing blood loss prevention of tranexamic acid (TXA) to epsilon aminocaproic acid (EACA) for corrective spinal surgery. BMC Surg. 2010; 10(1):13

17 Nonsurgical Pain Management

William Sullivan, Julie Hastings, and Bradley Gale

Abstract

Nonsurgical management of back pain in older adults is a complex task. Evidence-based treatments include medications, physical therapy, cognitive therapy, meditation and mindfulness, exercise, and complementary and alternative medicine. Also important is the treatment of comorbid conditions such as depression. Back pain and depression frequently co-occur and exacerbate each other. In older adults, chronic back pain has been associated with isolation, disability, reduced mobility, poor health-related quality of life, depression and anxiety, and sleep impairment. The causes of back pain are broad, and the management is complex, without one clear solution. There are many circumstances when surgical management of a patient's back pain may not be appropriate, such as when a specific pain generator cannot be identified, when the risk of surgery and medical comorbidities outweighs the potential benefits, or when a patient chooses not to undergo surgery. This chapter will outline treatment options that can be considered when providing nonoperative back pain management in older adults. Also addressed are unique considerations providers should be aware of when caring for older adults.

Keywords: Back pain, older adult, non-surgical, pain management

---

Key Points

- Back pain is the most common type of pain reported by older adults and offers unique challenges in both diagnosis and management.[1]
- Comprehensive assessment and thoughtful management is especially important in this population, as back pain has been found to be associated with substantial disability from reduced mobility, poor health-related quality of life, depression and anxiety, sleep impairment, and isolation.[2,3]
- The techniques available for nonsurgical treatment are pharmacology, physical therapy, pain psychology/mind-body-based interventions, and complementary and movement-based therapies.

17.1 Indications and Contraindications

There are many circumstances when surgical management of a patient's back pain may not be appropriate, such as when a specific pain generator cannot be identified, when the risk of surgery due to medical comorbidities outweighs the potential benefits, or when a patient chooses not to undergo surgery. Even when a patient is an appropriate surgical candidate, medical providers can greatly increase the likelihood of a successful outcome by utilizing adjunctive pain management techniques as described in this chapter.

17.2 Technique Descriptions, Benefits, Risks, Outcomes, and Evidence

17.2.1 Pharmacologic Therapies for Back Pain

Using medication for the management of chronic low back pain is often a trial and error process that takes time and multiple office visits. There is no single best agent that consistently works for all patients with back pain. Acute back pain will often resolve on its own with time, but the recovery can usually be facilitated and function improved if pain can be relieved in the interim. Pharmacologic management of back pain in the older adult population is complicated by age related physiologic changes, which lead to altered drug absorption and decreased renal excretion, sensory and cognitive impairments, polypharmacy, and multimorbidity.[4] Commonly prescribed medications for managing back pain include nonsteroidal anti-inflammatory drugs (NSAIDs), acetaminophen, serotonin and norepinephrine reuptake inhibitors (SNRIs), tricyclic antidepressants (TCAs), benzodiazepines, opioids, skeletal muscle relaxants, anti-seizure medications, and corticosteroids. When prescribing medication to any patient, it is important to consider medical comorbidities and other medications the patient may be taking. This is especially important in the aging adult population, in which polypharmacy is a common problem. The number of medical comorbidities that can alter metabolism or effectiveness are likely to increase with a patient's age. An important resource to use when prescribing for aging patients is the American Geriatric Society's (AGS) Beers Criteria for Potentially Inappropriate Medication use in Older Adults,[5] a guide created by the AGS to inform clinical decision making when prescribing medication to older adults.

Acetaminophen

Acetaminophen is a commonly-prescribed medication for pain management because of its general effectiveness for acute pain and relatively low risk profile. Acetaminophen was previously recommended as a first-line agent for the management of back pain.[6,7] However, more recent data has changed that recommendation and found that there is no significant benefit from using acetaminophen for chronic low back pain. Evidence is not available to make recommendations about the use of acetaminophen for acute or radicular low back pain.[8] Despite the widespread use of acetaminophen for pain, there are risks associated with its use, especially in older adults. Heavy alcohol use, liver pathologies, and other medications metabolized by the liver should also be noted prior to recommending acetaminophen, and the potential risks and benefits should be discussed.

Nonsteroidal Anti-Inflammatory Drugs

Nonsteroidal anti-inflmmatory drugs (NSAIDs) are another medication commonly used for pain management in the general population. Recent data continues to support the recommendation of NSAIDs as a first-line treatment for acute low back pain, with demonstrated pain relief, although the effect on function is inconsistent. The same is true for chronic low back pain, with NSAIDs being more effective than placebo for pain relief.[8] There are risks associated with NSAIDs, especially in the older adult populations. For example, other medications metabolized by the kidney can interact with NSAIDs, increasing the risk of kidney damage. Additionally, regular nonaspirin NSAID use is associated with a 4-fold increase risk of serious upper gastrointestinal tract disease.[9] The elevation in risk is dose-dependent and also rises with increasing age. Beers Criteria recommends avoiding chronic use unless other options are not effective.[5]

Opiates

Opiates and other mu-receptor agonist drugs are commonly prescribed for pain. There has been a steady rise in the prescription rate of opiates, paralleled by a rise in opiate overdose-related deaths.[10] Opiates can be effective pain relievers under the right circumstances, but evidence does not support the use of opiate and opiate-like medications for acute back pain.[8] Stronger opioids such as morphine and hydromorphone have been shown to provide some-short term relief for chronic low back pain, but evidence does not support their continued use or show any positive effect on function.[8] There are many potential adverse effects associated with opioid use, which include nausea, vomiting, constipation, somnolence, dry mouth, dizziness, and addiction. These risks are elevated in older adults with a slower drug metabolism rate. Additionally, the use of long-acting opioids in patients with chronic noncancer pain has been shown to significantly increase all-cause mortality, including the risk of death from causes other than overdose.[11]

Skeletal Muscle Relaxants

The phrase "Skeletal Muscle Relaxants" is a very broad term for medications that can have significantly different mechanisms of action. Skeletal muscle relaxant is a bit of a misnomer. Evidence for the use of these medications is mixed for acute low back pain. Some of these medications include cyclobenzaprine, tizanidine, orphenadrine, and carisoprodol. Cyclobenzaprine and tizanidine fall under the tricylic antidepressant (TCA) umbrella. Orphenadrine is an anticholinergic medication. Carisoprodol is a centrally-acting medication metabolized to meprobamate, an addictive substance in the carbamate class. There is evidence to support an improvement in short-term pain relief with the general class of skeletal muscle relaxants, compared with placebo. However, there is insufficient data to make any conclusions regarding changes in function. Evidence does not suggest a benefit on pain nor function in chronic back pain.[12,13] Beers Criteria strongly recommends against the use of skeletal muscle relaxants in older adults because of the risk of anticholinergic effects, sedation, and increased risk of fractures.[5]

Benzodiazepines

There is limited and inconsistent evidence regarding the use of benzodiazepines for acute, chronic, or radicular low back pain.[8] The American College of Physicians was unable to determine any magnitude of effect of benzodiazepines on pain or function based on the available research. Additionally, benzodiazepines were associated with an increased risk of central nervous system adverse effects including somnolence, fatigue, and light-headedness.[8] While the Beers Criteria does not comment on the use of benzodiazepines in back pain, they note that the medication should generally be avoided, except in certain disorders such as seizures, generalized anxiety disorder, or ethanol withdrawal.[5]

Antiseizure Medications

Anti-seizure medications such as gabapentin and pregabalin do not have strong evidence for acute, chronic, or radicular low back pain.[8,14] These medications are associated with a risk of adverse effects, including fatigue, dry mouth, difficulties with mental concentration, memory, or visual accommodation, and loss of balance.[14] Again, when combined with other medications that an older adult patient may be taking, these adverse effects may be exacerbated due to slowed drug metabolism.

Antidepressant Medications

Antidepressants have been gaining in popularity for pain management, as increasing research is supporting their use. Antidepressants most commonly used for pain management include tricyclic antidepressant (TCA), serotonin and norepinephrine reuptake inhibitor (SNRI), and selective serotonin reuptake inhibitor (SSRI) classes of medications. Specific to low back pain, duloxetine has been found to be of some benefit for the treatment of chronic low back pain after a 12-week course of treatment.[8,15] Again, there are risks associated with duloxetine, including, but not limited to, nausea, dry mouth, fatigue, diarrhea, hyperhidrosis, dizziness, and constipation.[15] Caution should also be taken when prescribing any of the antidepressant medications if a patient is already on other centrally-acting medications. Beers Criteria recommends caution in older adults, as TCAs, SSRIs, and SNRIs may cause or exacerbate the syndrome of inappropriate antidiuretic hormone secretion (SIADH) or hyponatremia.[5]

Corticosteroids

Systemic corticosteroids are often prescribed with the goal of reducing inflammation and subsequently reducing low back pain. As an oral formulation, they are easier to administer than a local steroid injection, however, available research does not support the use of systemic corticosteroid for acute or chronic low back pain in the general adult population.[8] Additionally, Beers Criteria recommends against the use of corticosteroid in older adults who are at risk for delirium or in conjunction with NSAIDs because it can increase the risk of GI bleeding or peptic ulcer formation.[5]

17.2.2 Physical Therapy

Physical therapy is a frequently utilized treatment for patients with low back pain. Physical therapists have specialized skills and treatment options that are beyond the scope of this section. The following physical therapy interventions are some of the more commonly used techniques for back pain and include identification and treatment of trigger points, motor control exercises, and the McKenzie Method of Mechanical Diagnosis and Treatment (MDT). Manual therapy is an additional technique utilized in the management of back pain by various practitioners, including physical therapists, and is described in detail in subsequent sections.

Motor Control Exercise

Motor control exercise (MCE) focuses on the activation and control of deep trunk muscles. Once this muscle control is established, the exercises focus on integrating functional tasks into muscle activation. MCE is unique from other forms of exercise because it is meant to target a direct cause of low back pain.[16] The theory behind MCE is that people with back pain tend to have a weak core that provides poor stabilization to the spine. This leads to the onset and perpetuation of nonspecific low back pain.[16] By targeting these stabilizing muscles, the patient can theoretically increase the support to the spine, and reduce the strain placed on it, leading to a reduction in pain.

MCEs require extensive training to ensure proper performance. Some methods used by physical therapists to ensure activation of the targeted muscles include palpation, ultrasound imaging, and pressure biofeedback. The goal is to teach patients how to isolate and contract specific muscles and muscle groups, build up strength and endurance, and eventually integrate the specific muscle contractions into functional tasks. MCEs differ from stabilization exercises because of this integration of functional tasks.

The utility and risks of MCE as it specifically pertains to older adults has not been extensively studied. The same risks that apply to most forms of exercise should be considered when recommending MCE. Providers should take into consideration the overall health of the patient before recommending more intensive physical activity. The evidence for MCE for the general adult population is mixed but suggests a clinically important effect when compared to minimal intervention for chronic low back pain,[16] and has been shown to be more effective than general exercise for addressing pain and function.[12]

Trigger Points and Dry Needling

Trigger-point treatments, including dry needling, are interventions that can be performed by a variety of providers, including physical therapists. Trigger points, in this context, are referred to as myofascial points that are pain-generating palpable zones of tense musculature. Trigger points have identifiable morphologic changes in muscle tissue under microscopic visualization.[17] Dry needling refers to the use of a high gauge needle inserted into areas of trigger points identified by the practitioner.[17] While physicians will often perform trigger point injections with medications (local anesthetics and/or steroids), physical therapists are increasingly using dry needling of trigger points as a treatment for trigger point-associated back pain. Trigger points can also be treated by physical therapists using manual techniques. Recent data shows that manual trigger-point therapy using an inflatable ball improved function and alleviated pain in older adults with chronic low back pain.[18] The purpose of acting on these trigger points, through manipulation, dry needling, or other techniques, is to disrupt to

pathologic muscle contractions, decrease tone, and reduce pain.[17]

The evidence in support of dry needling for the treatment of chronic low back pain has been growing in recent years, as the popularity of this intervention increases. More studies are being conducted to evaluate the effectiveness of dry needling as an adjunct to other treatments, as well as in comparison to other commonly used interventions. A 2005 Cochrane Review of the literature suggests that dry needling is an effective adjunctive therapy for chronic low back pain.[19,20] There is further review evidence suggesting that dry needling has a statistically significant effect on pain intensity and functional disability in the immediate postintervention period, but no statistically significant difference at follow up.[20] There is some controversy on whether dry needling is a form of acupuncture. Early training of physical therapists in dry needling was performed by acupuncturists, and there are some that consider this a type of acupuncture (Ahsi point acupuncture), though terminology varies in different regions of the world.

Dry needling does have its possible adverse effects that need to be considered in elderly patients. There are very few differences in risks when compared to the general population, but the provider should use caution with patients on anticoagulation due to increased risk of bleeding and hematoma formation. Other risks to be taken into consideration include infection, tissue damage, and injury to nearby structures.

The McKenzie Method of MDT

The McKenzie Method of MDT is a classification-based assessment and treatment system for low back pain. The technique was developed by physical therapist Robin McKenzie in 1981 and classifies patients with low back pain based on how their pain responds during the initial evaluation. The primary categories of classification are derangement, dysfunction, and postural. The classification is made by the physical therapists watching and evaluating a patient's pain response to various repetitive movements.

Centralization of pain and directional preference are key features in the McKenzie therapy. Centralization occurs when a patient's back pain moves from radiating more peripherally to a more central location in the spine. This occurs when a practitioner guides the patient to find positions, or directional preferences, that lead to this type of change in their pain. Studies show strong evidence indicating that back pain which centralizes has much better clinical outcomes when compared with back pain the does not centralize.[21,22] Once the practitioner identifies positions that are beneficial to the centralization of their patient's pain, they can instruct the patient on ways to incorporate those activities into their daily routine. This has been shown to reduce pain as well as lower incidences of pain recurrence.[23,24]

The effectiveness of MDT compared to other physical therapy techniques has been studied with mixed results. A 2006 meta-analysis found that MDT may be more effective than passive treatment for acute low back pain, although clinical significance was unclear.[23] Further research found MDT to be more effective than other treatments—including NSAIDs, education, strengthening exercises, back massage, and spinal mobilization—in short-term pain and disability.[24] Most available research agrees that there is limited evidence for improvement in pain in intermediate and long-term outcomes, or those with chronic back pain.[23,24]

17.2.3 Pain Psychology and Mind-Body Approaches

Chronic Back Pain and Depression

An association between depression and chronic, disabling low back pain has been established in the adult population including in aging patients. In aging patients, this association becomes increasingly complex due to physical and psychological changes associated with the aging process. Research focused on the community-dwelling older adult population has found that the presence of depressive symptoms was a strong and independent risk factor for the occurrence of disabling back pain, with studies suggesting that depression worsens both the severity of and the disability caused by chronic low back pain.[25,26,27] Findings suggest this is a bidirectional relationship, as it is widely recognized that chronic pain conditions can increase the risk of depressive symptoms.

There are several theories behind the relationship of depression and chronic pain, especially chronic nonspecific back pain, in the older adult population. One is that depressed older adults may be less likely to spontaneously report depressive symptoms and may instead communicate emotional distress by focusing on somatic complaints and describe feeling helpless or debilitated due to back or joint pain.[27] Another widely discussed theory is that pain-related disability in aging patients may be driven by pain "homeostenosis". This is described as a diminished ability to effectively respond to the stress of persistent pain due to the comorbidities of the aging process, including cognitive and physical impairments, increased sensitivity to suprathreshold pain stimuli, medical and psychological comorbidities, altered pharmacokinetics and pharmacodynamics, and increased social isolation.[26] Psychological similarities between patients with depression and patients with chronic low back pain have also been noted, including diminished mental flexibility and decreased self-efficacy with subsequent learned helplessness.[27]

Research looking at the neurochemical and neuromorphology of depression and chronic low back pain in the older adult population have also elucidated a relationship at this biological level. It has been proposed that neurochemical changes in serotonergic or noradrenergic function that occur as a consequence of depression have the potential to increase sensitivity to painful stimuli, rendering affected patients more susceptible to disabling chronic pain.[25] Several areas of the brain which modulate mood also process pain, including the dorsolateral prefrontal cortex, anterior cingulate cortex, periaqueductal gray, insular cortex, and hypothalamus. Data has demonstrated that older adults with chronic low back pain have pain morphology differences from pain-free individuals, including decreased gray matter volume in the posterior parietal cortex and middle cingulate white matter volume of the left hemisphere.[25]

This shared biology and psychology support a unified approach to treatment, including screening older adult patients presenting with chronic low back pain for depression. The Patient Health Questionnaire-2 (PHQ-2) is a commonly used and validated screening tool which is best utilized when the patient has no prior diagnosis of depression and no spontaneous report of depressive symptoms. Patients who screen positive with the PHQ-2 and those who already carry a diagnosis of depression or are spontaneously reporting depressive symptoms should be administered the Patient Health Questionnaire-9 (PHQ-9) or the 15-item Geriatric Depression Scale. Expert-based recommendations include following up the diagnosis of clinically significant depression with screening for comorbid psychiatric conditions, including anxiety, cognitive impairment, PTSD, and alcohol or other substance misuse.[27] The intent of treating depression and chronic low back pain in older adults as linked conditions is to encourage a holistic approach to treatment and prescribing which may spare the overuse of opioids in this population.

Fear Avoidance Beliefs and Pain Catastrophizing

Both fear avoidance beliefs and pain catastrophizing have been associated with persistent pain and disability in both middle-aged and aging patients with back pain. The fear-avoidance model as it relates to chronic pain has been widely studied since its introduction in 1983 by Letham et al, who theorized that fear avoidance may contribute to the development of adverse pain behaviors and subsequent pain experiences, including chronic pain and increased disability.[28] Research focused on the role of physical activity fear-avoidance beliefs in older American adults with low back pain have found these beliefs to be independently associated with self-reported disability and overall physical health.[29] Additional research has demonstrated that physical activity fear-avoidance beliefs were significantly associated with both self-reported and observed measures of disability even after controlling for other potential contributors to disability. Notably, psychological factors, including fear-avoidance beliefs, may be more predictive of disability in older adults with chronic low back pain than the pathology of the pain itself and its associated impairments. These researchers found an intervention consisting of general conditioning and aerobic exercise to improve fear-avoidance beliefs beyond reduction in pain.[28]

Pain catastrophizing has also been found to be predictive of pain-related outcomes in both surgical and nonsurgical patients. Pain catastrophizing has been described as an exaggerated negative "mental set" associated with pain and has been linked to increased perceived pain intensity and disability, which has been theorized to explain the relationship between fear-avoidance beliefs and increased low back pain associated disability in aging patients.[29] Research has found preoperative pain catastrophizing to be a unique predictor of postoperative pain intensity during activity and analgesic use after lumbar fusion surgery.[30] Research looking at the effect of pain catastrophizing in patients undergoing lumbar stenosis surgery found that pain catastrophizing predicted back pain intensity, pain interference, and disability. These researchers propose employing interventions such as TCAs and cognitive behavioral therapy (CBT), which have been utilized to address increased levels of pain catastrophizing in other patient populations.[31]

Cognitive Behavioral Therapy

CBT is a classification of therapy that is commonly utilized in the treatment of chronic pain. CBT aims to reduce the psychological distress and dysfunction associated with pain by teaching patients methods to challenge maladaptive thoughts and beliefs, decrease maladaptive behaviors, increase adaptive behaviors, and increase self-efficacy for pain management.[32] CBT can also include pain education and instruction in adjunctive techniques, such as progressive muscular relaxation. CBT has demonstrated clinical benefit for treatment of both depression and chronic low back pain and utilizes similar techniques for treatment of both conditions, including activity pacing, active coping and problem-solving skills, relaxation techniques, and involvement of spouses/caregivers.[27]

Cognitive Functional Therapy

Cognitive functional therapy (CFT) is a related behavioral approach to pain that encourages patients to both cognitively reconceptualize the pain experience and functionally normalize provocative movements and postures while discouraging pain behaviors. The aim of CFT is to address multiple dimensions of chronic pain, including fear-avoidance behaviors and catastrophizing. The intervention is behaviorally based and targets specific physical behaviors, such as pain behaviors, aggravating postures and activities, and muscle guarding while simultaneously addressing related psychosocial and/or cognitive behaviors.[33]

Research has shown CFT to have promise in reducing functional disability and reported pain amongst adult patients with nonspecific chronic low back pain.[33] However, this has yet to be looked at specifically in the older-adult population.

Mindfulness Meditation and Mindfulness-Based Stress Reduction

Meditation is a mind and body practice that has been in use for over 5,000 years. Practices focus on the interactions between the brain, mind, body and behavior and aim to support practitioners' learning to focus their attention as a way of gaining greater insight into themselves and their surroundings. There are many forms of meditation, each of which falls into one of two categories: mindfulness meditation and concentrative meditation. Mindfulness meditation focuses attention on breathing to develop increased awareness of the present, while concentrative meditation aims to increase overall concentration by focusing on a specific word or phrase. Most forms of meditation have four elements in common: a quiet location with minimal distraction, a specific comfortable posture, a focus of attention, and an open attitude.[34]

Mindfulness meditation aims to transform everyday activities, such as sitting and walking, into a meditation through nonjudgmental observation of physical sensations, thoughts, and feeling. Dr. Jon Kabat-Zinn has been credited with conceptualizing mindfulness meditation for a Western audience with his pioneering of the mindfulness-based stress reduction (MBSR) program at the University of Massachusetts Medical Center in 1979.[35] MBSR, in particular, focuses on increasing a detached observation and acceptance of experiences, including uncomfortable emotions and physical sensations.[36] Because it has been operationalized and standardized, MBSR has been studied in clinical trials for a variety of disorders and diseases, including chronic pain. Several neuroimaging studies have attempted to elucidate the mechanism of mindfulness meditation and have found increased cortical thickness in the prefrontal cortex and right anterior insula among long-term meditators compared with controls. The prefrontal cortex and occipito-temporal regions of the brain show a typical decline with age; however, studies have shown that long-term meditators aged 40–50 are more likely to maintain their cortical thickness.[26]

Research comparing a MBSR-based intervention to health education for community-dwelling adults aged 65 years or older with chronic low back pain demonstrated the MBSR intervention led to improved short-term function and improved long-term pain. This led researchers to conclude that the utility of the intervention could be increased by focusing on the durability of functional improvement.[37] Other research focusing on adults ages 20–70 with nonspecific low back pain has shown MBSR to be as effective as CBT in improving both pain and functional limitations, noting that MBSR-based interventions may be more accessible in populations where patient access to skilled CBT may be limited.[36]

17.2.4 Complementary Therapies

Complementary therapies, as defined by the National Center for Complementary and Integrative Health (NCCIH), include health care approaches developed outside of mainstream Western, or conventional, medicine. Other terms include "alternative" medicine and "integrative" medicine, which are often used interchangeably but, in fact, have different meanings. Complementary health approaches often, but not always, fall into the categories of either natural products (such as herbs and supplements) or mind-body practices (such as yoga, acupuncture, relaxation techniques, and movement therapies).[38] Complementary therapies are increasingly pursued by patients as adjunctive pain treatments, or when conventional treatments are not successful. A 2010 survey performed by the American Association of Retired Persons (AARP) and the National Center for Complementary and Integrative Health (NCCIH), looking at whether Americans aged 50 years and older discuss the use of complementary therapies with their health care provider, found that over half (53%) of respondents reported use of complementary therapies, while only a little over half of these respondents reporting having discussed their use of complementary therapies with their health care provider.[39] This highlights the importance of asking patients about their use of complementary therapies in order to assess for potential risks or contraindications as well as to facilitate the conversation about pain beliefs and management goals and expectations.

Acupuncture

Acupuncture is a 3,000-year-old technique of Traditional Chinese Medicine which utilizes the insertion of fine, sterile needles into the skin at specific anatomic sites, or acupuncture points, to release blockages in the flow of *qi* or energy. The theory is that the release of blocked qi encourages the balance of oppositional forces within the body, which improves function of the internal organs and promotes the body's natural healing response. Other methods used to stimulate acupuncture points, or acupoints, include manual pressure, moxibustion or heat therapy, electrical stimulation, and the application of topical herbal liniments.[40]

While acupuncture is traditionally used for various health conditions, there is significant research supporting the efficacy of acupuncture for a variety of pain conditions, including low back pain. Acupuncture has been shown to be most beneficial for reducing pain and improving function in chronic low back pain when used as an adjunct to conventional treatments. There is conflicting evidence over the difference in effect between acupuncture and sham acupuncture (superficial needle insertion at nonacupoints). It is possible that superficial needle penetration could potentially mediate analgesic placebo effects and that nonpenetrating acupuncture is a more reliable control.[38]

Acupuncture is considered to be a relatively safe procedure with serious complications, such as pneumothorax, being rare. The most common complications include bleeding, hematoma or ecchymoma formation, and insertion site pain.[41] Caution should be exercised when recommending acupuncture to patients with clotting disorders or on long-term anticoagulation.

Chiropractic Care

Chiropractic care is based on the belief that health is directly affected by the relationship between the body's structure (primarily that of the spine) and its function, as coordinated by the nervous system. Hands-on therapy is central to chiropractic care, with spinal manipulations, or adjustments, being a core mechanism of treatment. Additional approaches may include modalities such as heat and ice, electrical stimulation, ultrasound, rehabilitative exercise, and lifestyle counseling.[42]

Efficacy studies of middle-aged adults have established a therapeutic and restorative benefit of chiropractic care on functional abilities and relief of low back pain. Studies focused on the older adult population have also demonstrated chiropractic care to be beneficial with an observed protective effect of chiropractic care against declines in ADLs, IADLs, and declines in self-rated health.[43] Spinal manipulation therapy combined with home exercise has also been shown to lead to greater intermediate-term pain reduction than home exercise alone.[44]

A primary concern regarding chiropractic care is the risk of injury or adverse events. Because spinal manipulation involves application of physical force, there is a potential risk of traumatic injury, especially with patients particularly vulnerable to injury and/or if the manipulation is deficient in technical skill or precision. Risks identified by systemic review include arterial dissection, myelopathy, fracture, disk extrusion or herniation, cauda equina syndrome, and formation of hematoma.[45] While the rate of injury is considered to be low, ranging from 0.05 to 1.46 adverse events per 10,000,000 manipulations in a middle-aged population[46] to 40 incidents per 100,000 subjects in a population aged 66–99 years,[45] these injuries are associated with significant morbidity. When considering patients for chiropractic care, one should exercise extreme caution with regard to the provision of spinal manipulation in patients with long-term use of anticoagulation therapy or coagulation disorders, history of aortic aneurysm or dissection, or inflammatory

spondylopathy. Occlusion or stenosis of precerebellar arteries are contraindications to cervical spine manipulation, given the increased risk for vertebrobasilar stroke.[45]

Massage Therapy

Massage therapy is a treatment modality encompassing many different techniques, generally including therapists using manual pressure to manipulate and mobilize the muscles and other soft tissues of the body. The effectiveness of massage therapy in the treatment of back pain is challenging to establish, largely due to the lack of standardization of treatment, with the heterogeneity of massage therapy and the diversity of training acquired by practitioners. Popular modalities range from Swedish massage, which uses a variety of stroke techniques to promote relaxation, to myofascial release, which utilizes shear compression or tension and skin rolling with the goal of releasing adhered fascia and muscles.

Clinical evidence supports the use of massage therapy in adult patients to relieve the pain of acute, subacute, and chronic low back pain in the short term, but the benefit has not been established for long-term pain relief nor for improvement of function.[47] The most common adverse events include soreness in muscles, increased pain, and stiffness. Serious adverse events are rare.[48] Notably, the data on adverse events has not been established in the aging population.

Proponents of massage therapy for pain often cite the benefit of relaxation in the treatment of chronic pain, with evidence that massage therapy may at least temporarily reduce blood pressure.[49] It has also been argued that the emotional value of touch and its effect on mood has the potential to be beneficial in patients with comorbid pain and anxiety and/or depression.

17.2.5 Movement-Based Interventions

Exercise or physical activity is recommended as a first-line treatment for chronic nonspecific low back pain.[50,51] Exercise may look very different from patient to patient. This is especially true when caring for older adults with widely ranging physical limitations. Providers must consider the patient's medical comorbidities and what the patient is capable of doing safely prior to recommending a specific exercise plan or type of physical activity.

Exercise or physical activity has been shown to improve back strength, flexibility, and range of motion, as well as to lead to overall improvements in mood.[52,53] For acute and subacute low back pain, exercise versus no exercise or usual care is reported to have inconsistent effects on pain. However, for chronic low back pain exercise was associated with greater pain relief than no exercise.[12]

General Exercise Recommendations

The American College of Sports Medicine's (ACSM's) position statement on exercise and physical activity for the aging population recommends that all adults should be active. The recommended amount of moderate-intensity physical activity is 150 minutes per week. If a patient cannot perform 150 minutes of activity per week because of comorbid medical conditions, they should still continue to be as physically active as their bodies allow.[54] When prescribing exercise, the patient's initial level of fitness must be taken into consideration. Often, muscle strengthening and balance exercise will need to precede aerobic training for individuals who have previously been sedentary.[54] There is increasing evidence that the amount of time that someone is sedentary is also detrimental to their overall health. Repetitive, extended sedentary periods are harmful even to people who regularly meet the recommended physical activity standards.[55] Types of exercise are frequently grouped into four broad categories: aerobic or cardiorespiratory exercise, resistance or strength training, flexibility, and balance. In the following sections, we will discuss some specific forms of exercise and their utility in management of back pain in older adults.

Cardiorespiratory or Aerobic Exercise

Cardiorespiratory or aerobic exercise refers physical activity that is performed over an extended period of time at an elevated heart rate. A recent meta-analysis comparing various types of exercise for low back pain did not find a significant effect of aerobic exercise over other forms of exercise.[50] However, aerobic exercise is known to have numerous benefits on general health and includes many different activities that can be appropriate for aging patients, including walking, running, cycling, swimming or water-based activities. There is high-level evidence recommending aerobic exercise for older adults five or more days per week at moderate intensity for at least 30 minutes, or three or more days per week of vigorous exercise for at least 20 minutes. The exercise can be performed in one continuous session or in 10-minute intervals spaced out throughout the day.[56]

There are risks associated with initiating and maintaining an exercise regimen. Running may be difficult for someone with significant knee arthritis, but they may be able to walk briskly, without putting the same strain on their knees. If someone has concerns about their balance, cycling may not be the best option; however, it can be low impact, and a stationary bike can eliminate the concern about falling. Swimming or water aerobics can be especially popular among older adults wishing to exercise without placing significant strain on their joints. There is evidence to suggest that the addition of deep-water running, in addition to a multimodal physical therapy program, has better results at reducing low back pain when compared to physical therapy alone, though the difference is not significant.[57] The most common issues that arise when patients who are unaccustomed to physical activity start to exercise include muscle soreness, musculoskeletal injury, and attrition.[56]

Strength and Resistance Exercise

There is good evidence to suggest that back pain, without a specific identifiable pathology, can be associated with both trunk and extremity muscles that are weak and easily fatigued.[50] When comparing the broad categories of exercise listed above, the trials that measured the effect of strength and resistance training on improvements in low back pain had the largest effect size. Exercises that targeted multiple muscle groups were shown to have the largest effect on decreasing low back pain.[50] However, the data specific to using strength and resistance exercises to manage back pain in older adults is limited.

Strength and resistance exercise is a very broad term and includes activities such a weight lifting, body-weight exercises, elastic band exercises, and many others. Physical therapists can be an excellent resource to help a patient start an exercise routine, especially strength and resistance exercises. There are extensive benefits to strength and resistance exercises beyond the potential for improvement in low back pain. Similar to other forms of exercise, resistance training can improve health outcomes, including blood pressure, insulin sensitivity, and overall body composition.[56]

Yoga

The term yoga has been used in India for over 2.5 thousand years, with different meanings. Currently in Western culture, what is referred to as yoga is most often Hatha yoga, which usually involves holding the body in a sequence of postures, or *asanas*, accompanied by breathing, concentration, and meditation techniques. The National Center for Complementary and Integrative Health (NCCIH) defines yoga as "a mind-body practice that combines breathing, physical movements, and meditation or relaxation to benefit health and well-being."

Clinical trials have shown clinical effectiveness and cost-effectiveness of yoga in middle-aged adults with chronic low back pain, with outcomes including decreased perceived pain, decreased pain-related disability, improved balance, flexibility and back function, and improved pain self-efficacy.[58] Systematic review has found strong evidence for short-term effectiveness and moderate evidence for long-term effectiveness of yoga for chronic low back pain in the most patient-centered outcomes.[59] A challenge in studying yoga-based interventions is the inability to standardize yoga programs. Elements common to most yoga-based interventions include specific stretching, breathing, and relaxation exercises, with goals typically including building strength, improving flexibility, and promoting relaxation. The American Pain Society guidelines recommend that clinicians consider offering yoga to patients with chronic low back pain with this recommendation being limited to Viniyoga-style yoga.[7]

While there is data demonstrating the efficacy of yoga in reducing hyperkyphosis in the over-60 adult population,[60] there is minimal data on the role and usefulness of yoga on pain management in the older adult population. One factor to consider in the recommendation of yoga to older adults with chronic back pain is the increased risk of vertebral compression fractures (VCFs) in osteopenic patients with yoga spinal flexion based postures. It has been argued that improvement in the flexibility of the spine in older age can be both an advantage and an adversity as the spinal rigidity associated with aging may act as a protective mechanism that decreases the risk of spinal flexion in osteoporosis.[61] It should also be considered that causes of back pain that are more prevalent in the aging population—such as vertebral fracture, spinal degeneration, and osteoarthritis—may not be as amenable to yoga intervention as are causes of back pain in younger patients.[62] Given the movement-based nature of yoga, it is likely that a yoga intervention is not appropriate for all adults with chronic back pain and should be considered very carefully after evaluation of a patient's specific risk, with yoga being directed by a qualified yoga therapy instructor.

Tai Chi

Tai chi is an ancient martial and health art developed in China several hundred years ago. The movements of tai chi are gentle, flowing, and circular and are intended to move qi (the internal energy of the body) and train mind-body control via breathing exercises and meditation. Tai chi is a mild-to-moderate aerobic exercise, depending on the intensity, pace, frequency, and duration of the practice. In the United States, approximately 2.5 million individuals have participated in tai chi, with that number likely growing.[63]

Previous tai chi research has found evidence for improvements in postural control as demonstrated by increased body awareness, improved balance and reduced falls, improved muscle tone, and better kinesthetic control.[64] In particular, tai chi-based intervention has been shown to reduce risk of falls and fracture in the elderly[65] with tai chi frequently recommended to osteoporotic women and a safe and effective exercise for bone density maintenance and fall prevention.[63]

Tai chi has demonstrated potential to decrease pain intensity in patients with chronic nonspecific neck pain, with the reduction in pain intensity associated with several factors, including decreased anxiety and increased postural awareness.[64] Beyond the physical components of tai chi, the integration of cognitive and mindfulness-based components have been credited with promoting an individual's ability to exercise executive control over nociceptive input, including potential pain generators, and using learned imagery techniques and meditation to cope.[63]

Risk of injury with tai chi is fairly low and usually includes minor muscle and joint soreness at commencement of activity.[66] A potential concern when engaging aging people in tai chi is the higher prevalence of knee osteoarthritis (OA) in this population, as tai chi movements typically incorporate a flexed knee posture, which has been shown to produce increased load on the lower limbs, including the knee joint. Sun-style tai chi is a form of tai chi specifically developed for aging patients with knee OA, as it utilizes a higher stance, which reduces the torque on the knee joint.[67]

Pilates

Pilates is a form of exercise developed in the 1920s by Joseph Pilates and consists of a set of dynamic strength and flexibility exercises performed on a mat (without special apparatus) or on specialized equipment. The Pilates method is based on six principles—concentration, control, centering, flow, precision, and breathing—and aims to develop improved core stability, body awareness, and posture.[68]

Systematic review of available randomized controlled trials looking at middle-aged patients with low back pain have found Pilates to be more effective than minimal intervention for improving pain, disability, function, and global impression of recovery in the short term, and better pain intensity and disability outcomes at intermediate-term follow up.[69] This benefit has not been demonstrated in the comparison of Pilates with general exercise.[70]

There is minimal data supporting the use of Pilates for back pain in the older adult population; however, data does support the use of Pilates to increase bone mineral density, physical performance, and quality of life in postmenopausal women with osteoporosis with minimal risk of adverse events.[71]

17.3 Pitfalls, Complications and Avoidance

The potential risks associated with the above spine care management options are generally minimal. However, all interventions have potential complications. The American Geriatric Society's (AGS's) Beers Criteria for Potentially Inappropriate Medication use in Older Adults,[5] should be referenced when considering the risks various medications pose to older adults. Opiate medications pose a unique risk, especially when prescribed for chronic noncancer pain, as this has been shown to increase all-cause mortality.[11]

The treatments and modalities provided by physical therapists involve minimal risk when offered to patients who have been properly screened. The risks posed by movement-based interventions are also low, so long as the patients' medical comorbidities do not preclude exertion. Therefore, knowing your patients' medical history is essential to choosing the proper treatment while minimizing risk.

17.4 Conclusion

There are a variety of medications, modalities, and exercise techniques available for the treatment of appropriately diagnosed low back pain in the aging patient. An individualized approach weighing the risks and benefits of these treatments is appropriate. There is no one approach appropriate for all patients, and there remains a paucity of evidence for the majority of treatment options, especially data that is specific to the aging population.

Key References

[1] Carley JA, Karp JF, Gentili A, et al. Deconstructing Chronic Low Back Pain in the Older Adult: Step by Step Evidence and Expert-Based Recommendations for Evaluation and Treatment: Part IV: Depression. Pain Med. 2015; 16(11): 2098–2108

[2] Chou R, Qaseem A, Snow V, et al. Clinical Efficacy Assessment Subcommittee of the American College of Physicians, American College of Physicians, American Pain Society Low Back Pain Guidelines Panel. Diagnosis and treatment of low back pain: a joint clinical practice guideline from the American College of Physicians and the American Pain Society. Ann Intern Med. 2007; 147(7): 478–491

[3] Makris UE, Abrams RC, Gurland B, Reid MC. Management of persistent pain in the older patient: a clinical review. JAMA. 2014; 312(8):825–836

[4] Panel., A.G.S.B.C.U.E., American Geriatrics Society 2015 Updates Beers Criteria for Potentially Inappropriate Medication Use in Older Adults. JAGS. 2015; 63: 2227–2246

[5] Reid MC, Ong AD, Henderson CR, Jr. Why We Need Nonpharmacologic Approaches to Manage Chronic Low Back Pain in Older Adults. JAMA Intern Med. 2016; 176(3):338–339

[6] Searle A, Spink M, Ho A, Chuter V. Exercise interventions for the treatment of chronic low back pain: a systematic review and meta-analysis of randomised controlled trials. Clin Rehabil. 2015; 29(12):1155–1167

References

[1] Patel KV, Guralnik JM, Dansie EJ, Turk DC. Prevalence and impact of pain among older adults in the United States: findings from the 2011 National Health and Aging Trends Study. Pain. 2013; 154(12):2649–2657

[2] Reid MC, Ong AD, Henderson CR, Jr. Why We Need Nonpharmacologic Approaches to Manage Chronic Low Back Pain in Older Adults. JAMA Intern Med. 2016; 176(3):338–339

[3] Makris UE, Abrams RC, Gurland B, Reid MC. Management of persistent pain in the older patient: a clinical review. JAMA. 2014; 312(8):825–836

[4] By the American Geriatrics Society 2015 Beers Criteria Update Expert Panel. American Geriatrics Society 2015 Updated Beers Criteria for Potentially Inappropriate Medication Use in Older Adults. J Am Geriatr Soc. 2015; 63(11): 2227-2246

[5] Panel., A.G.S.B.C.U.E., American Geriatrics Society 2015 Updates Beers Criteria for Potentially Inappropriate Medication Use in Older Adults. JAGS. 2015; 63: 2227–2246

[6] Chou R, Huffman LH, American Pain Society, American College of Physicians. Medications for acute and chronic low back pain: a review of the evidence for an American Pain Society/American College of Physicians clinical practice guideline. Ann Intern Med. 2007; 147(7):505–514

[7] Chou R, Qaseem A, Snow V, et al. Clinical Efficacy Assessment Subcommittee of the American College of Physicians, American College of Physicians, American Pain Society Low Back Pain Guidelines Panel. Diagnosis and treatment of low back pain: a joint clinical practice guideline from the American College of Physicians and the American Pain Society. Ann Intern Med. 2007; 147(7): 478–491

[8] Chou R, Deyo R, Friedly J, et al. Systemic Pharmacologic Therapies for Low Back Pain: A Systematic Review for an American College of Physicians Clinical Practice Guideline. Ann Intern Med. 2017; 166(7):480–492

[9] Hernández-Díaz S, Rodríguez LA. Association between nonsteroidal anti-inflammatory drugs and upper gastrointestinal tract bleeding/perforation: an overview of epidemiologic studies published in the 1990s. Arch Intern Med. 2000; 160(14):2093–2099

[10] Okie S. A flood of opioids, a rising tide of deaths. N Engl J Med. 2010; 363 (21):1981–1985

[11] Ray WA, Chung CP, Murray KT, Hall K, Stein CM. Prescription of Long-Acting Opioids and Mortality in Patients With Chronic Noncancer Pain. JAMA. 2016; 315(22):2415–2423

[12] Chou R, Deyo R, Friedly J, et al. Nonpharmacologic Therapies for Low Back Pain: A Systematic Review for an American College of Physicians Clinical Practice Guideline. Ann Intern Med. 2017; 166(7):493–505

[13] See S, Ginzburg R. Skeletal muscle relaxants. Pharmacotherapy. 2008; 28(2): 207–213

[14] Atkinson JH, Slater MA, Capparelli EV, et al. A randomized controlled trial of gabapentin for chronic low back pain with and without a radiating component. Pain. 2016; 157(7):1499–1507

[15] Skljarevski V, Zhang S, Desaiah D, et al. Duloxetine versus placebo in patients with chronic low back pain: a 12-week, fixed-dose, randomized, double-blind trial. J Pain. 2010; 11(12):1282–1290

[16] Saragiotto BT, M C, Yamato TP, et al. Motor control exercise for chronic nonspecific low-back pain. (Review). Cochrane Database Syst Rev. 2016

[17] Liu L, Huang QM, Liu QG, et al. Effectiveness of dry needling for myofascial trigger points associated with neck and shoulder pain: a systematic review and meta-analysis. Arch Phys Med Rehabil. 2015; 96(5):944–955

[18] Oh SKM, Lee M, et al. Effect of myofascial trigger point therapy with an inflatable ball in elderlies with chronic non-specific low back pain. J Back Musculoskelet Rehabil. 2017

[19] Furlan AD, van Tulder M, Cherkin DC, et al. Acupuncture and dry-needling for low back pain: an updated systematic review within the framework of the cochrane collaboration. Cochrane Database of Systematic Reviews. 2005; 30 (8):944–963

[20] Liu L, Huang QM, Liu QG, Thitham N, Li LH, Ma YT, Zhao JM. Evidence for Dry Needling in the Management of Myofascial Trigger Points Associated with Low Back Pain: A Systematic Review and Meta-analysis. Arch Phys Med Rehabil. 2017

[21] Werneke M, Hart DL. Centralization phenomenon as a prognostic factor for chronic low back pain and disability. Spine. 2001; 26(7):758–764, discussion 765

[22] Aina A, May S, Clare H. The centralization phenomenon of spinal symptoms–a systematic review. Man Ther. 2004; 9(3):134–143

[23] Machado LAC, de Souza Mv, Ferreira PH, Ferreira ML. The McKenzie method for low back pain: a systematic review of the literature with a meta-analysis approach. Spine. 2006; 31(9):E254–E262

[24] Busanich BM, Verscheure SD. Does McKenzie therapy improve outcomes for back pain? J Athl Train. 2006; 41(1):117–119

[25] Reid MC, Williams CS, Concato J, Tinetti ME, Gill TM. Depressive symptoms as a risk factor for disabling back pain in community-dwelling older persons. J Am Geriatr Soc. 2003; 51(12):1710–1717

[26] Karp JF, Shega JW, Morone NE, Weiner DK. Advances in understanding the mechanisms and management of persistent pain in older adults. Br J Anaesth. 2008; 101(1):111–120

[27] Carley JA, Karp JF, Gentili A, et al. Deconstructing Chronic Low Back Pain in the Older Adult: Step by Step Evidence and Expert-Based Recommendations for Evaluation and Treatment: Part IV: Depression. Pain Med. 2015; 16(11): 2098–2108

[28] Camacho-Soto A, Sowa GA, Perera S, Weiner DK. Fear avoidance beliefs predict disability in older adults with chronic low back pain. PM R. 2012; 4(7): 493–497

[29] Sions JM, Hicks GE. Fear-avoidance beliefs are associated with disability in older American adults with low back pain. Phys Ther. 2011; 91(4):525–534

[30] Papaioannou M, Skapinakis P, Damigos D, Mavreas V, Broumas G, Palgimesi A. The role of catastrophizing in the prediction of postoperative pain. Pain Med. 2009; 10(8):1452–1459

[31] Coronado RA, George SZ, Devin CJ, Wegener ST, Archer KR. Pain Sensitivity and Pain Catastrophizing Are Associated With Persistent Pain and Disability After Lumbar Spine Surgery. Arch Phys Med Rehabil. 2015; 96(10):1763–1770

[32] Turner JA, Romano JM. Cognitive-behavioral therapy for chronic pain. In: Loeser JD, Bonica JJ, eds. Bonica's management of pain. Philadelphia, PA: Lippincott Williams & Wilkins; 2001:1751–1758

[33] O'Sullivan K, Dankaerts W, O'Sullivan L, O'Sullivan PB. Cognitive Functional Therapy for Disabling Nonspecific Chronic Low Back Pain: Multiple Case-Cohort Study. Phys Ther. 2015; 95(11):1478–1488

[34] Bramoweth AD, Renqvist JG, Germain A, et al. Deconstructing Chronic Low Back Pain in the Older Adult-Step by Step Evidence and Expert-Based Recommendations for Evaluation and Treatment: Part VII: Insomnia. Pain Med. 2016; 17(5):851–863

[35] Ludwig DS, Kabat-Zinn J. Mindfulness in medicine. JAMA. 2008; 300(11): 1350–1352

[36] Cherkin DC, Sherman KJ, Balderson BH, et al. Effect of Mindfulness-Based Stress Reduction vs Cognitive Behavioral Therapy or Usual Care on Back Pain and Functional Limitations in Adults With Chronic Low Back Pain: A Randomized Clinical Trial. JAMA. 2016; 315(12):1240–1249

[37] Morone NE, Greco CM, Moore CG, et al. A Mind-Body Program for Older Adults With Chronic Low Back Pain: A Randomized Clinical Trial. JAMA Intern Med. 2016; 176(3):329–337

[38] Cho YJ, Song YK, Cha YY, et al. Acupuncture for chronic low back pain: a multicenter, randomized, patient-assessor blind, sham-controlled clinical trial. Spine. 2013; 38(7):549–557

[39] AARP, N., Complementary and Alternative Medicine: What People Aged 50 and Older Discuss With Their Health Care Providers. Consumer Survey Report, 2010

[40] How Acupuncture Can Relieve Pain and Improve Sleep, Digestion and Emotional Well-being. 2017 [cited 2017 9/1/2017]; Available from: http://cim. ucsd.edu/clinical-care/acupuncture.shtml

[41] Chung KF, Yeung WF, Yu YM, Kwok CW, Zhang SP, Zhang ZJ. Adverse Events Related to Acupuncture: Development and Testing of a Rating Scale. Clin J Pain. 2015; 31(10):922–928

[42] Chiropractic: In Depth. 2012 [cited 2017 8/15/2017]; Available from: https:// nccih.nih.gov/health/chiropractic/introduction.htm

[43] Weigel PA, Hockenberry J, Bentler SE, Wolinsky FD. The comparative effect of episodes of chiropractic and medical treatment on the health of older adults. J Manipulative Physiol Ther. 2014; 37(3):143–154

[44] Maiers M, Bronfort G, Evans R, et al. Spinal manipulative therapy and exercise for seniors with chronic neck pain. Spine J. 2014; 14(9):1879–1889

[45] Whedon JM, Mackenzie TA, Phillips RB, Lurie JD. Risk of traumatic injury associated with chiropractic spinal manipulation in Medicare Part B beneficiaries aged 66 to 99 years. Spine. 2015; 40(4):264–270

[46] Gouveia LO, Castanho P, Ferreira JJ. Safety of chiropractic interventions: a systematic review. Spine. 2009; 34(11):E405–E413

[47] Furlan AD, Giraldo M, Baskwill A, Irvin E, Imamura M. Massage for low-back pain. Cochrane Database Syst Rev. 2015(9):CD001929

[48] Paanalahti K, Holm LW, Nordin M, Asker M, Lyander J, Skillgate E. Adverse events after manual therapy among patients seeking care for neck and/or back pain: a randomized controlled trial. BMC Musculoskelet Disord. 2014; 15:77

[49] Cady SH, Jones GE. Massage therapy as a workplace intervention for reduction of stress. Percept Mot Skills. 1997; 84(1):157–158

[50] Searle A, Spink M, Ho A, Chuter V. Exercise interventions for the treatment of chronic low back pain: a systematic review and meta-analysis of randomised controlled trials. Clin Rehabil. 2015; 29(12):1155–1167

[51] Qaseem A, Wilt TJ, McLean RM, Forciea MA, Clinical Guidelines Committee of the American College of Physicians. Noninvasive Treatments for Acute, Subacute, and Chronic Low Back Pain: A Clinical Practice Guideline From the American College of Physicians. Ann Intern Med. 2017; 166(7):514–530

[52] Rainville J, Hartigan C, Martinez E, Limke J, Jouve C, Finno M. Exercise as a treatment for chronic low back pain. Spine J. 2004; 4(1):106–115

[53] Hoffman MD, Hoffman DR. Does aerobic exercise improve pain perception and mood? A review of the evidence related to healthy and chronic pain subjects. Curr Pain Headache Rep. 2007; 11(2):93–97

[54] Chodzko-Zajko WJ, Proctor DN, Fiatarone Singh MA, et al. American College of Sports Medicine. American College of Sports Medicine position stand. Exercise and physical activity for older adults. Med Sci Sports Exerc. 2009; 41 (7):1510–1530

[55] Cortell-Tormo JM, S P, Chulvi-Medrano I, et al. Effects of functional resistance training on fitness and quality of life in females with chronic nonspecific low-back pain. J Back Musculoskelet Rehabil. 2017; 4

[56] Garber CE, Blissmer B, Deschenes MR, et al. American College of Sports Medicine. American College of Sports Medicine position stand. Quantity and quality of exercise for developing and maintaining cardiorespiratory, musculoskeletal, and neuromotor fitness in apparently healthy adults: guidance for prescribing exercise. Med Sci Sports Exerc. 2011; 43(7): 1334–1359

[57] Cuesta-Vargas AI, García-Romero JC, Arroyo-Morales M, Diego-Acosta AM, Daly DJ. Exercise, manual therapy, and education with or without high-intensity deep-water running for nonspecific chronic low back pain: a pragmatic randomized controlled trial. Am J Phys Med Rehabil. 2011; 90(7):526–534, quiz 535–538

[58] Combs MA, Thorn BE. Yoga attitudes in chronic low back pain: Roles of catastrophizing and fear of movement. Complement Ther Clin Pract. 2015; 21(3): 160–165

[59] Cramer H, Lauche R, Haller H, Dobos G. A systematic review and meta-analysis of yoga for low back pain. Clin J Pain. 2013; 29(5):450–460

[60] Greendale GA, Huang MH, Karlamangla AS, Seeger L, Crawford S. Yoga decreases kyphosis in senior women and men with adult-onset hyperkyphosis: results of a randomized controlled trial. J Am Geriatr Soc. 2009; 57(9): 1569–1579

[61] Sinaki M. Yoga spinal flexion positions and vertebral compression fracture in osteopenia or osteoporosis of spine: case series. Pain Pract. 2013; 13(1): 68–75

[62] Teut M, Knilli J, Daus D, Roll S, Witt CM. Qigong or Yoga Versus No Intervention in Older Adults With Chronic Low Back Pain-A Randomized Controlled Trial. J Pain. 2016; 17(7):796–805

[63] Peng PW. Tai chi and chronic pain. Reg Anesth Pain Med. 2012; 37(4):372–382

[64] Lauche R, Wayne PM, Fehr J, Stumpe C, Dobos G, Cramer H. Does Postural Awareness Contribute to Exercise-Induced Improvements in Neck Pain Intensity? A Secondary Analysis of a Randomized Controlled Trial Evaluating Tai Chi and Neck Exercises. Spine. 2017; 42(16):1195–1200

[65] Lauche R, Stumpe C, Fehr J, et al. The Effects of Tai Chi and Neck Exercises in the Treatment of Chronic Nonspecific Neck Pain: A Randomized Controlled Trial. J Pain. 2016; 17(9):1013–1027

[66] Kong LJ, Lauche R, Klose P, et al. Tai Chi for Chronic Pain Conditions: A Systematic Review and Meta-analysis of Randomized Controlled Trials. Sci Rep. 2016; 6:25325

[67] Song R, Lee EO, Lam P, Bae SC. Effects of tai chi exercise on pain, balance, muscle strength, and perceived difficulties in physical functioning in older women with osteoarthritis: a randomized clinical trial. J Rheumatol. 2003; 30 (9):2039–2044

[68] Di Lorenzo CE. Pilates: what is it? Should it be used in rehabilitation? Sports Health. 2011; 3(4):352–361

[69] Yamato TP, Maher CG, Saragiotto BT, et al. Pilates for Low Back Pain: Complete Republication of a Cochrane Review. Spine. 2016; 41(12):1013–1021

[70] Mostagi FQ, Dias JM, Pereira LM, et al. Pilates versus general exercise effectiveness on pain and functionality in non-specific chronic low back pain subjects. J Bodyw Mov Ther. 2015; 19(4):636–645

[71] Angın E, Erden Z, Can F. The effects of clinical pilates exercises on bone mineral density, physical performance and quality of life of women with postmenopausal osteoporosis. J Back Musculoskeletal Rehabil. 2015; 28(4):849–858

18 Interventional Pain Treatment Options

Eric A.K. Mayer and Ryan Zate

Abstract

In 2016, there were approximately 46 million Americans aged 65 and over. This number is expected to double by 2060, representing an increase from 15% of the population to 24%. CMS Data reports that lifetime prevalence of low back pain has been estimated to be as high as 84%.[1] According to the Medicare database, epidural injection utilization in Medicare populations rose 271–420% and use of facet joint injections increased 231–571% from 1995 to 2016.[2] Along with the growth of the aging population, a commensurate surge in medical utilization is expected. Procedural utilization has outpaced population growth logarithmically. Medical professionals will be tasked with treating a different pool of diagnoses with different outcome expectation (low likelihood for "return to work" metrics) in this older adult demographic. The goal of this chapter is a broad survey of common pathologies encountered in the aging population, of the continuum of interventional pain treatment options, and of the evidence underlying efficacious, individualized treatment recommendations.

Keywords: Interventional pain, spine interventions, epidural steroid injection, facet rhizotomy, sacroliliac joint injection

Key Points

- Determining the correct diagnosis is critical to performing successful interventional pain procedures.
- There is evidence that epidural steroid injections improve pain and function in spinal stenosis WITH neurogenic claudication.
- Indications for intervention include spinal stenosis, facet arthropathy and sacroiliac joint dysfunction.
- Interventional treatments rarely succeed without the concomitant use of physical therapy and exercise.
- Remember that time spent assessing for masqueraders of spine pain results in better outcomes and complication avoidance.

18.1 Indications and Contraindications

18.1.1 Lumbar Stenosis

Lumbar spinal stenosis (LSS) clinically presents with symptoms of neurogenic claudication (in the limbs). LSS is ALWAYS a clinical rather than a radiological diagnosis. This constellation of symptoms involves reduced walking distance tolerance and is difficult to differentiate from Peripheral Arterial Disease (PAD). Too often, patients with nonspecific, axial, mechanical chronic low back pain are misdiagnosed with LSS (though they have neither limitation in walking distance nor claudication symptoms in lower limbs). Surgical fusion MCID-adjusted success for nonspecific low back pain from (wrongly diagnosed LSS) has

been found to benefit approximately 1 in 6 individuals.[3] This erroneous radiological diagnosis may lead to ineffective treatment plans. When a physician takes time to listen to a patient with LSS, they usually describe clinical symptoms of "intermittent," "dull or achy" quality pain in a nondermatomal pain pattern starting in the buttocks/legs occurring ONLY during standing or walking and that follows a crescendo-type pattern (worsening as the patient stands and walks) that we term the "claudicant character" of pain. Most importantly, the patient's pain resolves rapidly (seconds to minutes) with a position change of leaning forward, sitting, or lying. The subjective quality of the pain may vary in description: aching, cramping, burning, or simply "heavy" limb fatigability. Care must be taken in differentiating neurogenic claudication from vascular claudication (See ▶ Table 18.1). Patients often note relief of symptoms shortly after sitting or with forward-flexed lumbar spine during ambulation (shopping cart sign). The pathophysiology of claudication is not fully understood, but the mechanism of repeated first-degree (neurapraxia), ischemic irritation of the intracanal nerve roots is hypothesized, with electrophysiological results to support this hypothesis.[4] Others hypothesize pathophysiological neuro-mechanical mechanisms related to narrowing around the nerve from ossified ligaments, joints, or discs consistent with a reduced dynamic cross-sectional area due to physiological bony arthritis in the spine.

For Lumbosacral stenosis, an assessment of ambulatory distance is a requisite part of the examination. The reflexes may be diminished, but most cases present with variable focal neurologic deficits. Having the patient stand in prolonged extension of the lumbar spine may be difficult in the geriatric population but can be helpful in reproducing "claudicant" symptoms.

Interventional treatment options include the interlaminar or transforaminal epidural steroid injection. There is no clear evidence supporting one approach over the other for this indication. Studies have demonstrated that epidural steroid injections are reasonable, 'short-to-medium term' treatment in patients with neurogenic claudication to improve function, walking distance, and pain.[5] Studies have demonstrated that 64% of patients deemed to be surgical candidates had subjective improvement in symptoms 1 year after epidural injection, with fewer patients in the treatment group electing for surgery.[6] More recent studies have demonstrated improvements in both numerical pain scores of pain and disability.[7]

Interestingly, this data also parsed response to anesthetic alone (vs. traditional combination of corticosteroid and

Table 18.1

Neurogenic Claudication	Vascular claudication
May be proximal or distal muscles	Distal >> Proximal Muscles
Symptoms not improved by standing still	Symptoms improve slightly by standing
Improved with flexion at waist	Cool extremities + /– pulses
Improved performance with biking/or activities with flexion at the waist	Symptoms are time-related and fatigue of legs happens at the same time as other positions.

anesthetic) and found no significant differences in response to treatment. Flexion-based exercise protocols may be recommended for patients with neurogenic claudication. Although active lifestyle and aerobic conditioning should be encouraged in all patients, there is inconsistent evidence that specific rehabilitation programs are effective in completely eliminating the return of symptoms. Given enough time in the best prospective cross-sectional study, nearly 7/10 patients randomly assigned to the nonsurgical group will opt to "cross-over" for surgical intervention to alleviate claudicatory symptoms within 5 years.[8] Different interventional approaches to delivering medication to the epidural space remain debated amongst specialists. In truth, comparing transforaminal vs. interlaminar epidural injection techniques has not reliably shown either approach to be significantly superior for treatment durability in symptomatic lumbosacral stenosis.

18.1.2 Facet Arthropathy

Facet arthropathy is anatomically ubiquitous in the aging population. Simultaneously, the prevalence of axial back pain is slightly greater than the prevalence in the general population, with the facet joint proposed to be a very common cause of axial back pain.[9] Seventy to 80% of the population will endure a "significant episode" of neck or back pain during adulthood.[10] Facet-mediated pain has been described as early as 1911 by Goldthwaitt and has been estimated to account for up to 45% of chronic spine pain. Clinically, painful facet arthropathy can be difficult to diagnose, as no *single* pathognomonic test, study, complaint, or physical exam maneuver has been reliably validated. Moreover, a number of twin-twin studies implicate genetics rather than stress/load-exposure as proximate cause of radiological changes.[11] Research has established that occupational spine-loading fails to demonstrate a causal link to intensity of spine pain or degree of radiological change observed by a physician.[12] The most rigorous evidence shows "activity-discordant" twin-twin studies in several countries. This body of evidence shows that the more "active" twin (presumed to have greater spine loading) had significantly lower risk of developing disabling spine-related pain in both short- and long-duration follow-up over multiple years.[13] Although diagnosing cervical or lumbar facet-mediated pain relies on the assimilation of clinical presentation and possibly invasive testing; treatment is incomplete if it fails to include physical activity. Moderately strong evidence shows that actively-resisted exercise with "directional preference" shows the greatest evidence for efficacy.[14]

Patients presenting with painful facet arthritis tend to present with axial back or neck pain that is worsened with prolonged static position and may be exacerbated during changing positions or weight bearing (standing, sitting in place, etc). There may be "pseudo-radicular" referral patterns into the proximal legs and buttocks that have been described and validated via intra-articular injection or electronic stimulation of respective sensory nerves in the lumbar spine.[15] Referral patterns in the neck have also been demonstrated through similar means, with referral patterns into the occiput, periscapular area, shoulder, posterior/lateral neck, and upper thoracic regions.[16]

As with the lumbar spine, cervical spondylosis is very common with increasing age and presence on imaging is found in a large number of asymptomatic patients. In the chronic neck pain population cervical facet pain prevalence is estimated to range from 49–61%. Presentation often includes referral patterns into the occipital region, traps, or proximal shoulders.[17]

[Insert Image #6 Here Cervical pain referral map]

Pain is typically described as aching, deep, dull, and exacerbated by movement. Examination is non-diagnostic and must be taken into context with presentation and imaging, though no focal neurologic deficits should be apparent.

As is seen in the lumbar spine exercise and therapy focusing on posture, flexibility, and strength is the mainstay of treatment. Interventional treatment for cervical facet pain may be performed as an intra-articular injection (into the joint capsule), or by blocking the cervical medial branch nerves. Since the C1 nerve root exits cephalad to the atlas (C1), the medial branches in the cervical spine each correlate to their respective level (C3 and C4 medial branch innervated the C3–4 facet joint). Radiofrequency ablation (RFA) for the facet-mediated cervical spine pain has demonstrated excellent outcomes when 'double block' diagnostic paradigm (described below) is followed.[18]

18.1.3 Sacro-Iliac Joint Pain

Like the above-mentioned facet joints, the sacro-iliac joint (SIJ) is an accepted source of low back, buttock, and proximal leg pain. Nevertheless, the etiology, epidemiology, and diagnostic criteria for SIJ pain is still debated among experts. Though the SI joint is diarthrodial like the facet joints; the SI afferent innervation is complex and continues to be a disputed topic with the lateral and ventral rami of the sacral spinal nerves both contributing to nociceptive and possibly neurogenic character of pain. Evidence supporting intra-articular mechanoreceptors within the joint complicates effective treatment.

Patients with SIJ-mediated pain often present with low back/buttock pain overlying the visible landmark of the posterior superior iliac spine (PSIS) and endorse referral patterns down the ipsilateral lateral and/or posterior-lateral thigh. Provocative joint injections reliably recreate concordant sclerotomal referral pattern that mimics patients usual pattern of exacerbation.[19] Numerous physical exam maneuvers exist. No particular maneuver possesses either high sensitivity or specificity, but a combination of several maneuvers are commonly employed in standard clinical practice to diagnose of SIJ mediated pain.[20] Some studies have suggested that if multiple exam maneuvers are positive (Gaenslens, distraction, compression, Patricks, Gillet's) the positive-predictive value increases, but this topic remains unsettled.

Currently, intra-articular delivery of medication into the joint is the favored diagnostic method. The 'gold standard' to diagnose SIJ pain is still intra-articular injection. The specificity of this procedure varies widely in literature (40–100%).[20] The addition of good physical therapy intervention aimed at lengthening/stretching the iliopsoas muscle, lengthening the adductors, and strengthening the gluteus and paraspinals are the "mainstay" of treatment. Radiofrequency ablation of the SIJ has mixed results in the literature and is not performed with nearly the frequency of facet RFA, likely due to incomplete understanding or access to the innervation of the joint.

18.1.4 Sagittal Balance

Kyphosis and Degenerative Scoliosis

Older patient's are often particularly sensitive to the appearance of kyphotic deformity "Dowager's Hump." The change in appearance may or may not have a painful, nociceptive component, but the cosmetic appearance can be a common reason that patients present to a spine specialist. It is important to remember that kyphosis and adult degenerative scoliosis are different entities from juvenile idiopathic scoliosis. The old biomechanical aphorism: "kyphosis begets kyphosis" remains true. At its most basic, physical training and physical fitness emphasizing extensor-muscle strength and endurance remains the 'core' to keep patient at full function. 'Perfect' radiological balance is less important than a patient's ability to perform advanced ADL's and maintain their independence. Often when degenerative scoliosis causes foraminal stenosis, judicious use of selective (transforaminal) nerve blocks and occasional micro-foraminotomies are safer than a large multi-level deformity surgery. A trans-disciplinary approach to deformity that starts with a shared functional goal with input from physical therapy, physical trainer, surgeon and interventional spine specialist can achieve greater functional outcomes with less harm to the patient.

18.2 Contraindications

The contraindications to interventional pain treatments can be divided into systemic and diagnostic. The systemic contraindications are as follows: allergy to iodinated contrast, or any other medication used in the intervention, kidney disease and poorly controlled diabetes. The diagnostic contraindications are treating the patient's pain without a clear understanding of the diagnosis from a clinical perspective. Extreme care must be taken to avoid interventions on a patient that do not match the patient's complaints. These so called "masqueraders" are discussed later in the "Pitfalls, Complications and Avoidance" section of this chapter. Additionally, no interventional pain technique should be employed without the addition of adjunctive physical therapy treatments to strengthen and improve the range of motion of the surrounding tissues.

18.3 Technique(s) Description

18.3.1 Midline Epidural Steroid Injection

Lumbar interlaminar injections are often safely performed but even in patients with no surgical history there are a number of anatomical considerations that must take place. The target for these injections is in the epidural space (fat pad) that can be seen on sagittal and axial imaging in T1 sequence (See example). Although this space is usually present at each level in the lumbar spine, it is not uncommon for it to be absent or exceedingly small. It is best avoided in patients with prior laminectomies. In the cervical spine the ligamentum flavum (often used to give tactile feedback when performing the injection) becomes discontinuous cephalad to the C7-T1 space. In addition, the epidural fat pad is also less common as you move cephalad. For these reasons, it is uncommon to perform

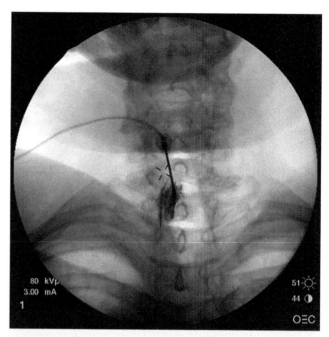

Fig. 18.1 Cervical Interlaminar Epidural Steroid Injection.

interlaminar epidurals above the C7-T1 level. Despite these limitations coverage of the entire epidural space has been demonstrated with as little as 3 mL of solution. Cervical interlaminar injections are the preferred method of delivering medicine into the epidural space and at their core are similar in technique to lumbar epidural steroid injections (Fig. 18.1).

For either cervical or lumbar epidural steroid injections, the patient is placed in a prone position and the target level is visualized under fluoroscopy. Frequently, the intensifier (X-ray) is obliqued slightly to the side to avoid passing through the interspinous ligaments. The needle is then placed in line with the beam and carefully directed back towards the midline. A lateral or "contralateral oblique" view is best taken well before the needle nears the ligamentum flavum to allow for a reference of depth. On this view the needle tip will be near the epidural space and ligamentum flavum when it is at the spinolaminar line (convergence of the spinous process and lamina). As this landmark is approached one usually notes a distinct sensation from the needle that a "fascial or firm" layer is breached. Contrast should be utilized looking for a thin line running cephalad to caudad along the epidural space in lateral or contralateral view. On the AP view a "bubbly" appearance is indicative of epidural placement.

18.3.2 Transforaminal Epidural Steroid Injection

Transforaminal epidural injections are another delivery method into the epidural space with studies by Derby and Bogduk suggesting it delivers more medication into the ventral epidural space.[21] This technique classically involves placing the tip of the needle into the superior foramina just above the exiting nerve root. Care should be taken when planning this procedure as severe foraminal narrowing or prior fusion surgeries can make it technically challenging or nearly impossible. Approaching this injection requires obtaining a more oblique view in which the superior articular process and pedicle are clearly visualized. If you recall looking for the "scotty-dog" on oblique X-ray in the lumbar spine you want to place the needle "under the dog's chin." The needle should be advanced towards the target and both lateral and AP views are helpful in precisely locating the needle. On the AP view you should avoid placing the needle tip medial to the pedicle at risk of puncturing the dura, with the lateral view allowing you to gauge depth and ensure that the needle tip is within the intervertebral foramen. Once satisfied

with the needle placement contrast is used and should demonstrate flow along the exiting nerve and superomedially past the pedicle into the epidural space (Figs. 18.2, 18.3).

18.3.3 Cervical Spine

Recently, the safety of transforaminal approach in the cervical spine has come into question by multiple case reports of catastrophic neurologic injury following cervical transforaminal epidurals.[22] For this reason, the authors do not recommend this approach in the cervical spine.

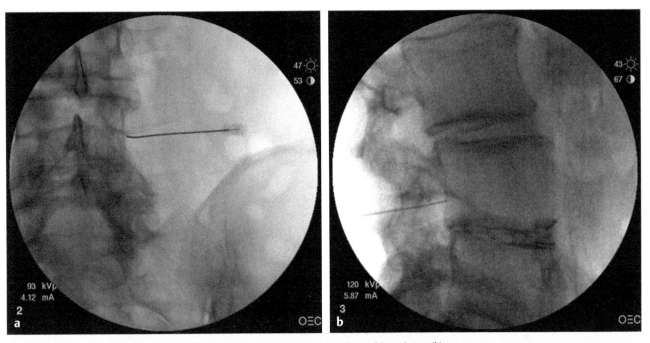

Fig. 18.2 Illustrated is an L4 transforaminal epidural steroid injection, AP view (**a**) and lateral view (**b**).

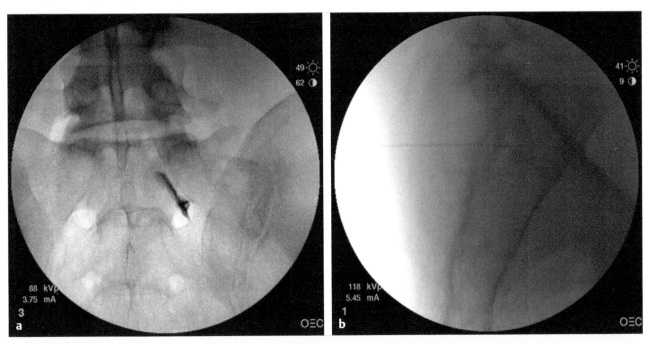

Fig. 18.3 Illustrated is an S1 transforaminal epidural steroid injection AP view (**a**) and lateral view (**b**).

18.3.4 Intraarticular Facet Injections

Intra-articular facet injections (IAF) involves breaching the joint capsule with a needle and placing medicine (intra-articular) within the joint, using a small volume of medication to anesthetize the joint. Intra-articular facet injections are very technically demanding,[23] have not reliably demonstrated long term superiority, and demonstrate higher false positive outcomes than medial-branch facet blocks adhering to strict protocols.[24]

The medial branches originate from the dorsal ramus of the spinal nerves and innervate the joint from above and below (Fig. 18.4). Due to the presence of the C8 nerve in the cervical spine, the thoracic and lumbar joint levels do not correlate with their respective medial branches (eg The L3 and L4 medial branches supply the L4–5 facet joint). The diagnostic value of a single intra-articular facet (IAF) injections and single facet joint blocks consistently demonstrates a high false positive rate because of multiple potential nociceptive sources (pain generators) near the facet itself, prompting work on more reliable diagnostic protocols to ensure efficacious treatments. Because of this diagnostic inaccuracy the so called "double block" paradigm has been described to improve diagnostic specificity. The technique requires the use of low injection volume, precise placement during facet blocks,[25] and use of contrast material during two separate sessions (separated in time). The "double block" paradigm has been demonstrated to vastly improve diagnostic specificity and provide commensurately better therapeutic outcomes.[26] If a patient demonstrates marked improvement in pain scores and function using the methods noted above they are eligible for radiofrequency ablation in which a lesion is created along the medial branch (or dorsal ramus) allowing for a more extended effect from the procedure. Careful technique during the RFA and adherence to the "double block" paradigm mentioned above have demonstrated better outcomes with 60% of the patients obtaining at least 90% relief of pain at 12 months, and 87% obtained at least 60% relief at the same time interval.[27]

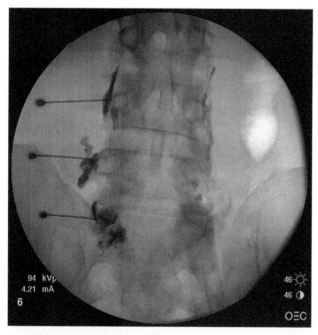

Fig. 18.4 Medial-branch facet block, AP view.

It is the authors recommendation that RFA only be pursued with strict adherence to the "double-block" paradigm, and reported > 80% improvement during the half-life of anesthetic with anesthetic medial branch block of facet(s).

18.3.5 Facet Radiofrequency Ablation

Radiofrequency ablation (RFA) can be performed in all segments of the spine, but is most commonly performed in the lumbar and cervical and will be discussed below only in these segments for the sake of brevity. The numbering system is discussed in the chapter above, but it is crucial to recall that below the cervical spine each joint receives half of its sensory innervation from the cephalad level (L3 and L4 medial branches supply the L4–5 joint.)

18.3.6 Lumbar Spine

The advent of new needle technology has allowed for differing techniques to ablate the nerve. The classic approach involves attempting to lie the needle as parallel as possible along the medial branches, in order to impart the largest ablation of the nerve. This is accomplished by lying the patient prone and tilting the fluoroscope caudal and oblique towards the side of interest. Using this approach the inferior to superior angle allows the needle to lie across the nerve imparting a larger lesion. The oblique trajectory is ideal when the view between the superior articular process (SAP) and transverse process ('scotty dog' ear and head respectively) is no longer acute ensuring the facet will not impede the trajectory of the needle. The needle tip is then directed just inferior to confluence between the SAP and the transverse process. Care should be taken not to slide over the target, towards the exiting spinal nerve. Placement of the needle for ablation of the L5 dorsal ramus is slightly different. Ideally, you will approach by again tilting the fluoroscope caudally, but the oblique angle is often limited by the ipsilateral iliac crest. The target for needle placement is the junction of the SAP and sacral ala.

Proper placement is ensured by checking the AP view to see that the needle terminates at the junction of the SAP and transverse process. On lateral view the needle should be seen near the midpoint of the SAP, and NOT inside the intervertebral foramen. Once the needles are in proper position motor stimulation is used to demonstrate mutlifidis firing (needles will twitch/bounce) and ensure no activation of the spinal nerve (movement/contraction of the leg). After proper and safe placement is confirmed radiofrequency ablation can commence.

18.3.7 Cervical Spine

The technique for cervical RFA typically involves two separate lesions as medial branches in the cervical spine are more variable than in the lumbar spine.[28] Generally speaking, the corresponding medial branch is targeted as it courses along the waist of the articular pillar (or just cephalad) just prior to innervating the corresponding joints. The patient is lying prone on the table with the fluoroscope tilted slightly caudally and slightly oblique towards the ipsilateral side. In this view the "waist" of each articular pillar should be visible and the needle placed in line with the beam, advancing so that it will contact at the waist.

The needle should contact bone at this structure, with a true AP view demonstrating the needle contacting bone at or just above lateral margin of the lateral mass. If the needle tip is seen medial to the osseous structure it may be too anterior or posterior. On a true lateral view the needle should be seen near the midpoint of the lateral mass in terms of depth, perhaps most critically the needle should not be too far anteriorly as the vertebral artery or spinal nerve could be contacted. Again motor stimulation is used once the needle tip is contacting bone and is in a safe position on multiple views. Although generally less dramatic than in the lumbar spine, the needles should be seen moving slightly with muscle contraction. No motor stimulation into the arm should be observed. After proper and safe placement is ensured, radiofrequency ablation can commence. Given the slight variability of the cervical medial branches a second lesion is frequently performed by slightly varying the position of the needle.

18.3.8 SI Joint

Successful Injection of the sacro-iliac joint (SIJ) can be one of the more demanding procedures for an interventionist as the posterior joint has variable anatomy. For the purposes of this chapter we will discuss the recommended starting approach to access the SIJ. When looking at an AP view of the pelvis, both the anterior (lateral on radiograph) and posterior (medial on radiograph) joint are seen however the inferior portion of the joint will demonstrate overlap. In most cases successful cannulation of the space can occur by slightly positioning the image intensifier in an oblique position looking for a "hyperlucent" region within the SI joint with sharp demarcation of bony landmarks. The needle is then placed in line with the beam and advanced into the joint, often times minor adjustments are required to access the space. A lateral view should demonstrate that the needle is ventral to the posterior sacrum, if the needle is not beyond the periosteum of the sacrum, it is not within the joint. The primary risk during this procedure is advancing the needle ventrally (or inferiorly) through the joint space into the pelvic cavity, which although unlikely, has been reported.

18.4 Benefits and Risks

Benefits of pursuing injection based therapy in appropriately selected patients can be seen as they are relatively low risk, have minimal to no recovery time, and possible reduction in use of daily analgesic medications/polypharmacy in the elderly cohort. Injections should also be performed in conjunction with an adequate physical therapy regimen to show durable benefit.

Serious complications from interventions can be minimized by thorough preparation (obtaining and personally reviewing advanced imaging) and use of multiview fluoroscopy to pinpoint the location of the needle at all times. Perhaps the most common intraoperative complication is vasovagal reaction, reported between 1–2% in multiple studies.[28,29,30] In these same studies minor complications such as increased localized pain and headaches with cervical injections are reported in under 6% of cases. Catastrophic complications are thankfully rare, and with good technique can be minimized but never fully eliminated. Epidural injections have slightly increased risk over facet or SI joint injections in regards for risk of dural puncture, CSF leak, or nerve damage. With studies of over 43,000 facet blocks no dural puncture or CSF leak was noted.[29] Dural puncture is more often seen with Interlaminar approaches, but still is frequently reported as less than 1% across all epidural approaches in the lumbar and cervical spine.[29,30,31] Though exceedingly rare, case reports of spinal cord injury or CVA from direct puncture or particulate steroid injection into the artery of Adamkiewicz (thoracolumbar) or cervical vasculature supply the brain have prompted recommendations by multiple societies to eliminate deep sedation during procedures and to strongly consider non particulate steroids for epidural injections. Another potential safeguard in the cervical spine is employed by initially injecting lidocaine only after obtaining an epidurogram and waiting 30–60 seconds. If inadvertent vascular uptake to the brain is present, the patient may complain of perioral numbness/metallic taste, or seizures could be seen. This should prompt abortion of the procedure prior to introduction of any particulate (or "non-particulate") steroid. The development of an epidural hematoma or infection is also a concern, but is again reported in less than 1% of injections. Clinically significant epidural hematoma is estimated to be as low as 1 in 190,000.[32] Finally, case reports of dropped head syndrome (cervical kyphosis) have been reported after cervical RFA.[33] A true incidence is hard to obtain, but this complication has led to requiring surgical stabilization and though exceedingly rare should be considered. The authors would recommend avoiding multiple levels, or bilateral procedures if possible to mitigate risk.

18.5 Outcomes/Evidence

18.5.1 Lumbar Stenosis

Studies have demonstrated epidural steroid injections are reasonable, 'short-to-medium term' treatment in patients with neurogenic claudication to improve function, walking distance and pain.[5] Studies have demonstrated 64% of patients deemed surgical candidates had subjective improvement in symptoms one-year after epidural injection and fewer patients electing for surgery in the treatment group.[6] More recent studies have demonstrated improvements in both numerical pain scores of pain and disability.[7]

Interestingly, this data also parsed response to anesthetic alone (vs traditional combination of corticosteroid and anesthetic) and found no significant differences in response to treatment. Flexion-based exercise protocols may be recommended for patients with neurogenic claudication. Although active lifestyle and aerobic conditioning should be encouraged in all patients, there is inconsistent evidence that specific rehabilitation programs are effective in completely eliminating the return of symptoms. Given enough time in the best prospective cross-sectional study, nearly 7/10 patients randomly assigned to non-surgical group will opt to 'cross-over' for surgery to alleviate claudication symptoms.[8] Different interventional approaches to delivering medication to the epidural space remain debated amongst specialists. Comparing transforaminal vs interlaminar epidural injection techniques has not reliably shown either approach to be significantly superior for treatment durability in symptomatic lumbosacral stenosis.

18.5.2 Facet Arthropathy

In general, interventions for axial back pain have less optimistic outcomes than for radicular or neurogenic pain. As noted above use of the double block paradigm can greatly enhance successful treatment in responders to medial branch blocks. There is a paucity of studies demonstrating therapeutic efficacy of intra-articular delivery of medication vs medial branch blocks (MBB), but for diagnostic purposes MBB has been validated whereas intra-articular approach has not.[34] Uncontrolled studies have noted therapeutic efficacy for the intra-articular approach.[35] As of now, some insurance carriers are now classifying intra-articular injections as "experimental."

18.5.3 SI Joint

As mentioned above the afferent innervation of the SIJ is complex and debate still exists as to treatment and potential generation of pain from the anterior joint, within the joint itself, or from posterior elements of the joint (posterior ligaments). In true spondyloarthropathies with sacroiliitis RCT's have demonstrated improvement and therapeutic benefit from intra-articular cortisone injections.[36] Although SIJ injection remains the gold standard for diagnosing all causes of SIJ pain (osteoarthritis, etc) data is limited on its therapeutic effect for non-inflammatory conditions.

18.6 Pitfalls, Complications and Avoidance

The authors of this chapter would like to impress upon readers that imaging alone fails to make a diagnosis in an aging spine. 'Physiological', age-related changes to the spine are ubiquitous and occur with equal frequency in painful and non-painful patient presentations. Multiple studies starting in the 1980's show the high prevalence of asymptomatic, canal narrowing, disk herniation, end-plate changes, fractures, and arthritic/spondylotic changes discovered incidentally during imaging-machine calibration. Use of imaging as the primary diagnostic tool in the elderly is often the fastest way to unnecessary, risky and expensive treatment options that lead unintended frustration for patient and provider. Results from 3 anatomical studies illustrate the problem of the 'imaging first' approach to spine care:

1. Cadaveric studies have shown facet joint arthritis to be present in 100% of cadaveric spines over 60 years old.[37]
2. In 938 participants aged 40–93 (Mean 66.3yrs) over 30% had radiographically "severe central stenosis" with only 17% having any symptoms.[38]
3. Degenerative Disc Disease is a misnomer and is found in over 90% of individuals over 65 regardless of if they have low back pain.[39]
4. Degeneration or bulging of a disc was seen in at least one lumbar level in all but one of 60 to 80 year-old subjects.[40]
5. Studies comparing twins with differing physical activity noted strenuous physical activity is protective for seniors even in those with similar genetics.[13]

The purpose of this paragraph is not to dismiss imaging findings entirely, but encourage the physician to listen to and

Table 18.2

Red Flags of Axial Spine Pain	Suggestive Etiology
- History of Violent trauma	Fractures, Instability, Prior Hardware
- Nonmechanical Nature of pain (Terrible Pain at night)	Tumor, Bony Pain
- History of Cancer	Metastasis, Compression fractures
- Long term corticosteroid use	Fractures
- Osteoporosis	Fractures
- Drug abuse (IV)	Infection
- Fever/Night sweats	Infection
- Severe restriction of pain with any ROM	Instability/Fractures
- Structural deformity	Mechanical/progressive pain
- Bowel/Bladder incontinence/ Saddle Anesthesia	Cauda Equina/conus medullaris
- Progressive Motor Weakness or gait disturbance	Systemic diseases, Spinal nerve injuries
- Recent falls/balance disturbance	Cervical stenosis/Myelopathy

examine the patient rather than assuming imaging findings are the 'gold standard' diagnostic tool in an aging patient. The authors offer the above stipulation to emphasize that spinal pathology in the aging patient requires greater 'contextualization' within a clinical examination than in younger, healthier spine. We would encourage healthcare providers to educate patients on the difference between hurt and harm, to allay the common patient concern after hearing that their back has "degenerated." When discussing physiological aging versus pathological 'painful' changes, the physician can turn the conversation from non-productive/harmfully aggressive treatment plans to engage them in a gradual, active, treatment approach to address both the nociceptive and neuropathic pain pathways. This active approach, shows strong results arresting the 'progression' of symptoms to the point that they are disabling.[41] Remember: Functional adults maintain a large physiological reserve due to physiological compensation to gradual onset of heterogeneous age-related radiological findings. Physicians should take the approach of 'Primum non nocere' and understand that 'words can hurt.' Physicians and their teams should refer to 'widespread spondylotic change' as "age-related changes" rather than spinal degeneration.

When treating the aging patient be mindful of other non-degenerative causes and masqueraders of pain. As illustrated in the following table (▶ Table 18.2), "Red Flag", questions are used as part of the history to provide indicators of more dangerous causes of pain such as fracture, tumor or infection. Importantly, cancer and infection, have increased prevalence in the aging population and the physician should have greater awareness based on gathering the patient's personal and family history.

18.6.1 Hip Arthritis

Hip osteoarthritis is thought to be prevalent in 7–24% of the aging population. With a known relationship between age and prevalence of OA, this likelihood that concomitant radiological findings of hip and spine pathology increases in the geriatric population. Classically hip related pain will be present with weight bearing, ambulation, and possibly flexion at the waist (putting socks on). Though hip pain presents with groin and anterior thigh pain, posteriorly referred pain has been commonly described (even distally down thigh or proximally to lumbosacral junction).[42] The authors of the chapter implore all providers to include a full hip examination in all patients presenting with low back pain.

18.6.2 Shoulder Arthritis

The shoulders should be examined in all patients with neck complaints. Examination of the pain referral (sclerotomal) maps for cervical facet and shoulder pain, you may see significant overlap between potential shoulder and neck pathology. Rotator cuff tears are common in the elderly and have increasing incidence with age. Prevalence of shoulder pain is estimated between 17–25% of the geriatric population.[43] Concomitant shoulder and neck symptoms (colloquially called "shneck" syndrome) may be found on a thorough physical examination and may enable recommendations to rehabilitate shoulder before committing to more invasive cervical treatments that will have reduced efficacy due to untreated shoulder pathology.

18.6.3 Myelopathy

The prevalence of nontraumatic cervical myelopathy is estimated at 1.6/100K people in North America, and incidence increases over the age of 50 years.[44] Unfortunately, this can often be a 'silent' cause of disability, because it is often not associated with pain. Cervical and Thoracic central stenosis will often present with complaints of non-specific 'unsteady gait' or difficulty ambulating (either C or T-spine), clumsiness with fine motor tasks of the upper extremity (C-spine), neck/back pain (due to spondylotic/arthritic changes rather than myelopathy), and possibly Lhermitte's sign (Intermittent, brief electric shocking sensation into the limbs). In addition, patients may also mention subjective sensory disturbances in the feet sometimes described as "walking on sand" or "walking on balled-up-socks." These symptoms could represent a variety of different etiologies in the geriatric population (peripheral polyneuropathy, motor neuron diseases, normal pressure hydrocephalus, chronic inflammatory demyelinating polyneuropathy, deconditioning, etc) but a thorough physical examination supplemented by appropriate confirmatory diagnostic testing is likely to help direct clinical decision making and avoid risk of surgery for the wrong reason.

Importantly, when assessing/planning for surgical decompression of lumbar spinal stenosis an appreciation of possible dual stenosis (simultaneous cervical and lumbar stenosis) is necessary by completing a thorough physical exam (tandem gait, Rhomberg, assessment for pathological reflexes).[45] Cases exist where undiagnosed cervical spondylotic myelopathy resulted in central-cord syndrome after 'forced' extension during surgical intubation for the surgery.[46]

Physical examination remains the most reliable tool for diagnosing cervical or thoracic stenosis by assessing poor proprioceptive feedback or upper motor neuron signs on exam. Proprioception and balance can be assessed by performing tandem gait testing or Rhomberg testing,[47] though elderly patients may have more difficulty with these tests due to reasons other than spinal pathology/etiology. In conjunction with a positive Hoffman's, upgoing babinski, increased tone on exam, and/or brisk reflexes the etiology may become more clear.

Epidural injections for myelopathy are not recommended. Patients should be monitored for progression of symptoms (every 6–12 months) with interdisciplinary communication between medical specialist and spine surgeon. Cervical or thoracic spondylotic myelopathy due to stenosis is not always progressive. The former recommendation for 'prophylactic' cervical or thoracic surgery to "prevent paralysis" in mild or asymptomatic cases of myelopathy is not supported by evidence.[48]

18.6.4 Polymyalgia Rheumatica

Polymyalgia rheumatica (PMR) should also be considered in patients with bilateral proximal pain/stiffness in the hip and/or shoulder region. Estimated prevalence ranges between 0.5–0.7% and is rarely seen in patients under 50 years of age. The pathophysiology is not fully understood but is inflammatory in nature and ESR/CRP are helpful in diagnosis. Any patient suspected of having PMR should also be questioned about temporal arteritis as there is a strong association between the two entities with stroke or blindness as potential imminent sequelae. A low threshold when patients present with multi-articular pain should trigger a thorough investigation to prevent a very poor outcome.

When planning treatments in this population, there are some key considerations that differentiate this population from the younger population. In general, the aging population is more heterogeneous than a younger population. At a population level, the 60–70 year old population cohort is more numerous and generally healthier than 50 years ago.[49] Paradoxically, the health burden at highest quartile is worse than 50 years ago (chronic diseases managed rather than being fatal).[50] For this reason, clearly stated, achievable goals to manage function, pain and deformity are the key. In general, physiologic reserve is decreased in this age cohort compared to others and avoiding prolonged convalescence is in the 'top 3' considerations when trying to differentiate how aggressive to be with treatment. If the same outcome is achievable at a lower risk, the less risky treatment should be chosen. Those seem like easy goals, but often can be forgotten in a busy clinic.

Morbidity and mortality are higher for all treatments (especially surgery) in the aging patient.[51] It has been reported that over 50% of patients over 70 years at autopsy have significant cardiovascular disease.[52] Appropriate screening for CV risk is important. Effective trans-disciplinary communication between PCP, cardiology, physical therapy and the spine team understand CV risk ensures good patient outcomes for the leading cause of preventable morbidity.[53] Non-invasive screening for PAD or thrombotic risk can be an additional consideration to confirm claudication causes, or to screen patients who have become newly sedentary or non-ambulatory due to spinal pathology. Elderly patients remain at risk for pulmonary complications and even simple procedures carry a greater risk with higher rates of obstructive, or constrictive diseases.[54] Unrecognized renal decline/compromise is often present.[55]

18.7 Conclusion

In conclusion, the aging population continues to grow geometrically in most developed countries with older adult patients today holding functional goals that are different (more active) from previous generations. There are good reasons to treat this older population distinctly in an effort to preserve function. Older patients will likely require more individual time and will have different expectations around both outcomes and risk-tolerance. Contextualizing function is most important and should be stressed to the patient. For aging patients who remain active in the community, spinal intervention may allow greater function and ambulatory distance for a period of time. Combined injection with therapy is paramount. Creating realistic, shared goals with the patient for function remains the key to choosing the proper intervention for an individual patient. While population-health economics/informatics continue to be a constant external pressure, individualized, tailored care specific to the patient should be the ethical standard for all spine specialists.

Key References

[1] Chou R, Huffman LH, American Pain Society, American College of Physicians. Medications for acute and chronic low back pain: a review of the evidence for an American Pain Society/American College of Physicians clinical practice guideline. Ann Intern Med. 2007; 147(7):505–514

[2] Cohen SP, Williams KA, Kurihara C, et al. Multicenter, randomized, comparative cost-effectiveness study comparing 0, 1, and 2 diagnostic medial branch (facet joint nerve) block treatment paradigms before lumbar facet radiofrequency denervation. Anesthesiology. 2010; 113(2):395–405

[3] Mailloux J, Finno M, Rainville J. Long-term exercise adherence in the elderly with chronic low back pain. Am J Phys Med Rehabil. 2006; 85(2):120–126

[4] Botwin KP, Gruber RD. Lumbar epidural steroid injections in the patient with lumbar spinal stenosis. Phys Med Rehabil Clin N Am. 2003; 14(1):121–141

[5] Friedly JL, Comstock BA, Turner JA, et al. Long-term effects of repeated injections of local anesthetic with or without corticosteroid for lumbar spinal stenosis: a randomized trial. Arch Phys Med Rehabil. 2017; 98(8):1499–1507.e2

[6] Weinstein JN, Tosteson TD, Lurie JD, et al. Surgical versus nonoperative treatment for lumbar spinal stenosis four-year results of the Spine Patient Outcomes Research Trial. Spine. 2010; 35(14):1329–1338

References

[1] "Physician-and-Other-Supplier." CMS.gov Centers for Medicare & Medicaid Services, 1 Mar. 2018, www.cms.gov/Research-Statistics-Data-and-Systems/Statistics-Trends-and-Reports/Medicare-Provider-Charge-Data/Physician-and-Other-Supplier.html

[2] Specialty utilization data files from Centers for Medicare and Medicaid Services. http://www.cms.hhs.gov/ (accessed 16 Mar 2018)

[3] Brox JI, Sørensen R, Friis A, et al. Randomized clinical trial of lumbar instrumented fusion and cognitive intervention and exercises in patients with chronic low back pain and disc degeneration. Spine. 2003; 28(17):1913–1921

[4] Haig AJ, LeBreck DB, Powley SG. Paraspinal mapping. Quantified needle electromyography of the paraspinal muscles in persons without low back pain. Spine. 1995; 20(6):715–721

[5] Botwin KP, Gruber RD. Lumbar epidural steroid injections in the patient with lumbar spinal stenosis. Phys Med Rehabil Clin N Am. 2003; 14(1):121–141

[6] Riew KD, Yin Y, Gilula L, et al. The effect of nerve-root injections on the need for operative treatment of lumbar radicular pain. A prospective, randomized, controlled, double-blind study. J Bone Joint Surg Am. 2000; 82-A(11):1589–1593

[7] Friedly JL, Comstock BA, Turner JA, et al. Long-term effects of repeated injections of local anesthetic with or without corticosteroid for lumbar spinal stenosis: a randomized trial. Arch Phys Med Rehabil. 2017; 98(8):1499–1507.e2

[8] Weinstein JN, Tosteson TD, Lurie JD, et al. Surgical versus nonoperative treatment for lumbar spinal stenosis four-year results of the Spine Patient Outcomes Research Trial. Spine. 2010; 35(14):1329–1338

[9] Mooney V, Robertson J. The facet syndrome. Clin Orthop Relat Res. 1976 (115):149–156

[10] Chou R, Huffman LH, American Pain Society, American College of Physicians. Medications for acute and chronic low back pain: a review of the evidence for an American Pain Society/American College of Physicians clinical practice guideline. Ann Intern Med. 2007; 147(7):505–514

[11] Battié MC, Videman T, Levalahti E, Gill K, Kaprio J. Heritability of low back pain and the role of disc degeneration. Pain. 2007; 131(3):272–280

[12] Videman T, Battié MC. The influence of occupation on lumbar degeneration. Spine. 1999; 24(11):1164–1168

[13] Hartvigsen J, Christensen K. Active lifestyle protects against incident low back pain in seniors: a population-based 2-year prospective study of 1387 Danish twins aged 70–100 years. Spine. 2007; 32(1):76–81

[14] Browder DA, Childs JD, Cleland JA, Fritz JM. Effectiveness of an extension-oriented treatment approach in a subgroup of subjects with low back pain: a randomized clinical trial. Phys Ther. 2007; 87(12):1608–1618, discussion 1577–1579

[15] Fukui S, Ohseto K, Shiotani M, Ohno K, Karasawa H, Naganuma Y. Distribution of referred pain from the lumbar zygapophyseal joints and dorsal rami. Clin J Pain. 1997; 13(4):303–307

[16] Fukui S, Ohseto K, Shiotani M, et al. Referred pain distribution of the cervical zygapophyseal joints and cervical dorsal rami. Pain. 1996; 68(1):79–83

[17] Dwyer A, Aprill C, Bogduk N. Cervical zygapophyseal joint pain patterns. I: A study in normal volunteers. Spine. 1990; 15(6):453–457

[18] Lord SM, Barnsley L, Wallis BJ, McDonald GJ, Bogduk N. Percutaneous radiofrequency neurotomy for chronic cervical zygapophyseal-joint pain. N Engl J Med. 1996; 335(23):1721–1726

[19] van Leeuwen RJ, Szadek K, de Vet H, Zuurmond W, Perez R. Pain pressure threshold in the region of the sacroiliac joint in patients diagnosed with sacroiliac joint pain. Pain Physician. 2016; 19(3):147–154

[20] Dreyfuss P, Dreyer SJ, Cole A, Mayo K. Sacroiliac joint pain. J Am Acad Orthop Surg. 2004; 12(4):255–265

[21] Derby R, Bogduk N, et al. Precision percutaneous blocking procedures by localization of spinal pain. Part 2. The lumbar neuraxial compartment. Pain Digest.. 1993; 3:175–188

[22] Scanlon GC, Moeller-Bertram T, Romanowsky SM, Wallace MS. Cervical transforaminal epidural steroid injections: more dangerous than we think? Spine. 2007; 32(11):1249–1256

[23] Schwarzer AC, Aprill CN, et al. The False-Positive Rate of Uncontrolled Diagnostic Blocks of the Lumbar Zygapophysial Joints. Neurosurg Q. 1995; 5(4): 287–288

[24] Dreyfuss P, Schwarzer AC, Lau P, Bogduk N. Specificity of lumbar medial branch and L5 dorsal ramus blocks. A computed tomography study. Spine. 1997; 22(8):895–902

[25] Cohen SP, Williams KA, Kurihara C, et al. Multicenter, randomized, comparative cost-effectiveness study comparing 0, 1, and 2 diagnostic medial branch (facet joint nerve) block treatment paradigms before lumbar facet radiofrequency denervation. Anesthesiology. 2010; 113(2):395–405

[26] Dreyfuss P, Halbrook B, Pauza K, Joshi A, McLarty J, Bogduk N. Efficacy and validity of radiofrequency neurotomy for chronic lumbar zygapophysial joint pain. Spine. 2000; 25(10):1270–1277

[27] Lord S, McDonald G, et al. Percutaneous radiofrequency neurotomy of the cervical medial branches: a validated treatment for cervical zygapophysial joint pain. Neurosurg. 1998; 8:288–308

[28] Botwin KP, Castellanos R, Rao S, et al. Complications of fluoroscopically guided interlaminar cervical epidural injections. Arch Phys Med Rehabil. 2003; 84(5):627–633

[29] Manchikanti L, Malla Y, Wargo BW, Cash KA, Pampati V, Fellows B. Complications of fluoroscopically directed facet joint nerve blocks: a prospective evaluation of 7,500 episodes with 43,000 nerve blocks. Pain Physician. 2012; 15 (2):E143–E150

[30] Manchikanti L, Malla Y, Wargo BW, Cash KA, Pampati V, Fellows B. A prospective evaluation of complications of 10,000 fluoroscopically directed epidural injections. Pain Physician. 2012; 15(2):131–140

[31] Waldman SD. Complications of cervical epidural nerve blocks with steroids: a prospective study of 790 consecutive blocks. Reg Anesth. 1989; 14(3):149–151

[32] Wulf H. Epidural anaesthesia and spinal haematoma. Can J Anaesth. 1996; 43 (12):1260–1271

[33] Stoker GE, Buchowski JM, Kelly MP. Dropped head syndrome after multilevel cervical radiofrequency ablation: a case report. J Spinal Disord Tech. 2013; 26 (8):444–448

[34] Kirpalani D, Mitra R. Cervical facet joint dysfunction: a review. Arch Phys Med Rehabil. 2008; 89(4):770–774

[35] Kim KH, Choi SH, Kim TK, Shin SW, Kim CH, Kim JI. Cervical facet joint injections in the neck and shoulder pain. J Korean Med Sci. 2005; 20(4):659–662

[36] Maugars Y, Mathis C, Vilon P, Prost A. Corticosteroid injection of the sacroiliac joint in patients with seronegative spondylarthropathy. Arthritis Rheum. 1992; 35(5):564–568

[37] Eubanks JD, Lee MJ, Cassinelli E, Ahn NU. Prevalence of lumbar facet arthrosis and its relationship to age, sex, and race: an anatomic study of cadaveric specimens. Spine. 2007; 32(19):2058–2062

[38] Ishimoto Y, Yoshimura N, Muraki S, et al. Associations between radiographic lumbar spinal stenosis and clinical symptoms in the general population: the Wakayama Spine Study. Osteoarthritis Cartilage. 2013; 21(6):783–788

[39] Hicks GE, Morone N, Weiner DK. Degenerative lumbar disc and facet disease in older adults: prevalence and clinical correlates. Spine. 2009; 34(12):1301–1306

[40] Boden SD, McCowin PR, Davis DO, Dina TS, Mark AS, Wiesel S. Abnormal magnetic-resonance scans of the cervical spine in asymptomatic subjects. A prospective investigation. J Bone Joint Surg Am. 1990; 72(8):1178–1184

[41] Mailloux J, Finno M, Rainville J. Long-term exercise adherence in the elderly with chronic low back pain. Am J Phys Med Rehabil. 2006; 85(2):120–126

[42] Offierski CM, MacNab I. Hip-spine syndrome. Spine. 1983; 8(3):316–321

[43] Chard MD, Hazleman R, Hazleman BL, King RH, Reiss BB. Shoulder disorders in the elderly: a community survey. Arthritis Rheum. 1991; 34(6):766–769

[44] Boogaarts HD, Bartels RH. Prevalence of cervical spondylotic myelopathy. Eur Spine J. 2015; 24(2) Suppl 2:139–141

[45] LaBan MM, Green ML. Concurrent (tandem) cervical and lumbar spinal stenosis: a 10-yr review of 54 hospitalized patients. Am J Phys Med Rehabil. 2004; 83(3):187–190

[46] Buchowski JM, Kebaish KM, Suk KS, Kostuik JP, Athanasou N, Wheeler K. Central cord syndrome after total hip arthroplasty: a patient report. Spine. 2005; 30(4):E103–E105

[47] Harrop JS, Naroji S, Maltenfort M, et al. Cervical myelopathy: a clinical and radiographic evaluation and correlation to cervical spondylotic myelopathy. Spine. 2010; 35(6):620–624

[48] Fehlings MG, Tetreault LA, Riew KD, et al. A clinical practice guideline for the management of patients with degenerative cervical myelopathy: recommendations for patients with mild, moderate, and severe disease and nonmyelopathic patients with evidence of cord compression. Global Spine J. 2017; 7(3) Suppl:70S–83S

[49] Sanders JL, Boudreau RM, Penninx BW, et al. Health ABC Study. Study. Association of a modified physiologic index with mortality and incident disability: the Health, Aging, and Body Composition study. J Gerontol A Biol Sci Med Sci. 2012; 67(12):1439–1446

[50] Hainer V, Aldhoon-Hainerová I. Obesity paradox does exist. Diabetes Care. 2013; 36 Suppl 2:S276–S281

[51] Turrentine FE, Wang H, Simpson VB, Jones RS. Surgical risk factors, morbidity, and mortality in elderly patients. J Am Coll Surg. 2006; 203(6):865–877

[52] Goldman L. Cardiac risks and complications of noncardiac surgery. Ann Intern Med. 1983; 98(4):504–513

[53] Fleisher LA, Beckman JA, Brown KA, et al. American College of Cardiology, American Heart Association Task Force on Practice Guidelines (writing Committee to Revise the 2002 Guidelines on Perioperative Cardiovascular Evaluation for Noncardiac Surgery), American Society of Echocardiography, American Society of Nuclear Cardiology, Heart Rhythm Society, Society of Cardiovascular Anesthesiologists, Society for Cardiovascular Angiography and Interventions, Society for Vascular Medicine and Biology, Society for Vascular Surgery. ACC/AHA 2007 guidelines on perioperative cardiovascular evaluation and care for noncardiac surgery: a report of the American College of Cardiology/American Heart Association Task Force on Practice Guidelines.... J Am Coll Cardiol. 2007; 50(17): e159–e241

[54] von Knorring J. Postoperative myocardial infarction: a prospective study in a risk group of surgical patients. Surgery. 1981; 90(1):55–60

[55] Lindeman RD, Tobin J, Shock NW. Longitudinal studies on the rate of decline in renal function with age. J Am Geriatr Soc. 1985; 33(4):278–285

19 Vertebral Augmentation for Insufficiency Fractures

Vincent J. Miele and Matthew Pease

Abstract

Vertebral compression fractures (VCF) are a common pathology in the aging osteoporotic spine. Percutaneous vertebral augmentation (PVA) after a reasonable trial of conservative treatment has been demonstrated to be an effective treatment option for vertebral body insufficiency fractures that frequently occur in older adults. The two types of PVA, vertebroplasty and kyphoplasty, both utilize cannulation devices to access the vertebral body and inject cement. Research published in 2009 suggested that the procedure was no more effective than sham, but these studies have been found to have serious methodological flaws. Numerous studies have been subsequently published that support the use of PVA in appropriately selected patients to reduce overall pain, narcotic use, and increase activity level. The procedure is well accepted and recommended by the guidelines of numerous specialty societies.

Keywords: kyphoplasty, vertebroplasty, compression fracture, osteoporosis, back pain, burst fracture, brace

Key Points

- Vertebral compression fractures (VCF) are a common pathology in the aging osteoporotic spine.
- Percutaneous vertebral augmentation (PVA) after a reasonable trial of conservative treatment has been demonstrated to be an effective treatment option for vertebral body insufficiency fractures that frequently occur in older adults.
- Research published in 2009 suggesting that the procedure was no more effective than sham but have been found to have numerous flaws. Numerous studies have been subsequently published that support the use of PVA in the appropriately selected patient and the procedure is well accepted and recommended by the guidelines of numerous specialty societies.

19.1 Indications and Contraindications

Common indications for percutaneous vertebral augmentation (PVA) are acute to subacute vertebral compression fractures (VCFs) that are resistant to conservative pain management strategies, without concomitant infection, anticoagulation, or other barriers to surgery. Typically, patients present with severe back pain that worsens with movements such as transferring from a bed or chair. The patients are often greater than 55 years old and have a history of osteopenia. They often have no history of trauma and rarely exhibit any neurological deficits. In some cases, the pain can be reproduced by pressure over the spinous process of the affected level.

PVA is not indicated for fractures causing minimal pain, even if they are proven to be acute. The role of this intervention in

stabilizing an asymptomatic fracture or in the prophylactic treatment of patients with osteoporotic vertebrae thought to be at high risk for fracture remains unproven. Similarly, younger patients with normal bone mineral density and traumatic VCFs are generally not considered candidates for PVA, as it is expected they will heal well without intervention. In patients less than 55 years of age with no history of trauma, or those with a known history of malignancy, PVA is not contraindicated, but further evaluation of the etiology of the fracture is warranted. A biopsy during the PVA can evaluate for a malignant etiology.

Imaging can help determine fracture acuity, allowing for proper patient selection. A good candidate for PVA has an acute or subacute fracture. In these patients, significant pain relief can be expected in 80–90% postprocedurally.[1,2,3] Plain radiographs or computed tomography (CT) imaging are excellent at identifying compression fractures through the loss of height of the vertebral body, but often do not provide information on the age of the fracture. Additionally, in many cases these studies demonstrate multiple compression deformities, making the localization of the symptomatic level difficult. Magnetic resonance imaging (MRI) is the best indicator of the age of the fracture along with the patient's pain history. Hypointensity on T1-weighted imaging and hyperintensity on T2-weighted imaging and short tau inversion recovery (STIR) is consistent with an acute or subacute fracture. This population tends to have a substantial improvement in pain with PVA.[4] If, however, the fracture is more chronic with minimal edema, the likelihood of substantial pain relief with treatment is much lower.[4,5] Bone scintigraphy, while less commonly used, is also very good at establishing the age of the fracture and in some cases may be more sensitive than MRI (▶ Fig. 19.1). It should be considered for patients unable to undergo MRI. Increased tracer activity at the level of a VCF is highly predictive of a positive clinical response to PVA treatment.

There is no clear guideline as to how long conservative treatments should be pursued before offering PVA. In general, most patients undergo conventional medical therapies for at least

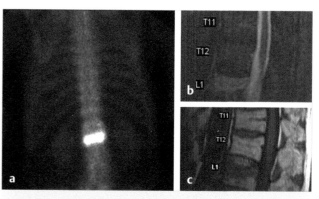

Fig. 19.1 A subacute L1 vertebral compression fracture that is activated by nuclear medicine skeletal scintigraphy (**a**), and hyperintense signal on T2-weighted MRI (**b**) and hypointense on T1-weighted MRI (**c**).

one month before undergoing the procedure. In patients who have uncontrollable pain causing them to be bedridden or remaining hospitalized, many advocate treatment as early as weeks or days following the injury.

Several contraindications to the procedure exist. One absolute contraindication is an active infection such as osteomyelitis, discitis, or epidural abscess. These are far more common in a patient with a history of intravenous drug abuse, diabetes, or alcohol abuse. Emergent performance of PVA is rarely, if ever, required, and treatment of patients with fever or sepsis should be postponed until they are afebrile and leukocytosis has resolved.

Another absolute contraindication for PVA is an uncorrectable coagulopathy, since it would significantly increase the risk of hematoma when placing the working channel in close approximation to the central canal and spinal cord. Likewise, patients must be able to be taken off of anticoagulant medications and have normal coagulation studies prior to the procedure.

A neurological deficit or severe spinal cord compression at the vertebral body level requiring treatment is an absolute contraindication to PVA. This stenosis can be due to degenerative changes or retropulsion of bone into the spinal canal. The latter most commonly involves the superior endplate. In a severely stenotic area, even a small amount of cement extravasation into the canal could create enough compression to cause permanent spinal cord injury. In this population, the procedure may be performed following decompression of the stenotic canal. Radiculopathy, although rare, can also occur with a VCF. While this is not a contraindication to the procedure, the patient should be counseled that their radicular pain is unlikely to improve. Fractures can involve the posterior cortical wall or the pedicle without resultant stenosis. While this is not an absolute contraindication to PVA, there is certainly an increased risk of cement extravasation into the central canal.

Fractures with greater than 70% loss of vertebral height can be technically difficult to treat. This is most commonly the result of difficulty in correctly being able to position the working channels in the remaining vertebral body. Similarly, fractures above the T5-T6 levels are more difficult to treat due to smaller pedicles as well as less favorable pedicle orientation. Compression fractures due to insufficiency tend to cluster at T12-L1 and to a lesser degree around T7-T8. These pedicles are usually large enough to accept the working needle safely for PVA. It is also much more common to find a single symptomatic fracture versus multiple fractures at any one time.

Compression fractures that are the result of malignancy have a far greater risk of complications in general. These are more likely to have involvement of the pedicle and posterior vertebral body and the resultant increased risk of extravasation of cement or tumor displacement into the central canal and neural foramina.

19.2 Technique Description

The first percutaneous vertebroplasty was performed in 1984 at the University Hospital of Amiens for a painful C2 hemangioma with excellent results. This case, as well as six others, were described in a 1987 publication.[6] The procedure was introduced in the United States in 1994 at the University of Virginia, and the results were subsequently published in 1997.[7]

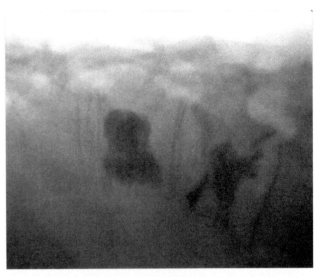

Fig. 19.2 A two-level bipedicular kyphoplasty with lateral radiograph showing the vertebral bodies after cement insertion. Note the cement extravasation into the disc space in the lower vertebral body.

The first kyphoplasty occurred one year later, in 1998, with excellent results.[8,9] With the exception of some minor technical differences, both procedures are minimally invasive procedures in which a working cannula is placed percutaneously into the vertebral body using fluoroscopic X-ray guidance(▶ Fig. 19.2).

The procedure can be performed under general anesthesia, light sedation, or local anesthesia depending on the patient's needs. Patients are placed in a prone position with a bolster placed under the sternum and pelvis. Care must be taken in patient positioning in the severely osteoporotic patient to avoid additional iatrogenic fractures. One or two fluoroscopic C-arms are placed so that anteroposterior and lateral imaging can be easily performed.

Needle placement is most commonly accomplished via a transpedicular route. This trajectory is in most cases the safest route of entry, since there are no structures within the pedicle that can be damaged during accurate transpedicular needle insertion. The pedicles also provide a discreet, easily identifiable target on imaging. This needle insertion pathway can be taken in the majority of cases.[2]

A second trajectory into the vertebral body is the transcostovertebral (or parapedicular) route. The entry site for this is the lateral vertebral margin and the needle enters above the transverse process and pedicle. Entry should not be performed below the transverse process and pedicle, as this could result in damage to the exiting nerve root and induce a postprocedural radicular pain syndrome. This placement technique can be used when the pedicle is very small or cannot be seen on imaging due to severe osteoporosis. It can also be used in patients in whom one or more pedicle(s) are destroyed by tumor involvement. This trajectory, while safe, does pose additional risks to nearby structures. In some patients, the lung may bulge beyond the lateral rib margin into the needle trajectory, and patients can get a periprocedural pneumothorax. This area also contains many arteries and veins that can be damaged, resulting in bleeding and hematoma. This problem can be compounded by the fact that there is no effective way to apply direct pressure to the underlying tissue. If bleeding does occur, it is much easier to control in the transpedicular approach, since direct pressure can be applied to the underlying tissue.

In most cases, vertebroplasty can be performed via a unipedicular or bipedicular technique. Kyphoplasty is most often performed with the bipedicular approach. When using a unipedicular approach, the needle is advanced more to the midline of the vertebral body on the anteroposterior view.

Once in place, in cases where the etiology of a compression fracture is in question, the working channel needle can be used to perform a vertebral body and pedicle biopsy. Then cement, most commonly polymethylmethacrylate (PMMA), is injected via the cannula into the trabecular bone under continuous fluoroscopic control. Early vertebroplasties utilized a cranioplastic acrylic cement that contained no radio-opaque agent, making tracing cement insertion challenging. Poly(methyl methacrylate) (PMMA), and other agents used for contemporary PVA, universally contain radio-opaque agents. Injection is halted when the PMMA reaches the posterior two-thirds of the vertebral body or there are any signs that it breached into an extraosseous space.

Some technical differences exist between vertebroplasty and kyphoplasty. For vertebroplasty, cement is injected directly into the bone without first creating any kind of a cavity. Since the cement must be forced into this cancellous bone surrounding the needle tip, it must be injected under a higher pressure. Thus, this is considered a high-pressure technique. Kyphoplasty, on the other hand, is a variation of a vertebroplasty that involves the creation of a cavity in the vertebral body for cement placement. Once working needles are in place, an inflatable balloon is used to create a void within the cancellous bone. The balloons are then deflated, removed and the cement injected into the newly created space. Since the cement is going into a void, it can be injected under a lower pressure at a higher viscosity. This is therefore considered a low-pressure technique. The balloon had several theoretical advantages. Its inflation could be used to restore some of the height of the collapsed vertebral body. While some studies have demonstrated a modest height restoration, its clinical significance seems to be negligible. Additionally, since a cavity is created by the balloon, and higher viscosity cement can be injected, there is a theoretically decreased risk of extravasation.

With either approach, the operator needs to remain cognizant that the vertebral body is not simply a box, as it appears on intraoperative imaging. Since it has a concave posterior margin, if cement extends to what appears to be the posterior margin on fluoroscopy, then it has likely already leaked beyond the true concave portion of the posterior wall into the central canal. This potentially serious complication can be minimized by halting placement of cement when it reaches the posterior quarter of the vertebral body.

Fracture morphology affects surgical technique and patient selection. The most common type is compression of the anterior superior endplate. These fractures are very amenable to PVA, and needle placement is fairly straightforward. Some compression fractures contain clefts or cavities. In general, these will fill preferentially with cement and provide substantial improvements in pain. Some fractures appear to be mobile on imaging, with changes in height during respiration or patient movement. This is a potential opportunity for height restoration when it is observed, and perhaps kyphoplasty would be preferable to vertebroplasty in this population. Regardless of the ability to restore height, these patients seem to have significant pain relief with PVA treatment. Importantly, the amount of vertebral body height loss from the fracture does not correlate to the amount of pain the patient experiences or how long pain will last with conservative treatment.

19.3 Benefits and Risks

The primary benefit of PVA is pain relief and stabilization of fracture that can lead to increased activity level and decreased dependence on opioids. The average patient who undergoes a PVA achieves an average of a 40-point reduction in a visual analog score for pain, with similar gains for other pain scales.[10,11] Upwards of 95% of patients achieve pain relief in the immediate postoperative period.[12] Similarly, opioid usage decreases by over 50%, and activity levels increase in 80% of patients.[13]

The mechanisms of PVA pain relief in osteoporotic fractures are not completely understood. Stabilization of the fracture likely plays a major role in the procedures success. As in fractures in other areas of the body, fixating the broken bone decreases motion and painful nerve stimulation. When PMMA polymerizes, it generates heat in an exothermic polymerization reaction. It has been hypothesized that the heat of polymerization causes thermal necrosis of neural tissue and pain relief. Whether enough heat is produced to cause such an effect is arguable. The PMMA monomer is also known to be cytotoxic. Whether the concentration present following a PVA procedure is high enough to cause significant damage to the surrounding tissue is also unknown. Histologic studies performed of the bone bordering the cement have demonstrated a zone of necrosis thought to be secondary to the toxic-thermic effect of PMMA used in the majority of cases. Another possibly etiology of this zone of necrosis is ischemia due to the cement destroying blood supply to tis area of bone.

The effectiveness of either the vertebroplasty or kyphoplasty technique has been demonstrated to be similar in most circumstances. Kyphoplasty does take longer to perform and is more expensive. In some circumstances, it does have a better ability to restore height.[14] This is especially true in fractures that appear to be mobile on imaging, with changes in height during respiration or patient movement. Whether this improves clinical outcome has not been proven. Vertebroplasty utilizes a smaller working channel that can be an advantage in cases of extreme vertebral body collapse.

In contrast to the benefits of pain relief, the risks of performing PVA are the following: failure for pain to improve, infection, hematoma, injury of surrounding structures by needle, extravasation of PMMA causing neural compression, embolization of PMMA, and adjacent VCF. Failure of the procedure to provide pain relief or additional pain relief compared to conservative measures is a common preoperative concern. Several studies have suggested high initial pain relief, with at least partial pain relief reported in up to 95 to 97% of patients in the immediate postoperative period, a result that diminishes with time.[1,10] While early randomized trials suggested that PVA did not provide significant pain relief compared to conservative management, these trials were plagued by methodological issues addressed below.[15,16] Additionally, the development of adjacent-level compression fractures, which may require additional PVA, is a concern. Recent studies indicate that the development of adjacent-level compression fractures may be as high as 8%.[2]

While infection from the procedure is uncommon, patients can experience localized perioperative pain and low-grade fever in the first 72 hours. This is usually due to local bruising and tissue irritation and resolves with mild analgesics. Hematoma and local irritation can be minimized by 5 minutes of manual compression over the incision following trocar removal as well as the postoperative injection of local anesthetic. This almost universally resolves within 24 to 72 hours. If fever persists, an infection workup should be initiated.

Although clinically significant symptoms induced through cement extravasation are rare, it is a common finding on postoperative imaging, occurring in up to 30% of postoperative images.[11,12] This can occur through defects in the surface of the vertebral body or flow into nearby vasculature. To minimize the risk of extravasation, cement should be viscous enough that flow ceases immediately when the injection ends. Leakage into the disk space is more common when treating vertebral bodies that are significantly collapsed. While it has been speculated that this increases the risk of adjacent level fractures, this has never been substantiated.

Other rare complications occurring in percutaneous augmentation are intercostal neuralgia or radiculopathy. This can occur secondary to irritation or damage to an adjacent nerve root or the extravasation of cement into a foraminal vein or the foramen itself. It often resolves without specific treatment. Patients with significant postoperative radicular pain may require a brief course of nonsteroidal anti-inflammatory drugs, oral steroids, or local steroid injections at the affected area. Significant extravasation into epidural veins or the spinal canal can result in spinal cord compression and paraplegia requiting emergent decompression.

Arterial hypotension has been reported with PVA. This is likely due to pulmonary emboli. These may occur from cement extravasation into the vasculature or the displacement of blood products and fat from the vertebral body during balloon inflation and cement injection. While usually asymptomatic or transiently symptomatic, they can cause significant problems, even cardiopulmonary failure, in patients with a limited pulmonary reserve such as those with chronic obstructive pulmonary disease or preexisting pulmonary hypertension. In these populations, minimizing the number of levels treated at one time to no more than two or three can decrease the risk. Another concern in treating multiple levels in a single session is the theoretical cardiotoxic effect of free methylmethacrylate monomer.

19.4 Outcomes/Evidence

Prior to 2009, over 500 publications demonstrated the effectiveness of the PVA procedure. The majority of these reports were case series, retrospective studies, and prospective, nonrandomized studies. This, combined with the excellent pain relief experienced in most patients and a low complication rate, resulted in the procedure becoming a well-accepted modality of treatment.[2,3,8,9,11,12]

This changed in 2009, when two studies published in the *New England Journal of Medicine* led to significant controversy surrounding the procedure.[15,16] These studies compared PVA to a placebo/sham procedure and reported no significant differences in treatment outcomes. The utilization of PVA dropped dramatically. Over the next several years, the articles were carefully evaluated, and numerous problems were discovered with the study's data collection and conclusions.[1,2,8,12,17,18] Both had difficulties in recruitment of potentially eligible patients, with only one-third of eligible patients participating. This resulted in one of the studies enrolling fewer patients than their power analysis originally required in order to reach significance. Problems with recruiting also caused a significant selection bias. Specifically, patients with more pain, who in practice would see the most benefit, declined to participate for fear of receiving the placebo treatment. Additionally, more patients in the control group chose to cross over to the vertebroplasty group at 1-month follow-up, which weakens the intention to treat measure used for this study. Another criticism of both studies was that their inclusion criteria did not match actual treatment patterns. Examples of this were including patients with very low visual analog scale (VAS) pain which would never be considered for the procedure outside of the studies and the inclusion of many patients with older, chronic compression fractures.

Following the controversial 2009 *NEJM* articles, numerous additional publications have once again demonstrated the effectiveness of PVA. The Fracture Risk Epidemiology in the Frail Elderly (FREE) study enrolled 300 patients in a randomized controlled trial over a 34-month period.[11] Inclusion criteria was much more similar to that seen in an actual treatment setting and included one to three VCFs, at least one of which had edema demonstrated by MR imaging and more than 15% height loss, and fracture age of less than 3 months. Of the patients that met these criteria, 49% agreed to participate. Kyphoplasty procedures were performed in 149 patients, and the remaining 151 patients were treated with medical therapy. The primary outcome measure was the improvement in the Short Form–36 (SF-36) physical component score from baseline to 1 month and was significantly greater for those patients treated with vertebral augmentation ($P < .001$). Secondary outcome measures of back pain and disability showed consistently superior and statistically significant results for the vertebral augmentation group as long as 1 year after treatment.

An open-label prospective randomized trial known as VERTOS II (Vertebroplasty versus conservative treatment in acute osteoporotic vertebral compression fractures) also supported the use of vertebroplasty.[18] The trial enrolled 202 patients over a 31-month period. Inclusion criteria included one to three VCFs, more than 15% vertebral height loss, bone edema on MR imaging, and fracture age of less than 6 weeks. Of those patients who met these criteria, 47% agreed to participate. Vertebroplasty was performed in 101 patients, and the other 101 patients were treated with medical therapy. The primary outcome measures were pain relief at 1 month and 1 year as measured by VAS, and a statistically and clinically significant improvement in pain relief was reported in the PVA group at all measured time points from 1 day through 1 year.

Population-based studies using medical billing claims have also been performed and demonstrate the benefits of PVA.[3] In 2010, a comparison of 5,766 vertebral compression fractures treated with or without kyphoplasty using a Nationwide

Inpatient Sample database. In this study, 15.3% of the patients with fractures underwent kyphoplasty. Despite the patients undergoing kyphoplasty having comorbidity indices equivalent to those treated nonoperatively, the treated group had a greater likelihood of routine discharge to home (38.4% vs. 21.0% for nonoperative treatment), a lower rate of discharge to skilled nursing (26.1% vs. 34.8%) or other facilities (35.7% vs. 47.1%), and a lower rate of in-hospital mortality (0.3% vs. 1.6%). The study also demonstrated that PVA via kyphoplasty was associated with a higher cost of hospitalization (mean $37,231 vs. $20,112).

Even larger populations have been studied using Medicare billing data. In 2011 and 2013, mortality studies were published on 858,978 VCFs. Of this group, 119,253 underwent kyphoplasty and 63,693 vertebroplasty. The studies concluded that the patients in the cohort that underwent PVA had a higher adjusted survival rate (60.8% compared with 50.0%) (p < .001), were 37% less likely to die [adjusted hazard ratio (HR) = 0.63, p < .001], and a median life expectancy 2.2–7.3 years greater than the nonPVA group.

The National Institute for Health and Care Excellence (NICE) provides evidence-based recommendations about which procedures represent the best quality care or which offer the best value for their money to the United Kingdom. Approval by the NICE organization mandates that funding be provided by the National Health Service for the provision of the services. This organization performed a review of the literature on PVA, which at the time consisted of 1,600 papers, including 27 randomized controlled trials. The organization concluded that the procedure is efficacious and its use was recommended.[19]

A consensus statement on PVA including both vertebroplasty and kyphoplasty was published in 2013 by the leading neurosurgical and radiological societies, including the Society of Interventional Radiology (SIR), the American Association of Neurological Surgeons (AANS), the Congress of Neurological Surgeons (CNS), the American College of Radiology (ACR), and the American Society of Neuroradiology (ASNR). The statement concluded that PVA is a "safe, efficacious, and durable procedure for the treatment of appropriate patients with pathologic fractures due to osteoporosis or neoplastic processes." These societies also stated that the procedure should be offered "only when nonoperative medical therapy has not provided adequate pain relief or pain is significantly altering the patient's quality of life."

19.5 Pitfalls, Complications, and Avoidance

As with most surgical procedures, the proper selection of patients is crucial to a good outcome. Knowledge of the time of onset of the fracture and, if needed, the use of bone marrow edema to determine the age and stage of healing of the fracture is very important in determining which patients are most likely to respond favorably to treatment. Many patients in this osteoporotic population have also had previous compression fractures. In this situation, the ability to determine which are new and symptomatic also often relies on the identification of edema. Thus, the imaging study of choice in a patient thought to have a symptomatic compression fracture but of unclear time course or location is MRI or bone scintigraphy. Acute and subacute fractures typically are hypointense in signal on T1-weighted images and hyperintense on T2-weighted and STIR sequences. Fractures that have been present for over a month commonly become isointense to normal bone marrow on T1- and T2- weighted sequences. When a fracture is completely healed, it's MRI findings will return to that of a normal vertebral body. If an MRI is obtained and findings are consistent with a healed fracture in a patient with continuing severe pain that correlates with the site of fracture, bone scintography may be considered, since in many cases this test is more sensitive than MRI. If the MRI findings are consistent with a healed fracture with associated sclerosis, computed tomography (CT) can be obtained to assess the degree of sclerosis. If it is significant, needle placement can be very difficult.

Compression fractures resulting in significant loss of height can be technically difficult to treat. The remaining vertebral body can be too small to accept the working channel. Fortunately, even in severe collapse, there is often lateral sparing of vertebral body height. This often allows for a lateral working channel insertion into the areas of preserved height. In this situation, a parapedicular approach or the use of smaller access needles and working channels may also be required. The needle trajectory also ought to be adjusted to a much flatter angle so that it parallels the endplates. If the working channel angle is steep, it will often not be possible to advance the working channel anteriorly without breaching the endplate. Cement extravasation into the adjacent disk space in severe compression fractures is more likely but rarely symptomatic.

Complications of either technique are rare and often related to the patient's preoperative condition. They are much more likely to occur in fractures of malignant etiology and those with a compromised posterior vertebral body cortical surface. Compression fractures resulting from malignancy are sometimes difficult to distinguish from those caused by osteoporosis. Findings more consistent with malignant VCFs include posterior element involvement or expansion of the contour of the vertebra. Likewise, if MRI demonstrates heterogeneous marrow signal, strong enhancement, or heterogeneous or diffuse vertebral hyperintensity on STIR and T2-weighted sequences, malignancy should be considered. In cases where the etiology of a compression fracture is in question, biopsy can easily be performed through the working channel prior to injection of cement.

19.6 Conclusion

Vertebral insufficiency fractures are becoming more common as our population ages. When traditional nonoperative managements such as pain relievers and functional rehabilitation with bracing fails, patients suffer from ongoing pain, progressive functional limitation, and loss of independence. PVA has been demonstrated to be an effective treatment in the appropriately selected patient and is relatively easy to perform, is inexpensive, and has few serious complications.

Key References

[1] Edidin AA, Ong KL, Lau E, Kurtz SM. Mortality risk for operated and nonoperated vertebral fracture patients in the medicare population. J Bone Miner Res. 2011; 26(7):1617–1626

[2] Farrokhi MR, Alibai E, Maghami Z. Randomized controlled trial of percutaneous vertebroplasty versus optimal medical management for the relief of pain and disability in acute osteoporotic vertebral compression fractures. J Neurosurg Spine. 2011; 14(5):561–569

[3] Klazen CA, Lohle PN, de Vries J, et al. Vertebroplasty versus conservative treatment in acute osteoporotic vertebral compression fractures (Vertos II): an open-label randomised trial. Lancet. 2010; 376(9746):1085–1092

[4] National Institute for Health and Care Excellence. Percutaneous vertebroplasty and percutaneous balloon kyphoplasty for treating osteoporotic vertebral compression fractures. NICE Technology Appraisal Guidance, 2013

[5] Wardlaw D, Cummings SR, Van Meirhaeghe J, et al. Efficacy and safety of balloon kyphoplasty compared with non-surgical care for vertebral compression fracture (FREE): a randomised controlled trial. Lancet. 2009; 373(9668): 1016–1024

[6] Zampini JM, White AP, McGuire KJ. Comparison of 5766 vertebral compression fractures treated with or without kyphoplasty. Clin Orthop Relat Res. 2010; 468(7):1773–1780

References

[1] Farrokhi MR, Alibai E, Maghami Z. Randomized controlled trial of percutaneous vertebroplasty versus optimal medical management for the relief of pain and disability in acute osteoporotic vertebral compression fractures. J Neurosurg Spine. 2011; 14(5):561–569

[2] Yang LY, Wang XL, Zhou L, Fu Q. A systematic review and meta-analysis of randomized controlled trials of unilateral versus bilateral kyphoplasty for osteoporotic vertebral compression fractures. Pain Physician. 2013; 16(4): 277–290

[3] Zampini JM, White AP, McGuire KJ. Comparison of 5766 vertebral compression fractures treated with or without kyphoplasty. Clin Orthop Relat Res. 2010; 468(7):1773–1780

[4] Park SY, Lee SH, Suh SW, Park JH, Kim TG. Usefulness of MRI in determining the appropriate level of cement augmentation for acute osteoporotic vertebral compression fractures. J Spinal Disord Tech. 2013; 26(3):E80–E85

[5] Spiegl UJ, Beisse R, Hauck S, Grillhösl A, Bühren V. Value of MRI imaging prior to a kyphoplasty for osteoporotic insufficiency fractures. Eur Spine J. 2009; 18(9):1287–1292

[6] Galibert P, Deramond H, Rosat P, Le Gars D. [Preliminary note on the treatment of vertebral angioma by percutaneous acrylic vertebroplasty]. Neurochirurgie. 1987; 33(2):166–168

[7] Jensen ME, Evans AJ, Mathis JM, Kallmes DF, Cloft HJ, Dion JE. Percutaneous polymethylmethacrylate vertebroplasty in the treatment of osteoporotic vertebral body compression fractures: technical aspects. AJNR Am J Neuroradiol. 1997; 18(10):1897–1904

[8] Yimin Y, Zhiwei R, Wei M, Jha R. Current status of percutaneous vertebroplasty and percutaneous kyphoplasty–a review. Med Sci Monit. 2013; 19: 826–836

[9] Denaro V, Longo UG, Maffulli N, Denaro L. Vertebroplasty and kyphoplasty. Clin Cases Miner Bone Metab. 2009; 6(2):125–130

[10] Röder C, Boszczyk B, Perler G, Aghayev E, Külling F, Maestretti G. Cement volume is the most important modifiable predictor for pain relief in BKP: results from SWISSspine, a nationwide registry. Eur Spine J. 2013; 22(10):2241–2248

[11] Wardlaw D, Cummings SR, Van Meirhaeghe J, et al. Efficacy and safety of balloon kyphoplasty compared with non-surgical care for vertebral compression fracture (FREE): a randomised controlled trial. Lancet. 2009; 373(9668): 1016–1024

[12] Zapałowicz K, Radek M. Percutaneous balloon kyphoplasty in the treatment of painful vertebral compression fractures: effect on local kyphosis and one-year outcomes in pain and disability. Neurol Neurochir Pol. 2015; 49(1):11–15

[13] Tolba R, Bolash RB, Shroll J, et al. Kyphoplasty increases vertebral height, decreases both pain score and opiate requirements while improving functional status. Pain Pract. 2014; 14(3):E91–E97

[14] Kong LD, Wang P, Wang LF, Shen Y, Shang ZK, Meng LC. Comparison of vertebroplasty and kyphoplasty in the treatment of osteoporotic vertebral compression fractures with intravertebral clefts. Eur J Orthop Surg Traumatol. 2014; 24 Suppl 1:S201–S208

[15] Kallmes DF, Comstock BA, Heagerty PJ, et al. A randomized trial of vertebroplasty for osteoporotic spinal fractures. N Engl J Med. 2009; 361(6):569–579

[16] Buchbinder R, Osborne RH, Ebeling PR, et al. A randomized trial of vertebroplasty for painful osteoporotic vertebral fractures. N Engl J Med. 2009; 361 (6):557–568

[17] Edidin AA, Ong KL, Lau E, Kurtz SM. Mortality risk for operated and nonoperated vertebral fracture patients in the medicare population. J Bone Miner Res. 2011; 26(7):1617–1626

[18] Klazen CA, Lohle PN, de Vries J, et al. Vertebroplasty versus conservative treatment in acute osteoporotic vertebral compression fractures (Vertos II): an open-label randomised trial. Lancet. 2010; 376(9746):1085–1092

[19] National Institute for Health and Care Excellence. Percutaneous vertebroplasty and percutaneous balloon kyphoplasty for treating osteoporotic vertebral compression fractures. NICE Technology Appraisal Guidance, 2013

20 Minimally Invasive Surgery in the Aging Spine

John Paul G. Kolcun, Jason I. Liounakos, and Michael Y. Wang

Abstract

The population of the United States and other developed countries is growing progressively older. Consequently, physicians of all specialties will see a greater incidence of age-related conditions in the coming decades, including degenerative disease of the spine. Spine surgeons should therefore be prepared to treat elderly patients, who may require specialized considerations unnecessary in younger patients. Minimally-invasive surgery is one major component in the successful treatment of these patients, reducing tissue damage, blood loss, and complication risk. In this chapter, we will discuss the indications for surgery, operative techniques, risks and benefits, and potential complications associated with minimally invasive surgery of the spine in elderly patients. At the conclusion of this chapter, the reader should recognize that minimally invasive surgery is a safe and effective approach to correct pathology in the aging spine.

Keywords: minimally invasive surgery (MIS), MIS posterior foraminotomy (MIS-PF), MIS transforaminal lumbar interbody fusion (MIS-TLIF), awake endoscopic MIS-TLIF, Enhanced Recovery After Surgery (ERAS)

Key Points

- The goal of minimally invasive surgery (MIS) is to provide comparable results to open surgery, while at the same time preserving as much normal human anatomy and physiology as possible.
- The appropriate indications for surgery and procedure selection are more important in the aging population because of the increased prevalence of medical comorbidities, higher incidence of osteoporosis, diminished functional mobility and increased fall risk, and reduced healing ability
- The surgeon's armamentarium for MIS includes the posterior cervical foraminotomy (MIS-PF), transforaminal lumbar interbody fusion (MIS-TLIF), mini-open anterior lumbar interbody fusion (ALIF), and percutaneous pedicle screw fixation.

20.1 Indications and Contraindications

Almost every surgical field is undergoing a transition from conventional, open surgery to more minimally invasive approaches. The goal of minimally invasive surgery (MIS) is to provide comparable results to open surgery, while at the same time preserving as much normal human anatomy and physiology as possible. This leads to decreased soft tissue trauma and intraoperative blood loss, as well as reduced postoperative pain and shorter hospital length of stay. Most importantly, this should accelerate a patient's return to their preoperative functional status.

MIS of the spine has gained particular interest amongst neurosurgeons and orthopedic surgeons. One reason for this is that spine surgeries, particularly fusion procedures with instrumentation, are typically regarded as cases with higher morbidity and longer recovery times. These procedures are often indicated in the treatment of degenerative processes that primarily afflict the aging patient, who themselves have a greater number of medical comorbidities and risk factors that must be taken into account.

Methods by which to minimize surgical morbidity while maximizing effectiveness should be considered. Life expectancy in the year 2000 was 66 years of age. Compare this to 45.5 years of age in 1950 and a projected 76 years in 2045. In addition, while 606 million people throughout the world were aged 60 or older in 2000, this number is projected to approach 2 billion by 2050.[1] As the global health burden shifts from acute illness to chronic and degenerative disease, the number of spine procedures performed will also grow.

The prevalence of spinal pathology increases with age. Consequently, the demand for spine surgery to relieve pain and functional impairment in our aging population has also increased. The appropriate indications for surgery and procedure selection are even more important in this subset of the population, given an increased prevalence of medical comorbidities, higher incidence of osteoporosis, diminished functional mobility and increased fall risk, and reduced healing ability.

As with other surgical fields, conventional techniques are being condensed into attractive MIS approaches that strive to accomplish the same goals with reduced morbidity. Therefore, the indications for surgery are generally the same, with some exceptions. Typical pathologies for which surgery is indicated include cervical spondylotic myelopathy, cervical radiculopathy, cervical deformity, lumbar stenosis with neurogenic claudication, lumbar spondylolisthesis, lumbar radiculopathy, and degenerative lumbar scoliosis. The number of MIS techniques is increasing, and the specific indications for selected techniques are discussed in the next section.

For cases such as short-segment cervical fusions, lumbar laminectomy, and simple lumbar fusion, the indications for surgery are generally straightforward and independent of age. For these smaller surgeries, the risk of postoperative complications may not be significantly different when comparing younger to older patients, but this is not likely the case with more extensive surgery. This is illustrated by a large retrospective cohort study reviewing Medicare claims from 2007, which found a significant increase in the incidence of life-threatening complications in complex fusion procedures compared to decompression alone.[2] For this reason, MIS has been proposed as a means to correct spinal deformity while minimizing surgical morbidity.

Clinical research related to the effectiveness of MIS in the treatment of spinal deformity has increased over the past several years. Current studies suggest that in properly selected patients, MIS is effective in both radiographic deformity correction and complication reduction, as compared to conventional open surgery.[3] Even so, dedicated, high-quality studies on the subject of MIS deformity correction in the aging population are lacking. It does stand to reason, however, that with proper patient selection, MIS may provide beneficial outcomes with a reduced complication profile compared to open surgery, particularly in aging patients with increased comorbidities. A recent retrospective review suggests the best clinical results from MIS deformity correction are obtained when correcting the pelvic incidence-lumbar lordosis (PI-LL) mismatch to within 10° and sagittal vertical axis (SVA) to less than 5 cm.[4] Conversely, it appears that patients with a fixed SVA > 6 cm, pelvic tilt > 25°, PI-LL > 30°, and/or thoracic kyphosis > 60° are poor candidates for MIS deformity correction.[5] Reoperation rates seem to be similar between MIS and open surgery for deformity correction, albeit for different reasons. Postoperative neurologic deficit appears to be a leading source of reoperation for open and hybrid MIS-open surgeries, whereas pseudoarthrosis is a leading cause in MIS.[6]

The surgeon's armamentarium for MIS includes the posterior foraminotomy (MIS-PF), transforaminal lumbar interbody fusion (MIS-TLIF), mini-open anterior lumbar interbody fusion (ALIF), and percutaneous pedicle screw fixation. While further high-quality studies with specific focus on patients aged 65 and older taking into account medical comorbidities are necessary, MIS remains an attractive option to avoid complex, open procedures in an aging population.

20.2 Technique Descriptions

20.2.1 Cervical Spine

In the cervical region the most commonly performed procedures for cervical stenosis and associated myelopathy and radiculopathy include the anterior cervical discectomy and fusion (ACDF) and posterior cervical laminectomy with or without instrumented fusion. While an MIS endoscopic alternative to the ACDF has been described,[7] the classic ACDF typically involves minimal soft tissue trauma and blood loss, and remains a surgical staple. The ability to perform MIS foraminotomies however, provides an excellent MIS alternative to the treatment of simple cervical radiculopathy that also allows for motion-preservation.

MIS posterior foraminotomies (MIS-PF) are indicated to treat cervical radiculopathy refractory to conservative management.[8] This is accomplished most effectively when the nerve root compression can be localized to the lateral aspect of or within the neural foramen, often as a result of an osteophyte or lateral disc herniation. A radicular distribution of symptoms should be identified and be supported by radiographic findings. This procedure may be performed bilaterally if indicated. Foraminotomies are not indicated for isolated neck pain. The main contraindications include concurrent cervical myelopathy, the presence of a central disc herniation, and significant instability. In these cases, the patient would likely benefit more from an anterior or posterior approach for decompression and stabilization.

Level 1 evidence suggests that while ACDF, cervical disc replacement (CDR) and MIS-PF are all effective in treating cervical radiculopathy, MIS-PF is associated with the lowest incidence of adverse effects.[9] MIS-PF has been shown to be effective in approximately 90% of cases and is associated with less blood loss, shorter operative time, and shorter hospital stay than open posterior foraminotomies.[10]

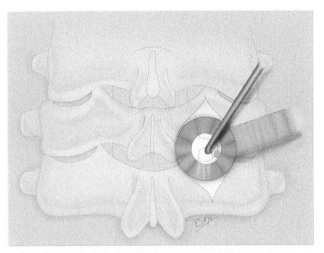

Fig. 20.1 MIS posterior microforaminotomy. View through working channel showing completed laminoforaminotomy. The exiting nerve root is free and decompressed.

The procedure is performed prone, with the head slightly flexed. After confirming the appropriate level with fluoroscopy, a paramedian incision is made, the fascia is opened sharply, and a blunt dilator is advanced and confirmed to be over the lateral mass of interest. Sequential dilators are then placed. Using the microscope and high-speed drill, followed by Kerrison rongeurs, a hemilaminotomy and medial facetectomy is performed. The ligamentum flavum is carefully removed, exposing the nerve root. If a soft lateral disc is the suspected culprit, careful discectomy is performed at this point. Decompression may be confirmed by palpating around the nerve root with a blunt nerve hook. ▶ Fig. 20.1 demonstrates a completed cervical laminoforaminotomy with the nerve root decompressed.

20.2.2 Lumbar Spine

MIS applications exist for most pathologies of the lumbar spine. MIS is typically performed through a tubular retractor system, either under loupe or microscopic magnification or via endoscopic assistance. In addition, a variety of "mini-open" procedures also exist, with the mini-open ALIF being the most common. This section will review a select number of MIS procedures, including tubular microdiscectomy, MIS-TLIF, and the awake endoscopic MIS-TLIF.

Lumbar Discectomy

The microdiscectomy remains the gold standard for unilateral lumbar radiculopathy with an identifiable radiographic disc herniation. Multiple variations exist, including the tubular microdiscectomy and endoscopic-assisted microdiscectomy. The classic indication for microdiscectomy is leg pain greater than back pain in a radicular distribution that is supported by MRI findings of a herniated disc with nerve root compression at the appropriate level, usually after a 6–8 week trial of conservative management. Acute indications include acute progressive neurologic deficit, as a result of the above, and cauda equina syndrome. Contraindications to microdiscectomy include symptoms that are not explained by imaging, a primary

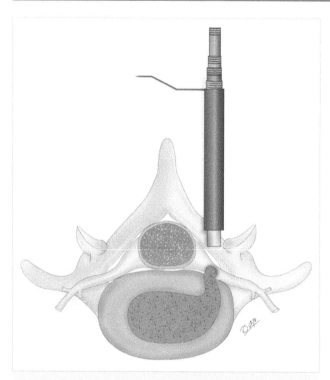

Fig. 20.2 Tubular microdiscectomy. Axial view showing placement of sequential dilators over the facet of interest with underlying disc herniation.

complaint of back pain, and cauda equina syndrome in the setting of a large central disc herniation not amenable to adequate decompression by an MIS technique alone.

Level 1 evidence supports equivalent outcomes between the standard microdiscectomy and the tubular MIS approach.[11] This procedure is commonly performed on an outpatient basis and typically under general anesthesia.

The tubular microdiscectomy (▶ Fig. 20.2) is performed on the Wilson frame to minimize lumbar lordosis and open the disc space. A line is drawn 1.5 cm parallel to midline, and a spinal needle is inserted to localize the disc space of interest. Centered on this point, a small incision is made, and a blunt dilator is passed through the incision, resulting in a "muscle-splitting" approach, until bone is contacted. Sequential dilators are inserted, and fluoroscopy confirms placement of the tubular system over the appropriate facet complex, in line with the disc space. Using microscopic magnification, the soft tissue is dissected off the bone, and a hemilaminotomy and medial facetectomy is performed. With the traversing nerve root retracted medially, the discectomy is performed.

Lumbar Decompression

Degenerative lumbar stenosis is a leading cause for spine surgery in patients over age 65. The most common indication for lumbar decompression is a moderate to severe lumbar stenosis at one or more levels with signs and symptoms of neurogenic claudication that is refractory to conservative therapy. Laminectomy is the gold standard for surgical treatment; however, advances in endoscopy have paved the way for MIS interventions such as the microendoscopic decompressive laminotomy first

described by Fessler et al in 2002.[12] Other variations of the same procedure exist, including a microscope-assisted approach.

Preliminary evidence reveals significant improvements in both Visual Analog Scale (VAS) scores for back and leg pain as well as Oswestry Disability Index (ODI) scores for elderly patients receiving MIS lumbar decompression.[13] Because of the favorable complication profile, this procedure is particularly attractive for the treatment of aging patients with multiple medical comorbidities who might otherwise not be candidates for open surgery. Another benefit of this procedure is that segmental stability should be adequately maintained.

Lumbar Fusion

The rate of lumbar fusion procedures has increased at a dramatic rate over the past 20 years. Data from the Healthcare Cost and Utilization Project Nationwide Inpatient Sample demonstrates a 137% increase in the number of spinal fusion hospital discharges from 1998 to 2008. Not unexpectedly, a significant increase in the mean age of surgery was also seen (48.8 to 54.2 years).[14] Lumbar fusion procedures typically represent the spinal surgeries with the greatest morbidity, intraoperative blood loss, length of hospital stay, and time until return to preoperative functional ability. Indications are widespread, from back pain to deformity correction. That being said, it is no wonder that the majority of MIS has targeted the lumbar spine.

MinimallyInvasive Transforaminal Lumbar Interbody Fusion

By combining the concept of the tubular retractor and the development of percutaneous pedicle screw instrumentation, the MIS-TLIF and other variations were born. The indications are the same as for open TLIF and include degenerative disc disease resulting in lower back pain with or without radiculopathy, often secondary to disc space collapse and foraminal stenosis, and segmental instability involving grade I or II spondylolisthesis. The MIS-TLIF may be performed in up to two levels reliably, and it is generally not indicated for deformity correction.

As first described by Foley et al,[15] the procedure is performed by first making a 2.5 cm skin incision centered over the disc space of interest, 4 to 5 cm lateral to midline on the side of the patient's worse symptomatology. Sequential dilator tubes (22 or 26 mm) are used to provide a surgical corridor centered over the facet joint. Using microscopic magnification, a complete facetectomy is performed, followed by discectomy (▶ Fig. 20.3). The disc space is then distracted either by placement of an interlaminar spreader or by placing contralateral percutaneous screws and rods. At this point the disc space is prepared with curettes and scrapers, and the interbody is placed. Percutaneous screws and rods are then placed ipsilaterally, followed by contralaterally, if not done so previously.

Awake Endoscopic Transforaminal Lumbar Interbody Fusion

General indications for the awake endoscopic TLIF include lumbar degenerative disc disease and low-grade spondylolisthesis causing back and/or leg pain. Contraindications include grade III or IV spondylolisthesis, more than two indicated levels, and > 90% central canal stenosis. Cases with a high risk of

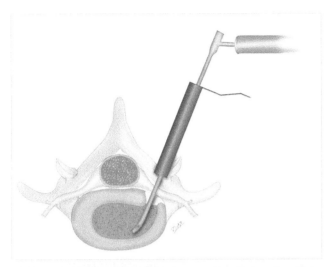

Fig. 20.3 MIS-TLIF. Axial image showing correct placement of working channel and access to the disc space after completed facetectomy.

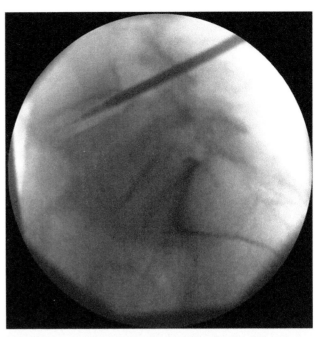

Fig. 20.4 Awake endoscopic TLIF. Lateral fluoroscopic radiograph showing initial dilator access to the disc space.

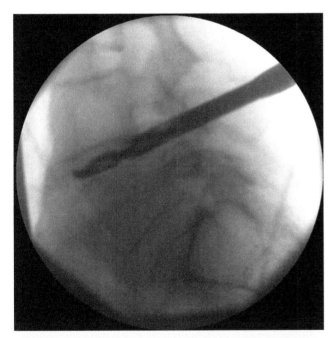

Fig. 20.5 Awake endoscopic TLIF. Lateral fluoroscopic radiograph showing discectomy being performed with specialized drill.

subsidence should also be excluded, as long-lasting indirect decompression is integral to the success of the procedure.[16]

In order to avoid general anesthesia, the authors have adopted an anesthetic technique that includes a continuous infusion of propofol and ketamine to achieve light to moderate sedation. Using fluoroscopy and a spinal needle, Kambin's triangle on the side of the primary pathology is localized, and sequential dilators leading to an 8 mm working channel are placed (▶ Fig. 20.4). The endoscope is inserted, and the traversing and exiting nerve roots at the level of interested are localized. Discectomy and thereby direct decompression is performed with a variety of specialized rongeurs, curettes, high-speed drill, and micro-osteotomies (▶ Fig. 20.5). Final disc

space preparation is achieved with specialized stainless steel-brushes. At this point, 2.1 mg of recombinant human bone morphogenic protein is placed into the anterior portion of the disc space and is followed by an allograft-filled meshed containment device. The interbody provides indirect decompression of the exiting nerve roots at that level. In order to achieve fixation, percutaneous pedicle screws and rods are then placed bilaterally, with the four-screw tracts having been injected with a total of 20 mL of bupivacaine to further assist with analgesia and recovery (▶ Fig. 20.6).

20.3 Benefit and Risks

The question of risk and benefit in spine surgery for aging patients is in many ways more complicated than in the general population. Older patients are constitutionally frailer than their younger counterparts and often carry medical comorbidities of greater severity and number. Further, a lower productive life expectancy can negatively impact the cost-effectiveness of surgical intervention (especially involving instrumentation), potentially limiting patients' access to otherwise beneficial procedures. However, the incidence of pathological alterations in spinal anatomy increases with age, and the progression of these changes often results in symptomatology for which surgery is warranted. A thorough examination of the risks and benefits specific to the aging population is then paramount to the sound practice of spine surgery in older patients.

The benefit of a given intervention in the aging cohort should be demonstrated with a high degree of confidence before offering surgery to these patients. Specifically, ideal procedures should minimize physiologic stress, shorten operative time, reduce exposure to potent anesthetic drugs, and optimize financial cost.

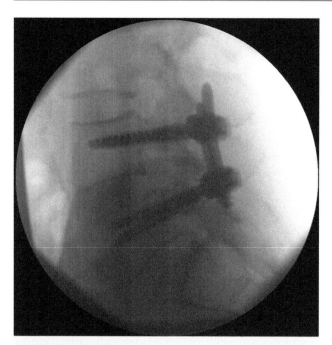

Fig. 20.6 Awake endoscopic TLIF. Lateral fluoroscopic radiograph demonstrating completed L4–5 TLIF with expandable mesh cage filled with demineralized bone matrix and percutaneous pedicle screw instrumentation.

Surgical procedures by definition involve a controlled trauma to the patient's body, including tissue damage, blood loss, and metabolic derangements. A growing body of literature supports the assumption that MIS approaches involve less injury to surrounding tissues when compared to conventional open surgery.[17,18] Significant reductions in blood loss have also been reported. This reduces the need for intraoperative transfusion, in turn reducing demand on hospitals' limited blood bank supply.[19] Reduced transfusion rates may be especially useful in elderly patients who may be immunocompromised, decreasing the risk of transfusion-related hypersensitivity reactions or infection.

In addition to direct surgical risks, the potential harm of anesthesia exposure should be addressed when considering older patients for surgery.[20] Extra care should be placed on protecting the airway, managing fluid balance, and maintaining ideal perfusion during surgery. Drug metabolism may be altered or impaired in patients with comorbid liver disease or chronic kidney disease, affecting medication choice and intraoperative dosing. In addition to these physiologic dangers, anesthesia exposure has been associated with cognitive decline in some elderly patients.[21] MIS techniques may allow for reduced drug administration, while still achieving operatively viable anesthesia.[22] Indeed, as we describe in this chapter, the endoscopic MIS approach has made awake surgery under conscious sedation a possibility in the lumbar spine.[16]

Spine surgery, especially involving instrumentation, can frequently require revision. Indications for reoperation include progressive degeneration, hardware failure, pseudoarthrosis, and adjacent segment disease. Older adults, therefore, not only carry the baseline risks for revision after a primary spine procedure, but also may require reoperation for surgeries performed years or decades earlier in life. In the case of primary surgeries performed in elderly patients, cases should be optimized to reduce the risk of reoperation in order to avoid subjecting frail patients to anesthesia and surgical stress a second time. In cases where revision is necessary, however, MIS approaches represent an effective means to accomplish the revision safely. The trajectories afforded by novel MIS approaches may be of particular benefit when revising a prior open surgery, as the native anatomy is typically distorted or replaced by scar tissue. Conversely, an MIS primary surgery should have less associated tissue destruction, and so may result in an easier approach if a subsequent revision procedure is required.

Efficient resource utilization allows more patients to be treated at lower cost. Therefore, determining the optimal course for patients and institutions requires a frank consideration of the price of a given surgical procedure. Cost can be especially relevant to elderly patients, whose care already may include treatments for a variety of age-related comorbidities, and the associated financial burden. As we discuss above, the frequency of spine surgery in elderly patients is projected to increase in the coming decades. This demographic trend should be seen as a call for not only more effective, but also more affordable techniques. MIS procedures answer that need. Independent financial analyses in Europe and America have demonstrated lower costs associated with MIS spine surgery as compared to open procedures.[23,24] These savings have been attributed primarily to a reduced postoperative hospital stay, including less pharmacy utilization and laboratory cost. MIS procedures have also been associated with fewer surgical site infections, a major driver of extended postoperative length of stay and increased cost.[25]

20.4 Outcomes/Evidence

To justify the profound investment of time and resources— as well as the associated risks of injury or death— surgeons and patients should reasonably expect a good and clinically significant postoperative outcome. This is a nontrivial consideration in older patients, whose frailty may limit the extent of intervention that can be safely achieved, ultimately affecting outcomes. Further, certain pathologies resulting from chronic progressive degeneration can be multifactorial, producing complex symptomatology that may not fully resolve even after a feasible procedure. It is then necessary to understand the realistic extent of improvement or clinical stabilization we can reach through surgery in aging patients, and to what extent MIS techniques can impact the degree of improvement.

It should first be understood that spine surgery in general, whether conventional or MIS, can be safe and effective in the aging population if proper attention is paid to patient selection.[26] This involves not only choosing patients for whom intervention is truly indicated, but also optimizing those patients (and their comorbidities) for the surgical stress and trauma necessary to achieve clinical improvement. Following these principles, spine surgery can be performed in these patients safely and beneficially. In recent years, however, a preponderance of literature has largely favored the utilization of MIS techniques in this population.[27]

MIS approaches to lumbar discectomy have found favor in patients of various ages and clinical conditions.[28,29,30] These studies demonstrate comparable safety and efficacy as compared to conventional techniques, with the added benefits of the MIS approach discussed previously (reduced tissue damage, blood loss, etc.). In particular, a large retrospective study of over 25,000 cases found a significantly lower complication rate with MIS compared to conventional open lumbar discectomy.[31] MIS techniques to treat adult spine deformity have also been investigated specifically in the aging population, with demonstrable safety and efficacy as compared to conventional deformity procedures.[32,33] Finally, clinical and radiological outcomes in aging patients undergoing MIS lumbar interbody fusion have been shown to parallel those achievable in younger patients, with significant qualitative improvements and good fusion rates.[34,35]

But in judging outcomes of MIS surgery for older patients, we must consider not only the direct clinical results of a single procedure, but the associated perioperative costs and benefits to patient and hospital. These chiefly include postoperative infection, analgesia consumption, and length of hospital stay.

As we discuss above, MIS techniques are associated with a lower risk of surgical site infection, reducing harm to patients and hospital costs.[36] This effect may be attributed to smaller incisions with less disruption of fascia and other subcutaneous tissue, which better maintains the body's physical barriers to infection. As we describe our awake endoscopic MIS-TLIF, our reduced administration of anesthesia includes an avoidance of potent opioid analgesics both during and after surgery, instead relying on long-acting local anesthesia, acetaminophen, and gabapentin.[16]

Previous authors have demonstrated a reduced postoperative length of stay (LOS) associated with MIS procedures.[37] However, this effect has not been reproduced in all studies.[38] This discrepancy likely reflects the multiple and disparate nature of the variables that together determine LOS, only one of which is surgical technique. In the aging population, spine surgeons should seek to optimize the remaining perioperative variables that determine LOS in order to expedite recovery and remove these susceptible patients from exposure to potential hospital-acquired infection or other complication during the postoperative period.

Enhanced Recovery After Surgery (ERAS) is one avenue to achieve this end. ERAS is a multidisciplinary approach to the surgical process pioneered by European anesthesiologists and colorectal surgeons.[39] The ultimate goal of ERAS programs is to reduce postoperative LOS by accelerating the recovery process. This is accomplished by a number of specific perioperative interventions, including the coordination of all teams caring for a given surgical patient from admission to discharge toward the ultimate goal of early discharge. Preoperative interventions include patient optimization and nutritional planning. Intraoperative interventions include the strong support of MIS techniques, as discussed here, and reduced administration of general anesthetics. Postoperative interventions include early mobilization, early oral feeding, and reduced consumption of opioids analgesics.

Recently, work has begun to develop ERAS protocols for major spine surgery.[40] In hand with the authors' development of the awake endoscopic TLIF, the authors' have published their experience with an ERAS pilot protocol for lumbar spine fusion.[41] Since establishing this program at our institution, we have seen excellent clinical results in our enrolled patients, with associated shorter LOS and reduced institutional costs.[42] We attribute these benefits not only to the limited soft tissue damage afforded by the MIS techniques employed, but the systematic interventions the ERAS program provides our patients.

Programs such as these would seem ideal in aging patients, whose frailty and comorbid conditions often require special perioperative considerations.

20.5 Pitfalls, Complications, and Avoidance

Complications in MIS spine procedures generally reflect those of conventional open procedures, including pseudoarthrosis, instrumentation failure, systemic complications during surgery, dural tear, nerve injury, and wound complications. In aging patients, wound and systemic medical complications may be more common.[26]

The technical and clinical benefits of MIS procedures we describe above (e.g. reduced blood loss) may include a reduced risk of common surgical complications. A recent national-level meta-analysis of over 25,000 cases concluded that MIS discectomy was associated with fewer major surgical complications and surgical site infections.[31] However, other studies have not replicated this effect, instead finding no difference in complication rates between conventional and MIS approaches.[11,43] Nonetheless, it can be reasonably concluded that MIS procedures do not confer additional risk of complication.

Current literature does characterize complications of MIS procedures specifically in aging patients. Successful fusion and complication rates appear to be similar to those seen in younger patients following MIS-TLIF.[44] Another study including a variety of MIS lumbar procedures (including laminectomy, microdiscectomy, and interbody fusion) identified a comparable complication rate and profile to that seen in conventional surgery.[45]

20.6 Conclusions

As the population of the United States continues to age, we have already begun to witness an increasing incidence of age-related degenerative spinal pathology. Consequently, more spine procedures will be performed in progressively older patients. As we have described, there are a number of MIS procedures available to spine surgeons that are safer and more affordable than conventional open procedures, while achieving equivalent or superior clinical outcomes. The increased demand for MIS procedures will require continued innovation to develop new and better techniques ideally suited to the aging spine.

Key References

[1] Deyo RA, Mirza SK, Martin BI, Kreuter W, Goodman DC, Jarvik JG. Trends, major medical complications, and charges associated with surgery for lumbar spinal stenosis in older adults. JAMA. 2010; 303(13):1259–1265

[2] Wang MY, Widi G, Levi AD. The safety profile of lumbar spinal surgery in elderly patients 85 years and older. Neurosurg Focus. 2015; 39(4):E3

[3] Shamji MF, Goldstein CL, Wang M, Uribe JS, Fehlings MG. Minimally Invasive Spinal Surgery in the Elderly: Does It Make Sense? Neurosurgery. 2015; 77 Suppl 4:S108–S115

[4] Barbagallo GMV, Raudino G, Visocchi M, et al. Restoration of Thoracolumbar Spine Stability and Alignment in Elderly Patients Using Minimally Invasive Spine Surgery (MISS). A Safe and Feasible Option in Degenerative and Traumatic Spine Diseases. Acta Neurochir Suppl (Wien). 2017; 124:69–74

[5] Lu VM, Kerezoudis P, Gilder HE, McCutcheon BA, Phan K, Bydon M. Minimally Invasive Surgery Versus Open Surgery Spinal Fusion for Spondylolisthesis: A Systematic Review and Meta-analysis. Spine. 2017; 42(3):E177–E185

References

[1] Fehlings MG, Tetreault L, Nater A, et al. The Aging of the Global Population: The Changing Epidemiology of Disease and Spinal Disorders. Neurosurgery. 2015; 77 Suppl 4:S1–S5

[2] Deyo RA, Mirza SK, Martin BI, Kreuter W, Goodman DC, Jarvik JG. Trends, major medical complications, and charges associated with surgery for lumbar spinal stenosis in older adults. JAMA. 2010; 303(13):1259–1265

[3] Kanter AS, Tempel ZJ, Ozpinar A, Okonkwo DO. A Review of Minimally Invasive Procedures for the Treatment of Adult Spinal Deformity. Spine. 2016; 41 Suppl 8:S59–S65

[4] Than KD, Park P, Fu KM, et al. International Spine Study Group. Clinical and radiographic parameters associated with best versus worst clinical outcomes in minimally invasive spinal deformity surgery. J Neurosurg Spine. 2016; 25(1):21–25

[5] Mummaneni PV, Shaffrey CI, Lenke LG, et al. Minimally Invasive Surgery Section of the International Spine Study Group. The minimally invasive spinal deformity surgery algorithm: a reproducible rational framework for decision making in minimally invasive spinal deformity surgery. Neurosurg Focus. 2014; 36(5):E6

[6] Hamilton DK, Kanter AS, Bolinger BD, et al. International Spine Study Group (ISSG). Reoperation rates in minimally invasive, hybrid and open surgical treatment for adult spinal deformity with minimum 2-year follow-up. Eur Spine J. 2016; 25(8):2605–2611

[7] Yao N, Wang C, Wang W, Wang L. Full-endoscopic technique for anterior cervical discectomy and interbody fusion: 5-year follow-up results of 67 cases. Eur Spine J. 2011; 20(6):899–904

[8] Papavero L, Kothe R. Minimally invasive posterior cervical foraminotomy for treatment of radiculopathy: An effective, time-tested, and cost-efficient motion-preservation technique. Oper Orthop Traumatol. 2017

[9] Gutman G, Rosenzweig DH, Golan JD. The Surgical Treatment of Cervical Radiculopathy: Meta-analysis of Randomized Controlled Trials. Spine. 2017

[10] Song Z, Zhang Z, Hao J, et al. Microsurgery or open cervical foraminotomy for cervical radiculopathy? A systematic review. Int Orthop. 2016; 40(6):1335–1343

[11] Clark AJ, Safaee MM, Khan NR, Brown MT, Foley KT. Tubular microdiscectomy: techniques, complication avoidance, and review of the literature. Neurosurg Focus. 2017; 43(2):E7

[12] Khoo LT, Fessler RG. Microendoscopic decompressive laminotomy for the treatment of lumbar stenosis. Neurosurgery. 2002; 51(5) Suppl:S146–S154

[13] Rosen DS, O'Toole JE, Eichholz KM, et al. Minimally invasive lumbar spinal decompression in the elderly: outcomes of 50 patients aged 75 years and older. Neurosurgery. 2007; 60(3):503–509, discussion 509–510

[14] Rajaee SS, Bae HW, Kanim LE, Delamarter RB. Spinal fusion in the United States: analysis of trends from 1998 to 2008. Spine. 2012; 37(1):67–76

[15] Holly LT, Schwender JD, Rouben DP, Foley KT. Minimally invasive transforaminal lumbar interbody fusion: indications, technique, and complications. Neurosurg Focus. 2006; 20(3):E6

[16] Wang MY, Grossman J. Endoscopic minimally invasive transforaminal interbody fusion without general anesthesia: initial clinical experience with 1-year follow-up. Neurosurg Focus. 2016; 40(2):E13

[17] Fan S, Hu Z, Zhao F, Zhao X, Huang Y, Fang X. Multifidus muscle changes and clinical effects of one-level posterior lumbar interbody fusion: minimally invasive procedure versus conventional open approach. Eur Spine J. 2010; 19(2):316–324

[18] Kim CW. Scientific basis of minimally invasive spine surgery: prevention of multifidus muscle injury during posterior lumbar surgery. Spine. 2010; 35 (26) Suppl:S281–S286

[19] Patel AA, Zfass-Mendez M, Lebwohl NH, et al. Minimally Invasive Versus Open Lumbar Fusion: A Comparison of Blood Loss, Surgical Complications, and Hospital Course. Iowa Orthop J. 2015; 35:130–134

[20] Roy RC. Clinical pearls in the anaesthetic management of elderly patients. Ann Acad Med Singapore. 1994; 23(6) Suppl:20–25

[21] Evered L, Scott DA, Silbert B. Cognitive decline associated with anesthesia and surgery in the elderly: does this contribute to dementia prevalence? Curr Opin Psychiatry. 2017; 30(3):220–226

[22] Buvanendran A, Thillainathan V. Preoperative and postoperative anesthetic and analgesic techniques for minimally invasive surgery of the spine. Spine. 2010; 35(26) Suppl:S274–S280

[23] Vertuani S, Nilsson J, Borgman B, et al. A Cost-Effectiveness Analysis of Minimally Invasive versus Open Surgery Techniques for Lumbar Spinal Fusion in Italy and the United Kingdom. Value Health. 2015; 18(6):810–816

[24] Wang MY, Lerner J, Lesko J, McGirt MJ. Acute hospital costs after minimally invasive versus open lumbar interbody fusion: data from a US national database with 6106 patients. J Spinal Disord Tech. 2012; 25(6):324–328

[25] Parker SL, Adogwa O, Witham TF, Aaronson OS, Cheng J, McGirt MJ. Postoperative infection after minimally invasive versus open transforaminal lumbar interbody fusion (TLIF): literature review and cost analysis. Minim Invasive Neurosurg. 2011; 54(1):33–37

[26] Wang MY, Widi G, Levi AD. The safety profile of lumbar spinal surgery in elderly patients 85 years and older. Neurosurg Focus. 2015; 39(4):E3

[27] Shamji MF, Goldstein CL, Wang M, Uribe JS, Fehlings MG. Minimally Invasive Spinal Surgery in the Elderly: Does It Make Sense? Neurosurgery. 2015; 77 Suppl 4:S108–S115

[28] Ahn SS, Kim SH, Kim DW, Lee BH. Comparison of Outcomes of Percutaneous Endoscopic Lumbar Discectomy and Open Lumbar Microdiscectomy for Young Adults: A Retrospective Matched Cohort Study. World Neurosurg. 2016; 86:250–258

[29] Cong L, Zhu Y, Tu G. A meta-analysis of endoscopic discectomy versus open discectomy for symptomatic lumbar disk herniation. Eur Spine J. 2016; 25(1): 134–143

[30] Gadjradj PS, van Tulder MW, Dirven CM, Peul WC, Harhangi BS. Clinical outcomes after percutaneous transforaminal endoscopic discectomy for lumbar disc herniation: a prospective case series. Neurosurg Focus. 2016; 40(2):E3

[31] Ohya J, Oshima Y, Chikuda H, et al. Does the microendoscopic technique reduce mortality and major complications in patients undergoing lumbar discectomy? A propensity score-matched analysis using a nationwide administrative database. Neurosurg Focus. 2016; 40(2):E5

[32] Barbagallo GMV, Raudino G, Visocchi M, et al. Restoration of Thoracolumbar Spine Stability and Alignment in Elderly Patients Using Minimally Invasive Spine Surgery (MISS). A Safe and Feasible Option in Degenerative and Traumatic Spine Diseases. Acta Neurochir Suppl (Wien). 2017; 124:69–74

[33] Park P, Okonkwo DO, Nguyen S, et al. International Spine Study Group. Can a Minimal Clinically Important Difference Be Achieved in Elderly Patients with Adult Spinal Deformity Who Undergo Minimally Invasive Spinal Surgery? World Neurosurg. 2016; 86:168–172

[34] Lee HJ, Kim JS, Ryu KS. Minimally Invasive TLIF Using Unilateral Approach and Single Cage at Single Level in Patients over 65. BioMed Res Int. 2016; 2016:4679865

[35] Nikhil N J, Lim JW, Yeo W, Yue WM. Elderly Patients Achieving Clinical and Radiological Outcomes Comparable with Those of Younger Patients Following Minimally Invasive Transforaminal Lumbar Interbody Fusion. Asian Spine J. 2017; 11(2):230–242

[36] McGirt MJ, Parker SL, Lerner J, Engelhart L, Knight T, Wang MY. Comparative analysis of perioperative surgical site infection after minimally invasive versus open posterior/transforaminal lumbar interbody fusion: analysis of hospital billing and discharge data from 5170 patients. J Neurosurg Spine. 2011; 14(6):771–778

[37] Lu VM, Kerezoudis P, Gilder HE, McCutcheon BA, Phan K, Bydon M. Minimally Invasive Surgery Versus Open Surgery Spinal Fusion for Spondylolisthesis: A Systematic Review and Meta-analysis. Spine. 2017; 42(3):E177–E185

[38] Mummaneni PV, Bisson EF, Kerezoudis P, et al. Minimally invasive versus open fusion for Grade I degenerative lumbar spondylolisthesis: analysis of the Quality Outcomes Database. Neurosurg Focus. 2017; 43(2):E11

[39] Ljungqvist O. ERAS–enhanced recovery after surgery: moving evidence-based perioperative care to practice. JPEN J Parenter Enteral Nutr. 2014; 38(5):559–566

[40] Wainwright TW, Immins T, Middleton RG. Enhanced recovery after surgery (ERAS) and its applicability for major spine surgery. Best Pract Res Clin Anaesthesiol. 2016; 30(1):91–102

[41] Wang MY, Chang PY, Grossman J. Development of an Enhanced Recovery After Surgery (ERAS) approach for lumbar spinal fusion. J Neurosurg Spine. 2017; 26(4):411–418

[42] Wang MY, Chang HK, Grossman J. Reduced Acute Care Costs With the ERAS® Minimally Invasive Transforaminal Lumbar Interbody Fusion Compared With Conventional Minimally Invasive Transforaminal Lumbar Interbody Fusion. Neurosurgery. 2017

[43] Zhang D, Mao K, Qiang X. Comparing minimally invasive transforaminal lumbar interbody fusion and posterior lumbar interbody fusion for spondylolisthesis: A STROBE-compliant observational study. Medicine (Baltimore). 2017; 96(37):e8011

[44] Lin GX, Quillo-Olvera J, Jo HJ, et al. Minimally Invasive Transforaminal Lumbar Interbody Fusion: A Comparison Study Based on End Plate Subsidence and Cystic Change in Individuals Older and Younger than 65 Years. World Neurosurg. 2017; 106:174–184

[45] Avila MJ, Walter CM, Baaj AA. Outcomes and Complications of Minimally Invasive Surgery of the Lumbar Spine in the Elderly. Cureus. 2016; 8(3):e519

21 Techniques for Spinal Instrumentation in the Aging Spine

Darryl DiRisio

Abstract

In this chapter, the challenges pertaining to instrumentation of the aged spine will be discussed, especially as it relates to osteoporosis, kyphosis, and increased pathologic complexity. Methods to fortify the integrity of constructs in this population, such as the use of bicortical and multicortical fixation techniques, utilizing multiple points of fixation, and triangulating screws on insertion aid to mitigate against instrumentation failure. Bicortical fixation is often felt to be dangerous in many areas of the spine, and is thus an underutilized technique. Safe methods for this type of fixation will be discussed in this chapter, by utilization of preoperative CT imaging and with the use of computerized stereotactic navigation techniques. Other methods to avoid complications in the aged population include instrumentation of the spine in an age-adjusted balanced state, and utilizing anterior load-sharing techniques so as to help off-load stresses on the screw-bone interface. Often times, instrumentation is not necessary when considering a decompression in an aged individual. Some of the decision-making processes that are necessary to consider stability in the aged population will be discussed, along with some of the evidence to back such decisions. Most evidence reported relates to instrumentation in degenerative conditions. Unfortunately, there is a paucity of evidence that exists in other pathologic entities, i.e., infection, trauma, and tumors with regards to instability and instrumentation necessity. Of course, the variable nature and presentations of these disease processes make it more difficult to obtain high level evidence.

Keywords: screw, osteoporosis, kyphosis, bicortical fixation, multiple points of fixation, cement augmentation, spine instrumentation

Key Points

- Aging leads to soft bone from osteoporosis, a higher incidence of kyphosis, and complex pathology.
- Successful instrumentation in this aging spine is accomplished by astute attention to bone quality, instrumentation indications, thoughtful preoperative instrumentation planning and adjusting plans based on intraoperative findings.
- The aging spine is biomechanically unique and requires careful instrumentation techniques to avoid hardware failure.
- Techniques include utilizing longer screws, applying bicortical fixation techniques, utilizing multiple fixation points, placing anterior load sharing implants and instrumenting the spine in balance.
- Additional fixation options include sublaminar wires and hook constructs.
- Methyl methacrylate within the osteoporotic bone of the spine can help to anchor instrumentation.
- Lastly, determining the necessity of instrumentation prior to embarking on surgical intervention can help avoid unneeded hardware complications.

21.1 Indications and Contraindications

21.1.1 Indication: Instability

Instrumentation of the aging spine is indicated when the spine is unstable. Overt instability often follows a traumatic event, and by definition is obvious. A cervical fracture dislocation is a good example of an overtly unstable condition. However, instability is not as clear in the setting of degeneration. In the aging individual who has lumbar spondylosis and degenerative glacial deformity, it is more difficult to define instability and the potential need for instrumentation. For example, in the setting of spondylolisthesis, an aging individual may have severe, incapacitating low back pain when upright, improved when supine. If imaging demonstrates a mobile spondylolisthesis, this would clearly indicate that instrumentation of the spine is a reasonable option. On the other hand, if an immobile spondylolisthesis is present with only neurogenic claudication symptoms, then the need for instrumentation may not be so obvious.

Preoperative assessments including dynamic radiographs (upright/supine or flexion/extension studies) may be helpful in determining whether instability exists. Identifying mechanical pain, pain that is worse in the upright position and improves in a supine position, that is associated with movement or deformity on the dynamic imaging, can help to identify instability. Anatomic factors such as the height of the disc space or the anatomic orientation of the facets should also be considered in the decision-making process when performing a decompression.

21.1.2 Contraindications: Osteoporosis, Kyphosis

Osteoporosis and kyphosis are relative contraindications to placement of spine instrumentation, as there is an increase in the likelihood of hardware failure. These contraindications should be balanced with the degree of instability and need for instrumentation to prevent pain and neurologic dysfunction.

Osteoporosis

Osteoporosis degrades the ability of instrumentation to engage the bones of the spine. The more osteoporotic the spine, the more likely hardware will fail to provide internal stabilization until the goal of bony fusion is achieved. The diagnosis of osteoporosis can be made by dual-energy X-ray absorptiometry (DXA) or quantitative computed tomography (CT). The most common method to test bone density is by utilization of the DXA scan, which provides a two-dimensional method to quantify bone density. It is accurate, inexpensive, safe, and normalizes the results to a distribution curve based on age and sex. A T score and a Z score is generated. The former normalizes one's score to a distribution curve of normal individuals of the same sex who are 30 years of age. A value between -1.0 to -2.5 indicates the presence of osteopenia, and scores below -2.5 are indicative of osteoporosis. The Z score normalizes an individual's score against the distribution curve of a group of individuals of the same age and sex. The Z score is not as useful in the elderly osteoporotic population. Though there is no absolute contraindication to instrumentation of the thoracolumbar spine with pedicle screws, a DXA score less than -2.5 is a relative contraindication to utilization of pedicle screws, especially for short segment fixation in the absence of anterior support.

Quantitative CT imaging can also be used to determine osteoporosis. Weiser et al designed a study to test fatigue strength in the setting of osteoporosis based on the quantitative CT diagnosis of osteoporosis. Twenty-one donors aged 12 to 96 had their T12 vertebrae evaluated with a quantitative CT protocol. The osteoporotic group had bone densities below 80 mg/cm3, and a normal group consisted of those with bone densities above 120 mg/cm3. Their vertebrae were then tested in a mechanical hydraulic testing machine with a single pedicle screw within the T12 vertebral body. The osteoporotic group achieved only 45% of the cycles to failure with only 60% of the fatigue load compared to the normal bone density group.[1]

Though this study potentially predicts a worse outcome with utilizing instrumentation in the setting of osteoporosis, this is not an absolute contraindication. Having the information enables the surgeon to alter his or her intraoperative strategy to decrease the risk of hardware failure.

Kyphosis

Kyphosis occurs with aging. Mean thoracic kyphosis is less than 30°in those under 30 years of age, and increases to 66°in the 75-year-old age group.[2] The pathogenesis of degenerative kyphosis is multifactorial and caused by either asymmetric disc collapse or vertebral body collapse. Hyperkyphosis is associated with overall impairment in physical function, worsening pulmonary function, worsening of gait, increasing falls, chronic pain, and fractures of all kinds. Pulmonary dysfunction associated with thoracic kyphosis greater than 40°results in increased mortality in the older population. In the elderly female population, the combination of hyperkyphosis and vertebral body fracture predicts a greater mortality compared to either condition alone.[3] In the aging population, worsening kyphosis results in weakening of the extensor musculature, further imbalance, and greater degeneration of the anterior discs. The sequela of worsening kyphosis results in an even greater degree of kyphotic deformity over time.

Thoracic kyphosis greater than 40°(T5 to T12) is associated with increased risks of proximal junctional kyphosis following spinal fusions[4] and is thus a relative contraindication to spinal instrumentation. The biomechanical forces on a screw–rod construct in the kyphotic spine are different than the nonkyphotic spine. Force vectors are often aligned with the pedicle screws when kyphotic individuals stand, thus creating less resistance to screw pull-out.

21.2 Technique Description

The poor bone quality in the aging spine patient necessitates the utilization of sound biomechanical principles for instrumentation. Techniques include engaging screws into cortical bone; utilizing multiple points of fixation, utilizing cross-connectors; triangulating screws on insertion; placing load-sharing interbody grafts; instrumenting the spine in balance; use of bone cement for anchors and use of wires and hooks aid in preventing screw backout and instrumentation failure.

21.2.1 Engaging Screws into Cortical Bone (Bi/multicortical Fixation Methods)

Pedicle screws engage the cortex of the pedicle and provide a powerful method to prevent construct failure. Pedicle screws can be utilized in the absence of laminae and can be placed in most of the thoracolumbar spine. Long pedicle screws engage and control all three columns of the vertebral body to provide a biomechanically superior cantilever beam construct. However, cancellous bone is weaker in the osteoporotic spine and provides a poor screw bone interface. Care should be taken to engage as much cortical bone along the trajectory of the screw as possible to prevent failure. Bicortical fixation is achieved by engaging the tip of the screw through the anterior vertebral cortex and can provide additional cortical purchase and biomechanical stability.

The utility and safety of performing bicortical screw purchase is specific to regional anatomy. Bicortical vertebral fixation of ventral constructs in the thoracic or thoracolumbar region have been found to significantly improve pullout strength. Engaging the promontory of the sacrum with sacral screw fixation in osteoporotic individuals has also proven to be a useful method to prevent pullout (▸ Fig. 21.1). The following paragraphs will discuss regional variation for bicortical screw fixation.

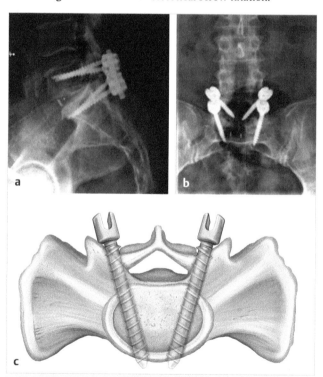

Fig. 21.1 (a) Lateral and (b) AP radiographs demonstrating bicortical sacral fixation, just lateral to the promontory of the sacrum. (c) Demonstrates an ideal screw length and trajectory into the promontory. This cartoon demonstrates the biomechanical principles of triangulation, and multicortical fixation.

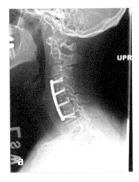 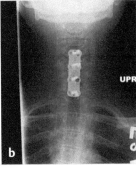 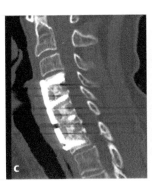

Fig. 21.2 **(a)** Lateral and **(b)** AP radiographs in the postoperative period in a 70-year-old who presented with severe myelopathy. Please note the bicortical nature of the screws in the end-vertebrae. **(c)** Note the fusion present at 2 years postoperatively as seen on a lateral CT with sagittal reconstruction

Cervical Spine

In the cervical spine there are advantages to using longer screws in those individuals with osteoporosis, and in cases spanning three or more motion segments. In the past when performing anterior cervical reconstructions with the early, non-locking plates, bicortical fixation was necessary. Fluoroscopy was utilized to verify bicortical purchase. Additionally, measurements on a sagittal reconstructed CT scan can determine an ideal screw length so as to be able to engage the posterior cortex (▶ Fig. 21.2). This becomes an important part of one's armamentarium when considering long constructs (three or more motion segments), and when performing multilevel corpectomies, especially in the osteoporotic individual. Biomechanical studies have shown that C1 screw fixation is optimized by engaging both cortices (▶ Fig. 21.3). Care must be taken to avoid extending the screw tip beyond 1 to 2 mm from the distal cortex to avoid injury to retropharyngeal structures. The anterior portion of the C2 vertebral body contains weaker cancellous bone. Therefore bicortical fixation should be considered at the cephalad end of the construct when performing an anterior cervical reconstruction that will include the C2 vertebral body (▶ Fig. 21.4).

Thoracic Spine

In the thoracic spine, safe havens for bicortical purchase exist. Ventral to the vertebral bodies of T1 and T4, no critical structures exist that create a significant danger for bicortical fixation. Structures anterior to the upper thoracic spine include the esophagus, segmental vessels, the mediastinal structures, the sympathetic chain, the phrenic and vagus nerves. The trachea lies much more anteriorly within the mediastinum, and the aortic arch is positioned closer to the T4 level. The aforementioned structures are difficult to injure with bicortical fixation utilizing the classically-described entry points and trajectories for thoracic pedicle screw placement (▶ Fig. 21.5). When considering bicortical fixation lower in the thoracic spine, the position of the aorta on the left side of the vertebra must be considered. A left-sided vertebral body screw with an entry point near the costovertebral joint and a trajectory which crosses the vertebral body provides a method for bicortical fixation at any segment of the thoracic spine (▶ Fig. 21.6).

The thoracic extrapedicular technique is an excellent example of multicortical screw fixation in the thoracic spine. By choosing an entry point within the pedicle, at the level of the costotransverse joint, one can pierce the pedicle laterally, and then regain entry through the costovertebral joint, and gain access into the vertebral body. This technique, originally described by Dvorak et al, provides sound biomechanical fixation of the thoracic spine (▶ Fig. 21.7).[5] Pullout testing between traditional pedicle screws and the extrapedicular technique reveals no significant differences, though longer screws are able to be utilized with the extrapedicular technique.[6]

Lumbar Spine

The lower lumbar spine contains wider pedicles, allowing more variation in trajectory. The screw trajectory can either be maintained in the sagittal plane or begin more laterally, thus applying triangulation. The cortical bone can be engaged in the pedicle, along the superior endplate and through bicortical purchase of the anterior vertebral body. Determining the optimal size and trajectory of the screw is accomplished by preoperative planning to select the optimal diameter and length for pedicle screws. Measuring the pedicle diameter and selecting the appropriate screw diameter can provide optimal engagement of the pedicle screw threads with cortical bone. Care must be taken not to oversize the screw, as this risks pedicle fracture. The long axis of the screw should be aimed in close approximation to the rostral endplate of the vertebral body (▶ Fig. 21.8). This will engage the long axis of the screw to the cortex of the superior endplate to optimize cortical bone engagement.

Design changes to pedicle screws that aid to prevent pullout include changes to the thread shape (v-shaped as opposed to rectangular shape), as well as the thread depth. Dual lead-threaded screws have been reported to help in settings of osteoporosis. However, biomechanical studies reveal that the optimal way to make a significant difference on screw pullout is to use a screw that abuts the internal cortex of the pedicle.[7] The thread pattern does not seem to matter.

A variation of lumbar pedicle screw placement, called the cortical trajectory, provides another option for lumbar fixation. This technique involves beginning the screw at the inferomedial portion of the pedicle, and applying a trajectory towards the superolateral portion of the pedicle (▶ Fig. 21.9). This screw trajectory engages more of the cortical bone as the screw passes obliquely through the pedicle. At the pedicle level, a safe haven exists just behind the transverse process for bicortical purchase. Further posteriorly along L5, one has to be careful to avoid the

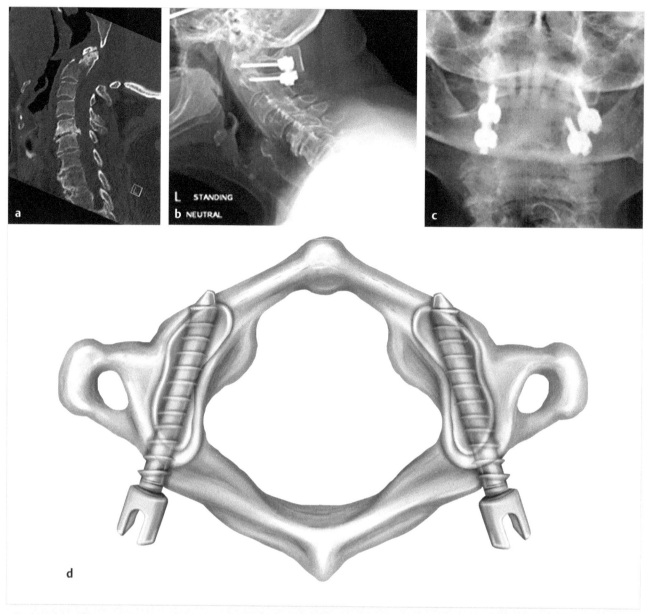

Fig. 21.3 **(a)** C2 fracture in a 70-year-old female with renal failure. **(b)** Lateral and **(c)** AP radiographs demonstrate the reconstruction. Notice that the C1 screws do not quite penetrate the entire C1 lateral mass. **(d)** Schematic depiction of proper bicortical C1 fixation

femoral nerve and the traversing L4 nerve root. Similarly, anterolateral to the sacrum, one has to be careful to avoid the L5 nerve root.

A tricortical fixation technique has been described for fixating the sacrum, which proves useful when performing multilevel fixation. Aiming the sacral screw through the sacral promontory, provides better fixation, especially in severely degenerated cases.[8] Fixation of the sacrum through the more densely calcified superior articular process (as opposed to an entry point more lateral) tends to provide better fixation of the sacrum.[2]

Finally, an underutilized region to engage cortical bone is the anterior portion of the inferior vertebral body in the setting of spondylolisthesis. For instance, in the setting of an L4–5 degenerative spondylolisthesis, the L5 vertebral body will

often have a separation with the iliac vessels of 5 mm or more (▶ Fig. 21.10). Engaging the anterior cortex in this setting is safe.

The preoperative CT scans can be used to plan appropriate trajectories and screw lengths. The axial view provides the best method to measure for an appropriate screw length. By measuring the distance between the transverse process/superior articular process border and the midline/ventral portion of the vertebral body, by adding 5 mm to that distance, one is able to obtain a very accurate screw length that can provide bicortical purchase. The potential for error or complications varies by the vertebral body level. For instance, when placing bicortical ventral vertebral body screws (ventral fixation) from the left side of the spine at the L2 level there are rarely critical structures to injure, even if one is 5 mm longer than intended. On the other

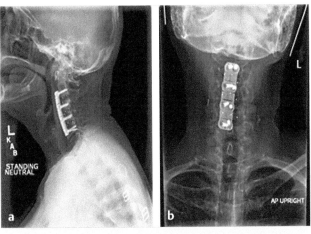

Fig. 21.4 Postoperative **(a)** lateral and **(b)** AP radiographs of a 65-year-old female with severe polyradiculopathy and cervicalgia. Note the presence of bicortical C2 screws.

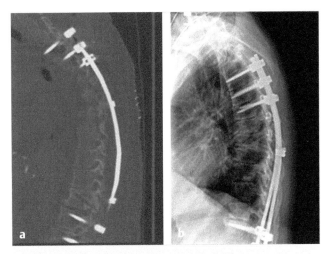

Fig. 21.5 Bicortical screws in the vertebral body of T3, as demonstrated on the reconstructed CT scan **(a)** and the plain radiograph. Note the location of the aortic arch in the lateral radiograph **(b)**.

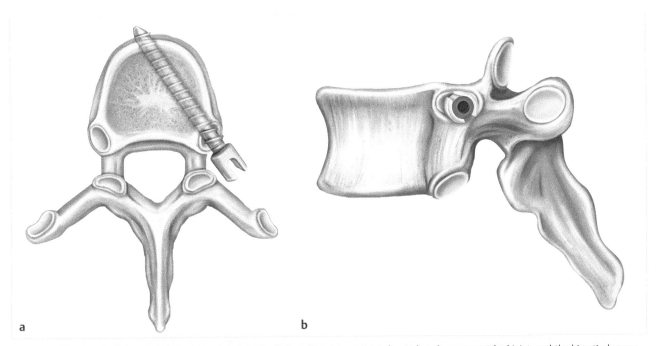

Fig. 21.6 This reveals the cross-thoracic, bicortical screw technique. The entry point is located at the costovertebral joint, and the bicortical screw often traverses from left to right. Above the T4 level, one can place a screw from either side.

hand, a mid-cervical vertebral body screw should not pierce the posterior cortex by more than 1 or 2 mm. Practice can be obtained either by the use of cadavers, or by attempting to predict with unicortical screws, the resulting correspondence between the intraoperative radiograph and the predicted depth of the screw. It is very important to consider that the manufacturer of the instrumentation is an important variable when one intends to utilize the preoperative CT scan measuring technique. Some manufacturers only utilize the screw shaft length, where others utilize the head/shaft length to determine screw length.

Technology is playing a larger role in the ability to precisely and accurately place pedicle screws. Three-dimensional (3-D) computerized navigation technology can be utilized to obtain exact trajectories for screw placement. Other advantages include the ability to precisely determine screw length so as to be able to apply a bicortical technique, or the ability to place a screw in a specific region of the pedicle for optimal screw purchase. Importantly, soft tissue structures can be visualized and avoided with 3-D navigation. Disadvantages include cost, patient radiation exposure, as well as additional time requirements.

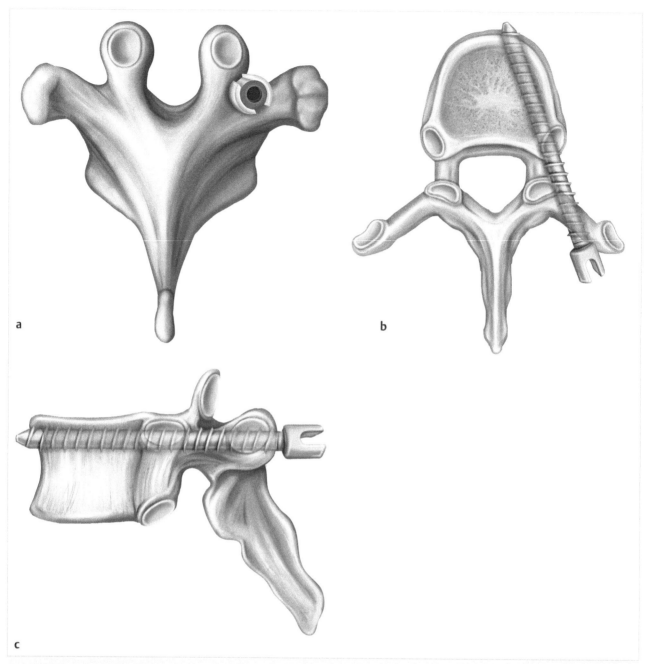

Fig. 21.7 The trajectory for a multicortical thoracic pedicle screw as demonstrated in the axial view of the thoracic vertebral body, and the entry point along the transverse process demonstrated on the AP view

An ineffective technique, hubbing, refers to the placement of the entire screw, including the head, into the bone (▶ Fig. 21.11). Hubbing results in weakening of the screw-bone interface by damaging the bone as it engages the screw threads. This results in a loss of up to 40% of pullout strength.[9]

21.2.2 Multiple Points of Fixation

In the osteoporotic spine, multiple points of fixation increase the bone/metal surface area, thus preventing construct failure. When placed at multiple levels, pedicle screw–rod constructs are the most effective constructs in resisting motion in all planes. Utilization of hooks and laminar wiring help to stabilize the spine by this method, though laminar, transverse process and pedicle fractures have been reported. The utilization of a laminar hook just above a pedicle screw is a very effective method to prevent backout in the case of osteoporotic bone.

Thoracic pedicles have a large sagittal diameter, but a smaller axial diameter, and are morphometrically smallest at the T4 level. In the lumbar spine, the pedicles can be small at the upper segments, but are often capacious at L4 to S1. Though it is possible to place screws at every level of a long construct, this is often times unnecessary, as the rod that connects the proximal

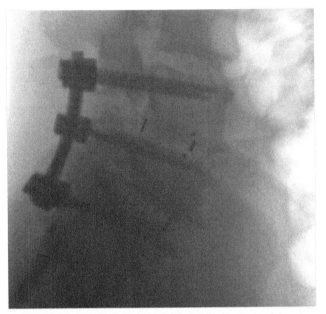

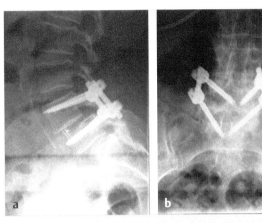

Fig. 21.10 **(a)** AP and **(b)** Lateral radiographs of a 75-year-old female who underwent lumbar reconstruction at L4,5 for spondylolisthesis. Please note the significant separation of the calcified iliac vessels (blue arrow) with the anterior aspect of L5.

Fig. 21.8 Note the position of the pedicle screws closely parallel to the superior endplates of L4 and L5 on the lateral radiograph. This allows the screw to engage another cortical surface to optimize fixation.

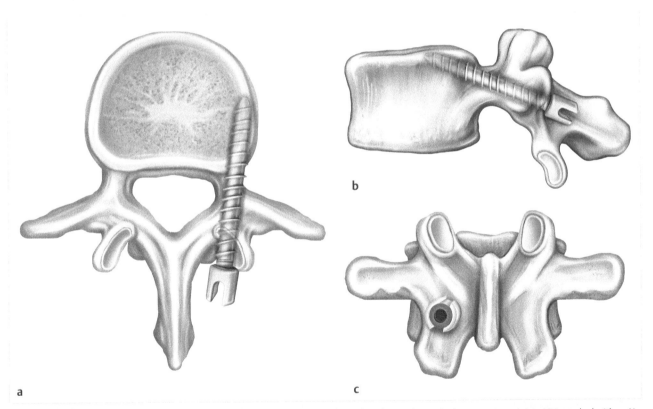

Fig. 21.9 Cortical screw trajectory, as seen in the axial and the sagittal view. In the dorsal view, the cortical screw entry point on L5 is marked with an X

and terminal screws has contact to the laminae in between. In traumatic situations, a construct engaging a minimum of two segments above and two below with dual intervening rods and a cross-connector provides adequate stability for most thoracic fractures (▶ Fig. 21.12). In these cases, it is important not to end a construct at a spine junction or the apex of a curve. When utilizing long instrumentation to the lumbar spine, anchoring the distal screws into the pelvis provides a powerful method to support a construct.

21.2.3 Cross-Connection and Triangulation

Cross-connectors applied to a construct increases stiffness and rotational stability. Screws applied above and below an unstable segment enhance the stability, but not in all planes. For instance, vertebral body screws placed in L2 and L4 in the case of severe instability can create stability in lateral bending and perhaps in the axial plane. However, rotation around the screws is still allowed to occur. The instability in this particular plane can be mitigated by multiple methods. Cross connectors enhance stability in the plane at the right angle to screw insertion. This prevents a parallelogram type of deformity (▶ Fig. 21.13). Other commonly used methods to enhance the stability in all planes include the utilization of multiple points of fixation. A third or even fourth set of screws increase stability by enlisting the help of the anchoring adjacent segments.

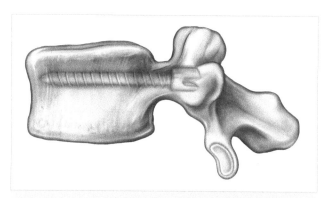

Fig. 21.11 Hubbing refers to deep insertion of a pedicle screw

Further stability is also obtained by utilization of a triangulation technique. Inward angulation of the screws helps to prevent backout in the plane of screw insertion, and also helps to prevent the parallelogram deformity from occurring in the right angle to screw insertion (▶ Fig. 21.14). The combination of all three methods— multiple points of fixation, triangulation, and the use of cross-connectors—enhance the stability of the construct in all planes.

21.2.4 Anterior Load Sharing

An additional consideration when instrumenting the elderly osteoporotic spine should be extended toward utilizing anterior load sharing in addition to dorsal instrumentation. Biomechanically, by applying an anterior strut, axially directed loads will be applied both through the instrumentation and through the ventral strut. This decreases the load on the instrumentation and the stresses at the bone-metal interface, which helps to prevent screw fracture and screw wear within the vertebral body.

21.2.5 Instrumenting the Spine in Balance

Degenerative kyphoscoliosis increases with age. Evidence exists demonstrating that worse health related-quality of life (HRQOL) outcome measures is related to poor sagittal balance in the elderly population. An unbalanced spine leads to postural changes, which require energy expenditure to balance the torso over the pelvis and the pelvis over the feet.[2] Compensatory mechanisms to maintain balance in the absence of lumbar lordosis include straightening of the thoracic spine and retroverting the pelvis (increasing the pelvic tilt). Our pelvic incidence is set after skeletal maturation. As our thoracic portion of our spine tends to become fixed with age, the major compensatory mechanism for maintaining balance in the elderly is through rotating the pelvis more posteriorly. By doing this, the pelvic tilt increases (the angle between a line connecting the femoral heads to the midpoint of the superior portion of a sacrum, and the vertical plumb line), the sagittal slope decreases (the angle of a line through the superior endplate of the sacrum and the horizontal). In order to further rotate the pelvis more posteriorly, the elder will often bend his or her knees, which is impossible to do

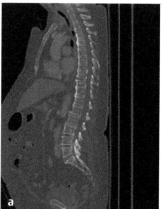
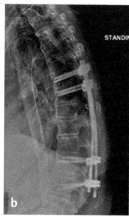
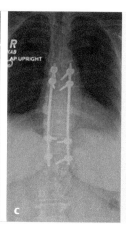

Fig. 21.12 (a) A Reconstructed sagittal CT scan demonstrates an extension injury in an 83-year-old female, who was unable to be mobilized. Postoperative (b) AP and (c) lateral plain radiographs reveal four points of fixation utilized in the reconstruction.

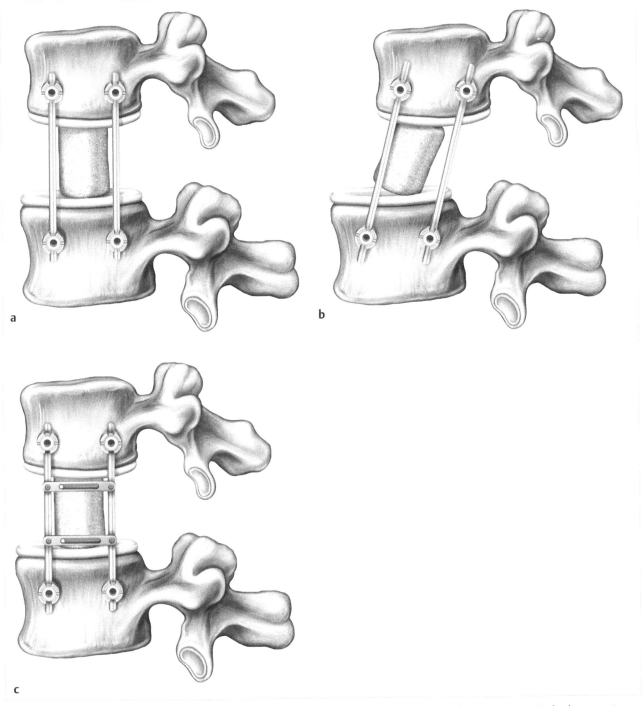

Fig. 21.13 (a) An artist's depiction of parallelogram deformity, with kickout of the graft anteriorly, as can be seen in an anterior lumbar corpectomy and reconstruction. In **(b)**, stabilization is provided with the use of dual cross-connectors.

for long periods without pain due to muscle fatigue and can lead to flexion contractures of the musculature surrounding the hips. Once the compensatory mechanisms are no longer possible, then the sagittal vertical axis (the distance between the vertical line extending from the mid-portion of the C7 vertebral body to the posterior superior endplate of the sacrum) begins to increase. Assistive devices (walker, wheel chair) are then often required for standing.

Appropriate balance of the spine should be considered to limit undue stresses on the bone metal interface and instrumentation failure. Many studies on adult spinal deformity demonstrate that instrumenting an elder spine in balance, whereby the pelvic tilt is less than 25°, the spino-pelvic mismatch is less than 10°, and the sagittal vertical axis is less than 50 mm results in better HRQOL outcomes. However, the complication rate increases with greater degrees of sagittal realignment[10,11]

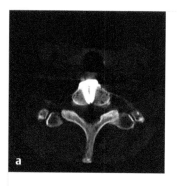

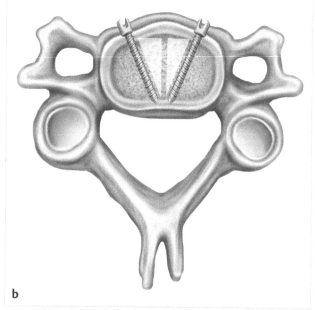

Fig. 21.14 (a) Represents an axial CT demonstrating triangulation and bicortical fixation of the cervical spine. In (b), the blue triangular regions represent the area of bone present to resist instrumentation "pullout".

Alignment overcorrection in the elderly is associated with greater rates of proximal junctional kyphosis (PJK), and undercorrection is associated with worse HRQOL outcome scores. Age-adjusted realignment results in optimal outcomes with an improved rate of PJK complications.[12]

21.2.6 Cement-Aided Screw Fixation

The use of bone cement (methyl methacrylate) to help with pedicle fixation in poor bone quality has been extensively described. Despite the reported complications, using methyl methacrylate improves fixation. Pullout test results have demonstrated 200% to 500% improvement in pullout strength with screws augmented with Polymethyl methacrylate.[13] Using as little as 1 mL of methacrylate in each pedicle screw hole has been found to incur significant benefit in the osteoporotic individual.

Four different techniques can be utilized to instill the methyl methacrylate. In the most basic technique, the surgeon creates a pilot hole in the pedicle and then injects the methyl methacrylate into the vertebral body. This is then followed immedi-

ately by placement of the screw. Downsides to this technique include the fact that extravasation of the methyl methacrylate out of the tapped hole creates a loss of the substance, and a loss of bone fusion surface area. A second technique is described whereby the screw is inserted by utilizing a traditional method. The methyl methacrylate is then added into the vertebral body through a separate hole lateral to the pedicle screw. The downside is that additional time and effort is necessary for the methyl methacrylate injection. More recently, perforated, cannulated screws have been developed so that the methyl methacrylate can be injected through the screw after placement.

Recently, a technique has been described whereby methyl methacrylate is placed into vicryl mesh, and is then tamped into a previously created pedicle screw hole. The benefit of this technique is that the methyl methacrylate is less likely to spread to unintended locations. The pullout strength with the use of this novel technique is found to be similarly increased as compared to using methacrylate alone.[14]

21.2.7 Sublaminar Hooks, Cables

Sublaminar hooks can be effective in providing stabilization in the aging spine. In cases where bone quality is poor, hooks are advantageous, as the mechanism of action relies on contact between the hook and cortical bone (▶ Fig. 21.15). Hitchon et al compared pullout strength of pedicle screws, sublaminar hooks, and sublaminar wires. He found that the sublaminar cables translated significantly when subjected to the pullout forces, that the pullout resistance of pedicle screws was greater than hooks, and that hook pullout resistance was greater than wire.[15]

Failure that occurs with cables and hooks is different from that occurring with pedicle screws. Laminar fracture, pedicle fracture, and separation of the posterior element connection to the vertebrae are the most common modes of hook failure. Cables fail by cutting through the lamina, laminar fracture and separating from the rod.

21.3 Benefits and Risks

In the aging individual with overt spinal instability, significant benefit is incurred with instrumentation. Immediate mobilization allows for improved pulmonary, gastrointestinal, circulatory, and musculoskeletal function. Skin integrity is maintained with mobilization, by decreasing the local pressure and thus improving skin circulation. When the patient is mobile, circulatory proteins, and other circulatory inflammatory components are decreased, allowing improved healing to occur.

Compromised pulmonary function in the aging individual is common. In an immobilized state, circulation to various portions of the lungs is altered. Changes occur in ventilation status when in a supine position for a prolonged period of time, resulting in atelectasis, higher rates of aspiration, impaired mobilization of secretions, and higher rates of infectious pneumonia.

Rapid stabilization with instrumentation has the added benefit of improved pain control, which in turn results in less narcotic usage. Narcotics can have dramatic effects on aging individuals, by causing constipation, instability, dizziness, blood pressure changes, and mental status impairment. Mobilization

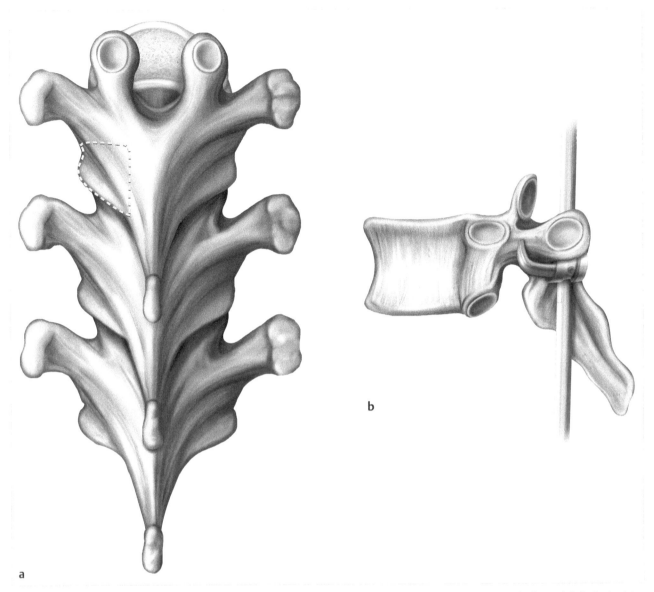

Fig. 21.15 Artist's rendition of hook placement. The inferior articular process is removed either with an osteotome or a high-speed drill. The hook is then placed underneath the removed inferior articular process towards the pedicle as depicted on the sagittal view below.

helps pain by multiple mechanisms: peripheral muscle firing stimulates afferent neurons, which connect to the nucleus raphe of the midbrain. This results in increased synthesis of norepinephrine, enkephalins, and dopamine, which all directly help to attenuate pain. Changing the position of the joints and muscles directly decreases inflammation in these regions, by rapidly changing the circulatory pattern.

Immediate stabilization has its risks as well. In order to stabilize the spine, large operative interventions are often necessary, with the potential for significant blood loss, blood pressure alterations, as well as cardiac and pulmonary complications. Screw backout, instrumentation pullout, and vertebral body fractures can all occur when attempting to stabilize the aging spine, which can all lead to repeat surgical procedures, and additional cardiac, pulmonary, neurologic stresses inherent to complicated surgical procedures.

21.4 Outcomes and Evidence

Most of the outcomes published pertain to lumbar degenerative disease. Outcomes analyses pertaining to other pathologic entities (tumor, infection, trauma) are more difficult to define because of the varied baseline characteristics of the patient populations.

The evidence that exists to determine whether instrumentation is necessary in the setting of spondylolisthesis is not straight forward. Ghogawala compared two cohorts of aged patients with mobile spondylolisthesis, with a single level disease. One group had a decompression alone, and in the other group, a decompression and stabilization was performed. The patients who were instrumented were found to have a significantly improved physical function outcome (physical component of the SF-36) and less reoperations compared to those who were decompressed without pedicle screw instrumentation.[16] The same journal (*New England Journal of Medicine*) concurrently published a Swedish study (looking at the outcomes of two cohorts of patients with lumbar spondylosis (some with a spondylolisthesis and some without). The patients with spondylolisthesis were randomized into two groups. One group had an instrumented fusion, at 1 or 2 levels, and in the second cohort, no instrumentation was utilized. Similar outcomes were reported in these two groups of patients.[17]

The outcomes in these studies were slightly different. However, the two studies had different baseline patient populations, different outcome measurements, and differed in the number of levels which were allowed to be fused. In the Forsth study, flexion/extension films were not utilized preoperatively to help determine instability. In patients who did not have a spondylolisthesis, some were randomized to receive instrumentation. In this study, they did separately review the cohort of patients who did demonstrate a spondylolisthesis preoperatively. No differences were found in the outcomes of this subgroup. Also, in the study by Ghogawala, no statistically significant difference in the Oswestry Disability Index was found in comparing the decompression group with the instrumented fusion group.

21.5 Pitfalls, Complications, and Avoidance

21.5.1 Complications of Bicortical Techniques

Multiple complications have been described with screws perforating the cortex in long constructs. Recently, vertebral failure has been described with bicortical fixation at the upper instrumented vertebral body in thoracolumbar reconstruction cases.[18] Risk factors include an increased length of construct, advanced patient age, and poor bone quality.

Vascular injury, though very rare in the acute setting, has been well described in the literature. Mechanistically, pulsation of the aorta is thought to create vessel damage. Endovascular graft placement to repair pseudoaneurysms of the aorta have been recently described.[19] With this mechanism of repair, screw removal is often times unnecessary. Bicortical fixation of the atlas has been found to be associated with carotid artery injury, as this vessel tends to be located near the anterior ring of C1, slightly lateral to midline. Bicortical fixation with lateral mass screws is associated with nerve root injury and vertebral artery injury. This technique is rarely performed today, as not much additional biomechanical advantage is gained by this method.

21.5.2 Complications of Methyl Methacrylate

Complications with the use of methyl methacrylate augmentation to assist pedicle screw fixation in osteoporotic bone have been well described. Cement leakage, which can result in intravascular injection through the epidural venous plexus, has been described, along with injection into the spinal canal. Though cement leakage has been reported as high as 60%, significant clinical adverse events are reported to be less than 4%.[14] Radicular symptoms have been reported in less than 1% of cases.[20]

21.5.3 Pathologic Complexity

Complex degenerative changes in aging patients require thoughtful operative planning. In the lumbar spine, facet hypertrophy, which advances with age, changes the location of the pathologic compression of nerve roots. For instance, with advancing age, degeneration and disc bulging, along with hypertrophy of the joints, create more of a central stenosis in the sixth and seventh decades of life.[21] However, with further aging, more settling occurs at the disc space level. Additional joint hypertrophy creates more of a lateral recess narrowing, which may necessitate complete facetectomy for appropriate decompression.

The preoperative decision-making is more complex. In the case of the very elderly, where there is near ankylosis of the motion segment, simple decompression even with facetectomy is often adequate. If abnormal motion exists on dynamic films, then consideration needs to be extended towards fusing the level with instrumentation. In these cases, especially when factoring in comorbidities such as diabetes, osteoporosis, COPD, and smoking status, the quality of the bone becomes a significant factor. In some of these individuals, delaying surgery to improve the bone status may be an essential step. Even in the aging population, this can be accomplished by changing habits (diet, smoking cessation, alcohol cessation, exercise), or adding medications (Vitamin D, teriparatide, bisphosphonates).

21.6 Conclusion

Instrumentation of the aging spine requires an understanding of the expected consequences of aging in the spine, a patient's particular pathology, spine stability and a knowledge of appropriate instrumentation techniques. Identifying instability will provide clear indications as to whether spinal instrumentation is necessary. Many aging spines may appear deformed but are not unstable. If instrumentation is needed then identification and preoperative treatment of osteoporosis may help improve the likelihood of successful surgery.

Utilizing techniques to engage screws into cortical bone, performing multiple points of fixation, utilizing cross-connectors, triangulating screws on insertion, placing load-sharing interbody grafts, instrumenting the spine in balance, using bone cement for anchors and using wires and hooks can aid in preventing instrumentation failure.

Key References

[1] Weiser L, Huber G, Sellenschloh K, et al. Insufficient stability of pedicle screws in osteoporotic vertebrae: biomechanical correlation of bone mineral density and pedicle screw fixation strength. Eur Spine J. 2017; 26(11):2891–2897

[2] Hitchon PW, Brenton MD, Black AG, et al. In vitro biomechanical comparison of pedicle screws, sublaminar hooks, and sublaminar cables. J Neurosurg. 2003; 99(1) Suppl:104–109

[3] Aydogan M, Ozturk C, Karatoprak O, Tezer M, Aksu N, Hamzaoglu A. The pedicle screw fixation with vertebroplasty augmentation in the surgical treatment of the severe osteoporotic spines. J Spinal Disord Tech. 2009; 22 (6):444–447

[4] Martín-Fernández M, López-Herradón A, Piñera AR, et al. Potential risks of using cement-augmented screws for spinal fusion in patients with low bone quality. Spine J. 2017; 17(8):1192–1199

[5] Liu FY, Wang T, Yang SD, Wang H, Yang DL, Ding WY. Incidence and risk factors for proximal junctional kyphosis: a meta-analysis. Eur Spine J. 2016; 25 (8):2376–2383

[6] Försth P, Ólafsson G, Carlsson T, et al. A Randomized, Controlled Trial of Fusion Surgery for Lumbar Spinal Stenosis. N Engl J Med. 2016; 374(15): 1413–1423

[7] Ghogawala Z, Dziura J, Butler WE, et al. Laminectomy plus Fusion versus Laminectomy Alone for Lumbar Spondylolisthesis. N Engl J Med. 2016; 374(15): 1424–1434

References

[1] Weiser L, Huber G, Sellenschloh K, et al. Insufficient stability of pedicle screws in osteoporotic vertebrae: biomechanical correlation of bone mineral density and pedicle screw fixation strength. Eur Spine J. 2017; 26(11):2891–2897

[2] Ailon T, Shaffrey CI, Lenke LG, Harrop JS, Smith JS. Progressive Spinal Kyphosis in the Aging Population. Neurosurgery. 2015; 77 Suppl 4:S164–S172

[3] Kado DM, Lui LY, Ensrud KE, Fink HA, Karlamangla AS, Cummings SR, Study of Osteoporotic Fractures. Hyperkyphosis predicts mortality independent of vertebral osteoporosis in older women. Ann Intern Med. 2009; 150(10):681–687

[4] Liu FY, Wang T, Yang SD, Wang H, Yang DL, Ding WY. Incidence and risk factors for proximal junctional kyphosis: a meta-analysis. Eur Spine J. 2016; 25 (8):2376–2383

[5] Dvorak M, MacDonald S, Gurr KR, Bailey SI, Haddad RG. An anatomic, radiographic, and biomechanical assessment of extrapedicular screw fixation in the thoracic spine. Spine. 1993; 18(12):1689–1694

[6] Fürderer S, Scholten N, Coenen O, Koebke J, Eysel P. In-vitro comparison of the pullout strength of 3 different thoracic screw fixation techniques. J Spinal Disord Tech. 2011; 24(1):E6–E10

[7] Bianco RJ, Arnoux PJ, Wagnac E, Mac-Thiong JM, Aubin CE. Minimizing Pedicle Screw Pullout Risks: A Detailed Biomechanical Analysis of Screw Design and Placement. Clin Spine Surg. 2017; 30(3):E226–E232

[8] Luk KD, Chen L, Lu WW. A stronger bicortical sacral pedicle screw fixation through the s1 endplate: an in vitro cyclic loading and pull-out force evaluation. Spine. 2005; 30(5):525–529

[9] Paik H, Dmitriev AE, Lehman RA, Jr, et al. The biomechanical effect of pedicle screw hubbing on pullout resistance in the thoracic spine. Spine J. 2012; 12 (5):417–424

[10] Lafage R, Schwab F, Challier V, et al. International Spine Study Group. Defining Spino-Pelvic Alignment Thresholds: Should Operative Goals in Adult Spinal Deformity Surgery Account for Age? Spine. 2016; 41(1):62–68

[11] Lafage R, Schwab F, Glassman S, et al. International Spine Study Group. Age-Adjusted Alignment Goals Have the Potential to Reduce PJK. Spine. 2017; 42 (17):1275–1282

[12] Scheer JK, Lafage R, Schwab FJ, et al. Under-Correction of Sagittal Deformities Based on Age-Adjusted Alignment Thresholds Leads to Worse HRQOL While Over-Correction Provides No Additional Benefit. Spine. 2017. DOI: 10.1097/b rs.0000000000002435

[13] Aydogan M, Ozturk C, Karatoprak O, Tezer M, Aksu N, Hamzaoglu A. The pedicle screw fixation with vertebroplasty augmentation in the surgical treatment of the severe osteoporotic spines. J Spinal Disord Tech. 2009; 22 (6):444–447

[14] Schmid SL, Bachmann E, Fischer M, et al. Pedicle screw augmentation with bone cement enforced Vicryl mesh. J Orthop Res. 2017. DOI: 10.1002/jor.236 31

[15] Hitchon PW, Brenton MD, Black AG, et al. In vitro biomechanical comparison of pedicle screws, sublaminar hooks, and sublaminar cables. J Neurosurg. 2003; 99(1) Suppl:104–109

[16] Ghogawala Z, Dziura J, Butler WE, et al. Laminectomy plus Fusion versus Laminectomy Alone for Lumbar Spondylolisthesis. N Engl J Med. 2016; 374(15): 1424–1434

[17] Försth P, Ólafsson G, Carlsson T, et al. A Randomized, Controlled Trial of Fusion Surgery for Lumbar Spinal Stenosis. N Engl J Med. 2016; 374(15): 1413–1423

[18] Park YS, Hyun SJ, Choi HY, Kim KJ, Jahng TA. Association between bicortical screw fixation at upper instrumented vertebra and risk for upper instrumented vertebra fracture. J Neurosurg Spine. 2017; 26(5):638–644

[19] Zerati AE, Leiderman DB, Teixeira WG, et al. Endovascular Treatment of Late Aortic Erosive Lesion by Pedicle Screw without Screw Removal: Case Report and Literature Review. Ann Vasc Surg. 2017; 39:285.e17–285.e21

[20] Martín-Fernández M, López-Herradón A, Piñera AR, et al. Potential risks of using cement-augmented screws for spinal fusion in patients with low bone quality. Spine J. 2017; 17(8):1192–1199

[21] Yong-Hing K, Kirkaldy-Willis WH. The pathophysiology of degenerative disease of the lumbar spine. Orthop Clin North Am. 1983; 14(3):491–504

Index

Note: Page numbers set **bold** or *italic* indicate headings or figures, respectively.